I was then [illegible] looking
at the heap[illegible] days
told that they had been visited
by the Cyclones of existence whose
mocking bottles of death gave rest,
just by the side of all these lifeless
bones I saw those [illegible] of thousand
which proved to be the skulls
of fallen generals The Livingston
of the Africa's of life, Cook &
Columbuses of the oceans
[illegible] with nothing on head
stone but "Explorer" ~~Causer~~ Discoverer
no trophies, no evidence that they
had found any thing that looked
like law or remedy. again the
question arose Does the God
of all creation play "hide and
go seek" with his creatures?

A. T. Still

From the Dry Bone
to the Living Man

The living human body is the work of a trustworthy Creator, and all the mysteries concerning health and disease disappear in proportion to your acquaintance with this sacred product.

John Lewis

9 June 2017

JOHN LEWIS

A.T. Still

From the Dry Bone to the Living Man

DRY BONE PRESS • *Blaenau Ffestiniog*

Dry Bone Press
2 Bowydd View
Blaenau Ffestiniog
Gwynedd LL41 3YW

www.atstill.com

A catalogue record for this book is available from the British Library.

ISBN 978-0-9572927-0-3

Cover design and typesetting by www.droplet.co.uk

Printed by TJ International Ltd., Padstow, Cornwall.

For all who seek

harmony with nature

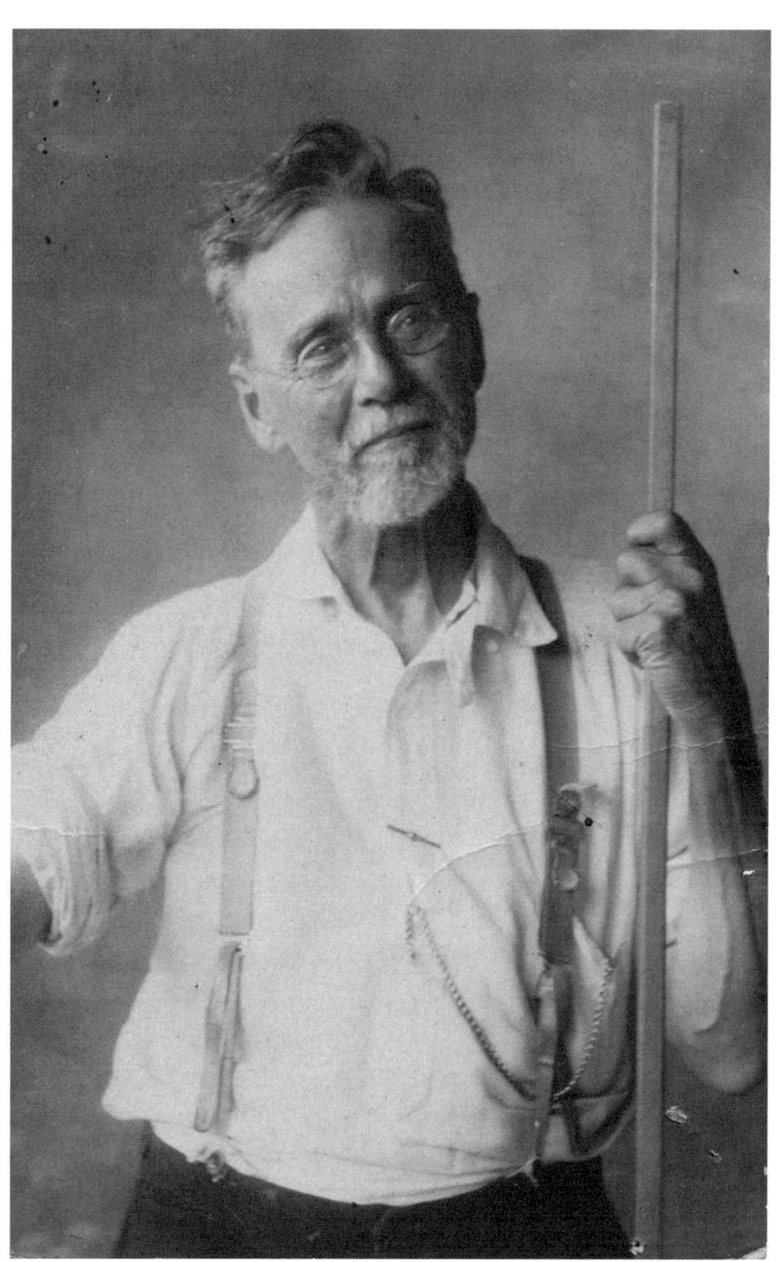

Contents

Illustrations

Maps

My life has been freely spent in the pursuit of knowledge. I have been pleased to take truth from the rich or poor, learned or ignorant, old or young, dead or alive, from the elements above me or the ground beneath me. I read, as a rule of life, all I see written by the hand of God or man in all the leaves of His book, whose lessons no mortal can number. Our forefathers have read this book of Nature during all ages, and it is more entertaining now than ever before. Read this book, for each day lost can never be regained. It is your fault if you do not improve it.

A. T. Still

Andrew Taylor Still made one of science's great discoveries, one equal in importance to Newton's laws of gravitation and Darwin's observations on evolution. A discovery capable of benefiting every human being, with the potential to help mankind more than any other achievement.[1] So his followers believed. He anticipated the science of immunity by a generation and, by marrying anatomy and physiology with principles more often associated with mechanics, developed a drugless medicine both preventative and curative across the whole disease spectrum. In 1905 he won a readers' poll in a major New York publication for nomination as a candidate for the Nobel Prize in Medicine or Physiology but, by dint of politics, his name was not put forward. His portrait hangs at the Smithsonian Institution, Washington D.C., in recognition of his contribution to medicine, yet his name remains obscure.

When he tried to interest the medical profession – his own profession – in what he had found they failed to investigate it. Instead they fought him bitterly and ridiculed it as a fad, a cult, quackery. Ironically, what he had worked out – a biological explanation of the cause of disease[2] – was in the strictest sense pure medicine, based on the latest scientific knowledge. But his conclusions undermined the very foundations of the regular system, challenging not only the drugs of the day but its whole approach to health and disease. He fought an epic David and Goliath battle with this powerful institution and emerged victorious through the legislatures.

Insistent that his method should stand or fall solely on results, he published nothing in any mainstream journal, never advertised, and employed no press agent. He evaded notoriety, demanded no plaudits, and was not even possessive of his findings. He did not attach himself to the faculty of a university to secure credentials for his rating in the world of scholarship, but remained in the remote Midwestern town he had made his home.[3]

Hiding the depth of his thought behind a rough exterior, he appeared unlike a regular doctor in both manner and dress. Scorning convention and custom, challenging the hierarchical structure of society, he rejected the cultural assumption that supposed authorities – doctors, scientists, ministers – know best. "The explorer for truth must first declare his independence," he asserted. "He must establish his observatory on hills of his own; he must establish it above the imaginary high planes of rulers, kings, professors of schools of all kinds and denominations. He must be the Czar of his own mental empire."[4] Provocative, outspoken, at times mercilessly critical, he refused to let fear prevent him expressing his truth. He held the prestigious medical universities of New York, Boston and Philadelphia in disdain, denigrating them "fossils of the East," bastions of habit, tradition and wrong philosophy.

Still grew up far from these great urban centers. Born in Virginia the third of nine children, he passed his formative years in undeveloped and sparsely settled Missouri, where the European and indigenous worlds met, and nature established its own rhythmic harmony. As a teenager he learned medicine by apprenticeship and entered practice on a Shawnee Indian reservation in Kansas where his preacher-physician father was sent as a missionary. As a young man he fought against slavery in the Civil War and came to regard his later battle with medicine as a struggle for emancipation from the bondage of drugs – though he fought not against physicians personally but against a way of thinking.

Already questioning the safety and efficacy of the nineteenth century's harsh remedies, it took a devastating personal tragedy to convince him that medicine needed not just reform but a revolution.[5] Believing there must be a better way of healing the sick than introducing toxic substances into the body, he embarked on a lifelong quest to decipher the riddles of life and death, health and disease.

Reading widely – from medicine to philosophy, geology to astronomy, the Bible to evolutionary biology – he took the observations and researches of others and subjected them to his own critical analysis, collating, correlating, synthesizing, and drawing new conclusions. And, filtering all through a mind dismissive of "undemonstrable theories," he made connections between disciplines kept discrete by science.

To find health should be the object of the doctor, he declared in a much quoted phrase. *Anyone can find disease.* Behind it lie two divergent approaches to medicine founded upon two radically different worldviews.

The new "scientific medicine" demanded that all phenomena of living organisms, including the mind and the body's mysterious animating power, be explained in terms of physical or chemical laws. Sill fervently believed in science, but as a preacher's son retained a conviction of the individual as a soul or spirit. His personal struggle mirrored that of late nineteenth-century Western civilization generally: two great social forces, religion and science, battling for ascendancy. Seeing truth in both, he not only retained the word *life* but also employed terms not usually associated with a physician: truth, spirit, soul, wisdom, love, God. He never challenged an established scientific fact, but found science's materialist foundation wanting when applied to the living being.

He eventually named his system *osteopathy,* perhaps too narrowly. The word – literally "bone suffering" – stands for more than a system of manual medicine. "Osteopathy was not a mere spinal treatment," one of his graduates explained. "It was not a method of treatment at all. It was a principle upon which all treatment might be based."[6] That principle was at once simple and profound: the human organism innately possesses all the agencies required for its own healing.

Still experienced at first hand the hardship and persecution faced by those who dare challenge orthodoxy and powerful vested interests. He encountered monumental obstacles, endured fifteen years of ridicule, abuse and ostracism, and suffered the desertion of most of his patients, family and friends. But, convinced he had discovered a great truth, it merely strengthened his resolve to complete the work he felt was his to do, and, one by one, through sheer force of results, those who had scoffed and jeered came to believe in him and finally see him win through to nationwide love and acclaim. His victory was nevertheless bittersweet for, even during his lifetime, those who came after him progressively diluted his teachings.

Still died from a stroke in December 1917, aged eighty-nine, and was buried a stone's throw from the institution he founded in the small rural community of Kirksville, Missouri. Afterwards his associates lauded him in glowing epithets: a sober, industrious and absolutely honest man, good natured, sociable and generous to a fault.[7] A doctor who gave his best to every patient regardless of sex, color or social position.[8] A philanthropist who "could have been one of the wealthiest men of his day, but he had no time for making money, he had a greater work to do."[9] A visionary but also a battler, "the man who saw the truth, who had the mind to conceive it, the indomitable will and courage to put it over in the face of bitter opposition, poverty and social ostracism, and an abiding faith in its ultimate triumph."[10] The minister who conducted his funeral went as far as to describe him as "one of the world's great men."[11] Today he remains a well-loved if rather distant mythological figure.

Still could not have anticipated the great changes the twentieth century brought to medicine: the saving of life by antibiotics, the sophistication of modern pharmacology, the march of technology. But while medicine continually discards old remedies and practices in favor of newer ones, his method remains timeless. To him osteopathy was not an *advance* – a word belonging to man's transient endeavors – but an *improvement*, a closer harmony with nature's unchanging laws.

He did not invent a system of healing. Like the force of gravity, osteopathy was always present, something familiar to everyone, waiting for a perceptive mind to unlock its secrets. "Millions of people before Newton and Galileo had seen apples fall and pendulums swing," an anonymous hand wrote:

> but practically none of them taught the world what those simple and familiar phenomena meant. So it was with Dr. Still. Millions of people had seen the same things as he had seen and one of them even announced the law, 'Nature heals,' but practically none before Dr. Still had ever learned to work with Nature and never against her in the healing art."[12]

1

PICTURES, EVENTS, FORCES, WHOLES

A life spent on frontiers, physical and mental, began in a one-room log cabin two miles west of Jonesville, Virginia. The settlement lay on the Wilderness Road, the trail blazed by Daniel Boone two generations earlier, a final stop for supplies and wagon repairs before the steep climb towards the Cumberland Gap, and through it passed a stream of pioneers heading to new and uncertain lives in the opening West. All around the forested mountains of the Appalachian chain fractured into a complex maze of ridges, plateaus, narrow valleys and deep gorges.

The scraps of family history that remain tell that Andrew Taylor Still's paternal great-grandfather Samuel Still emigrated from England sometime in the eighteenth century, fought the British in the Revolutionary War, and fathered eight sturdy boys. Andrew's grandfather Boaz, described as the "runt" of this litter, married Mary Lyda, "a good frontiers-woman known to have killed the fiercest of wild beasts with her rifle." Of mainly German ancestry, Mary had a Cherokee grandmother, a pedigree that made Andrew, whose skin was mildly dusky, one-sixteenth American Indian.[1]

As the ill-defined boundary of white settlement advanced haphazardly westward, squatters could claim ownership of one hundred acres for every one planted in corn, and Boaz held eight hundred near present day Asheville, North Carolina. Here Andrew's father Abram Still was born in 1796, one of fifteen children. Frontier life was hard, danger from Indians, wild animals and disease ever present, and lawlessness common. To fill the moral and spiritual vacuum the Methodist Church instigated an itinerant ministry and Boaz, a hard-drinking slaveholder who gambled on horses and fighting cocks,[2] typified the "lax morals" they targeted.

Abram chose a different path. During his childhood the Great Revival swept the western territory, ushering in the era of camp meetings and charismatic traveling preachers. When he was fifteen one of his father's black slaves influenced him to convert to Methodism and, three years later, convinced of a calling to preach, he served an apprenticeship as an exhorter before being admitted by the Holston Conference as a "circuit rider."[3]

These traveling ministers, messengers of Christ's saving gospel, rode horseback itineraries of up to four hundred miles that took four to six weeks to complete. Strict rules demanded unquestioning loyalty to the Church, absolute obedience to superiors, and forbearance of pomposity, self-ambition and personal vanity. Commonly regarded as zealots and deluded fanatics, their dogged perseverance was reflected in a phrase spoken during stormy weather: *There is nothing out today except crows and Methodist preachers.*[4] Exposed to the elements, often sleeping out in the woods, over half died before the age of thirty.

Circuits were assigned annually and Abram served a succession of appointments in the Holston country, a mountainous region that cut across the state boundaries of Virginia, Georgia, Tennessee, and the Carolinas. While riding the remote Tazewell circuit in 1821 he befriended converts James and Barbara Taylor Moore, farmers and horse breeders in the fertile bottom land of Abb's Valley near present-day Pocahontas, Virginia, and courted their daughter Martha. The idyllic setting, at 2550 feet elevation between the forested slopes of the Blue Ridge and North Mountain, belied the hardships that settlement of this region had entailed and trouble with Indians gave many families, including theirs, tragic histories.

Abram and Martha married in 1822 and had their first child, Edward, in January 1824. For a circuit rider the start of a family generally signaled "location" – preaching to a settled community – and in 1825, the year he was ordained presiding elder, Abram located to Jonesville, purchasing the cabin and five hundred acres of virgin soil for $200. He farmed, preached, operated a grist and saw mill, and held the occasional camp meeting under the brush arbors of the Jonesville Campground, established on his land. To supplement a meager salary of $60 per annum he emulated Methodist founder John Wesley by studying medicine, obtaining an MD degree from Rush Medical College, Knoxville, Tennessee.[5] A second son James was born in 1826, followed by Andrew on 6 August 1828.

When Drew, as they called him, was old enough they sent him to Jonesville's log schoolhouse. In this "place of torture" he learned to read and write, studied grammar and arithmetic, and lived in fear of the teacher, an old man named Vandeburgh, who kept a dozen canes to "thrash the boys and girls, big and little" until they "would not have sense enough to recite their lessons," and for his poor spelling made Drew sit on a horse's skull. This cruel regime came to an end in 1834 when Abram accepted a new appointment across the state line in New Market, Tennessee.[6]

They took a comfortable new house and farm, and the boys attended Holston Seminary, a good Methodist school taught without brutality. New Market proved less harmonious for Abram, though, as Church factions squabbled over the "vexed question" of slavery. Britain, Argentina, Central America, and Mexico had already emancipated their slaves and in New York a national Methodist Antislavery Society had been organized, but with the economies of Southern states dependent upon slave labor Tennessee enacted laws to prevent the distribution of abolitionist literature. John Wesley had vehemently opposed slaveholding, but the state's Methodist Conference, bowing to political and economic pressure, finally insisted its ministers toe a proslavery line.[7]

This Abram refused to do. He disagreed with those who argued that the Bible justified human slavery, and his preaching that the practice was "not of Divine origin"[8] provoked hostility and unpopularity. Other forces were working in him, too. The erection of permanent churches signaled the passing of the frontier and the era of camp meetings, and he longed for the freedom of circuit riding. In 1837, when a national financial collapse prompted many to head west to acquire cheap land, he requested a transfer to the Missouri Conference.[9]

Drew was eight, Ed and Jim thirteen and eleven, and three younger siblings, Barbara Jane, Thomas and John, six, four and two. In early March they piled their belongings onto two horse drawn wagons and embarked on a seven-week journey, fording streams and camping out at night, with strictly no travel on the Sabbath. They passed over the Cumberland Gap and traversed the blue grass country of Kentucky, where Shawnee Indians had twice captured Daniel

Boone, but that danger had passed since President Andrew Jackson's 1831 Indian Removal Act, when the entire indigenous population was forcibly relocated to reservations west of the Mississippi River. The Stills crossed the Ohio River by horse-drawn ferry to Cairo, Illinois, and drove north in heavy rain, hiring pilots to avoid straying from the flooded road and sinking into a perilous mire. They crossed the Mississippi by steam ferry to St. Louis, Missouri, and in nearby St. Charles sought out the local Methodist minister, a Reverend Harmon, to rest over the Sunday and wash caked black mud from clothes, wagons and horses.[10]

Abram was carrying nine hundred dollars in gold and silver – fifteen times his annual salary – the proceeds of selling the farm and livestock plus a stipend from the Church to establish a new mission. Harmon prevailed on his good nature to make an unsecured loan of seven hundred dollars, promising repayment with interest at the next meeting of the Missouri Conference, six months ahead.

They likely followed the Great Trail, an Indian trade route that ran along the divide between the Missouri and Mississippi watershed, and arrived at Bloomington, seat of newly organized Macon County, Missouri, on May 2, barely an hour after commissioners had begun driving its boundary stakes into the ground.[11] The embryonic community boasted a courthouse (a two-room log cabin) and a small store, but had no school, church or newspapers. North towards the Iowa line much was unmapped and unsurveyed, with no roads save the timeless trails of animals and the resident Sac and Fox Indians. The previous year nomadic Sioux had camped on the nearby Chariton River during the hunting season.[12]

With his remaining money Abram purchased a squatter's claim in nearby Barnesville, a mix of woods and prairie with a natural spring. He bought two cows,[13] then they dipped into Martha's $350 savings. The Conference came and went, and Harmon failed to repay the loan. It shocked Drew to learn that unlike his scrupulously honest father, "some preachers were not of God, but dirty liars, just the same as some other people are."[14]

Harmon's confidence trick threw them into a radical, raw existence, one that the seventh child Mary, born in September 1838, described as a life of "happiness yet of great privations," their "hard-earned home made sacred by years of self-denial."[15] Little currency circulated. Raccoon skins were legal tender and taxes were paid in wolf scalps.[16] Everyone was poor, but this was a poverty with no sense of degradation, for what mattered on the frontier was not money but practical results, achieved through self-sufficiency and hard physical work. Embracing the motto *necessity is the mother of invention,* the family prepared as best they could for the frigid Midwest winter.[17]

They dug a well, felled trees to make tables, chairs and bedsteads, and planted a garden with potatoes, pumpkin, squash and beans. With an old flintlock rifle Ed, Jim and Drew brought home deer, turkey, prairie chicken, duck, quail and squirrel. Nothing was wasted. Meat was preserved in the smokehouse, deerskins tanned and fashioned into moccasins, breeches and jackets,[18] and fox, raccoon, mink and beaver pelts crafted into hats.[19] The boys milked the cows, churned butter, and that first spring helped their father clear the land and plant a crop of corn before he embarked on a six-week circuit that allowed only brief visits home. Abram helped with the reaping, but left to the boys the laborious task of husking and cribbing before the onset of winter.[20] To grind flour for cornbread they carted the crop to Hannibal, one hundred miles each way.[21]

As the farm became established they constructed their own grist and saw mill, and split fence rails to make enclosures for horses, mules, cattle, hogs and sheep. Sundown was a time of anxiety, when everything needed securing not only against bear, wolf and mountain lion but also against the local Indians[22] who, though generally on good terms with the whites, commonly stole possessions and killed livestock.[23] Even in old age Still would never be able to enjoy the beauty of a sunset, the onset of dusk prompting an uncharacteristic coldness of manner and a surprising deadness to his usually springy gait.[24] The greatest danger, though, came from rattlesnakes. During the summer the timber and prairie were alive with them, and everyone carried a club the size of a walking stick for protection. One year a neighbor was bitten while helping with the harvest, the poison passing directly into a vein, and he collapsed dead after only a few steps.[25]

At age ten Drew made what he later called his "first discovery in osteopathy." Suffering from one of his frequent nauseous headaches, he tied a plow line between two trees to make a swing, hoping to rock away the pain, but swinging proved too painful so he lowered the rope to a few inches above the ground, spread the end of a blanket over it, and lay down with his neck supported by this "swinging pillow." He soon relaxed and fell asleep and to his surprise woke to find the headache gone. For the next thirty-five years this method and a home-made wooden rack with a notch for his neck, built for the same purpose, became his standard headache remedy.[26] On an early milling trip to Hannibal he adapted the principle to treat a four-year-old girl with a sore back. He took a bottle, placed it under the sore spot, and rolled her around over it.[27]

In spring 1840 Abram took an appointment in newly organized Schuyler County and they moved to an eighty-acre tract near present-day Queen City.[28] Two years later he was assigned the nearby Edina circuit,[29] and that year they built a small log schoolhouse seven feet high with a dirt floor.[30] During their first five years in Missouri the children had received only one three-month term of formal classes, the winter before they left Macon County, but they were by no means uneducated. When not traveling, ministers were expected to spend five hours a day in prayer, meditation and study,[31] with a list of recommended books that included John Wesley's *Sermons,* his *Philosophy* and *Notes,* and a host of other volumes on theology, philosophy, history, geography and grammar. The children perused these works and, as they grew older, studied their father's medical texts and his copy of Milton's *Paradise Lost*, a sourcebook favored by preachers for its graphic depictions of hellfire, damnation and the depravity of man.[32]

During the summer months farming took precedence and, with Abram absent for long periods, Martha oversaw the work – something she did "just as well as father," Drew considered, "or a little better." She taught the boys to handle the teams and manage the machinery from planting to harvest. On a homemade spinning wheel she twisted knitting yarn and on a card loom wove cotton cloth for jeans and brightly colored linsey-woolsey hunting shirts that in time supplanted their rude buckskins. Martha brought discipline to the family and occasionally resorted to the rod, but only in a "homeopathic way."[33] Drew admired his mother, her strength, determination and practicality engendering in him a lifelong conviction that women should have equality to men.[34]

He was more ambivalent towards Abram. "My father was a good man," he wrote, before adding in parentheses, "(or tried to be)."[35] Abram brought to the family the gifts of "generosity, honesty, untiring perseverance and practical good sense."[36] Though generally patient and mild, on one thing he was strict: religion.

"Know your disease! Know your cure!" John Wesley had exhorted. "Ye

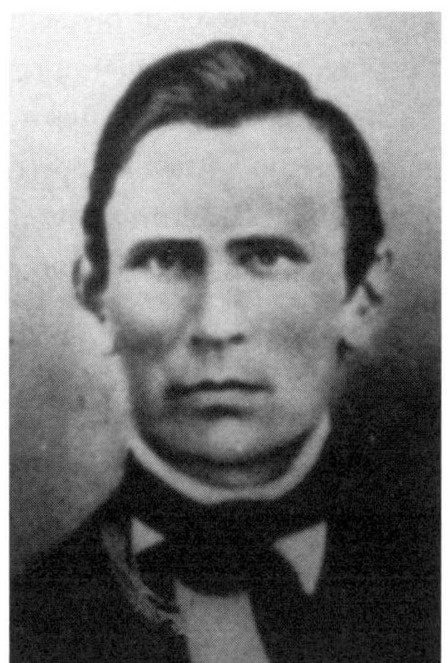
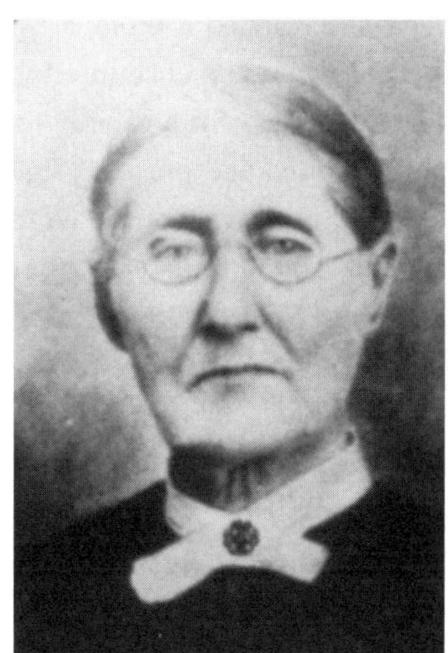

Reverend Abram and Martha Still.

were born in sin, therefore ye must be born again, born of God. By nature ye are wholly corrupted; by grace ye shall be wholly renewed. In Adam ye all died; in the second Adam, in Christ, ye are all made alive."[37] Ministers urged congregations to observe their moral responsibilities, do good works, and live in a state of unconditional love towards God and neighbor. Only by expelling "the love of the world, the love of pleasure, ease, honour and money, together with pride, anger, self-will, and every other evil temper," could they transform the "earthly, sensual, devilish mind into the mind that was in Christ Jesus" and "go on to perfection."[38]

Salvation, reserved solely for believers, was to be attained through *justification* and *sanctification*: a forgiveness of sins and a simultaneous blessing conferred by the Lord upon his pardoned child. With personal experience of God's saving grace a change took place in the heart and will, and the sinner was "born again," born of the Spirit, into a new life of "holy living." Complete sanctification was a lifelong process; the flesh continued to lust against the Spirit and constant vigilance was required to avoid backsliding.

Even on a bitterly cold day Abram would don his heavy bearskin coat, tie a beaver hat under his beard, and set off perhaps fifty miles on horseback.[39] In his saddlebags he carried a Bible, a hymn book and a wallet of medicines in sections of canes,[40] and on encountering settlers invited them to an impromptu service in the woods or in a cabin,[41] to sing a hymn or two and listen to one of his "plain, pointed and practical"[42] sermons peppered with self-deprecating humor and vivid portrayals of the wrath of God. When he returned home the family gathered around to listen to the stories of his travels and the success of his ministrations.

Abram expected – insisted – that before entering their teens his children convert to Methodism by a formal profession of faith in Christ the Savior.[43] When John and Mary showed no inclination of doing so he even organized a special camp meeting to produce the desired result. For Mary it proved dramatic. "Some unseen presence did enter my soul,"[44] she wrote of her conversion, "I can't tell how, and change it." She described the evangelical fervor of the time:

> It was a sight never to be forgotten to see one of those encampments after nightfall, with a half-dozen bonfires, and hear the melody of sacred song as it floated out upon the evening air. The people humbled themselves before God. And in answer to their consecration and prayer, God manifested His presence. People, while listening to the preaching of the word, would fall powerless, seized upon by the Holy Spirit, and continue in that condition for hours, and when they would come to consciousness it would be with such a perceptible 'death to sin' and a new life in Christ, they would shout and give glory for hours.[45]

Mary became a minister herself, but for Drew this fundamentalism inspired more fear than religious zeal. His father made him memorize lengthy passages from the Bible, under threat of a beating for any lapse, and he recited them as he walked behind the plow. These verses were never forgotten; fifty years later he could still repeat whole chapters from memory.[46] Drew lived in dread of the Day of Judgment, alert for the signs and half-signs that might herald the impending catastrophe. The millennial prophet William Miller had even predicted its date – 21 March 1843 – and his followers held frenzied camp meetings in preparation.[47]

The world did not end, but what did, the following year, was the unity of the Methodist Church. Festering discord over the issue of slavery led to a schism and the formation of a new proslavery organization, the Methodist Episcopal Church South, in direct competition with the parent Church, with state conferences left to decide their affiliation.

Missouri was a slave state. Carved from the vast region acquired by the United States in 1803 by the Louisiana Purchase, its admission to the Union in 1821 was accompanied by a series of measures designed to preserve an equal number of free and slave states. Under the terms of the Missouri Compromise all Louisiana Purchase territories south of Missouri's southern border became slave and all to its north free, with the exception of Missouri itself.

The Missouri Conference voted six to one in favor of the new proslavery Church South. The parent Church, lacking sufficient members, suspended organized activities in the state and Abram found himself stranded without an appointment.[48] In spring 1845 he took the family back to Macon County.

Much had changed. Bloomington, Callao and Macon City[49] had become centers of a thriving new tobacco industry with plantations and factories worked by slave labor. To prevent "race degeneration" the state legislature had enacted statutes pronouncing marriages between whites and "negroes or mullatoes" illegal and void, and passed new laws with stiff penalties for spreading abolitionist literature – a heavy fine and up to two years in jail for a first offence, up to life imprisonment for a third.[50] Those who openly criticized slavery were branded insurrectionist and subjected to persecution or violence. Abram nevertheless continued to preach that slavery was a sin, until the Church South finally issued him with a warning: change his affiliation or be expelled from Missouri. In response he attached himself to the antislavery Iowa Conference and was placed in charge of the handful of Missouri ministers who remained loyal to the parent Church.[51]

Drew was sixteen, and by his own admission "awkward, ignorant, and slovenly." He refused to attend a local school taught by a G. B. Burkhart, "as he and I did not agree," and took lodgings in La Plata, twenty miles north, to study at a school run by the Cumberland Presbyterian Church.[52]

He did not know what he wanted to do or be. He disliked farming, despising the tedium of long hours spent in the corn field and the boredom of arduous, repetitive chores like milking cows, churning butter and carrying slop to the hogs. He entertained a half-hearted notion of becoming a circuit rider, but was beginning to question the Christian concept of God and to develop his own ideas about "that unknown intelligence, call it what you please."[53] In 1847, at the height of the Mexican-American War, he desperately wanted to enlist in the army, but was underage and Abram refused to consent.[54]

One trait shone through, though: when something interested Drew it absorbed his whole attention. An "uncommon successful hunter," he brought home venison, turkey, prairie chicken and other game.[55] He was a good judge of dogs, too, if no businessman; instructed to sell good pups for $1 each, he usually gave them away.[56] Above all he enjoyed applying his ingenuity to practical problems, whiling away hours in his father's workshop repairing and maintaining the farm machinery, designing and making tools and implements, and crafting buckets, barrels, furniture, and other objects.[57]

Martha had early recognized in him a rare inquisitiveness, in particular a keen curiosity about nature.[58] "My mother used to say of me," he wrote cryptically, "that she felt sure that someday I would dig my toes into the opposite bank and come back with some of the clay sticking to them."[59] Game was more than food for the table. Martha would find him absorbed in primitive dissections of squirrels, rabbits, chickens, and other animals, examining bones and muscles and organs, even tracing the courses of nerves and blood vessels.[60] A habit of asking *how* and *why* was forming.

He brought home bones and tried to fathom reasons for their size and shape. He examined birds. The turkey vulture possesses a tongue "wonderfully constructed for cutting and tearing flesh," he noted, "otherwise his head and beak are formed just as a common turkey."[61] On finding the carcass of a swan, eager to learn how it made its "enchanting call," he plucked the neck feathers and made an incision to "see the construction of that great and natural music box." He laid bare the windpipe and followed its course to the breastbone, where it divided into two sack-like tubes, each extending to a lung. "Those sacks seemed to be the musical part of the bagpipe of the swan," he concluded, though much remained beyond the ken of this budding investigator. "When I took the windpipe out of the lungs with the musical bags I had a trachea five foot long. Why this wonderfully long pipe ran backward and forward doubling itself so often until it got into the mouth of the bird I cannot tell, I can only say this, that the softest and most melodious sound I ever heard came from that bird."[62]

In quiet moments he drew caricatures, gathering the sketches in a book he called his "commentary." One drawing depicted a quack doctor whose remedy for measles was ram's head soup, the patient trying to swallow the head whole, the horns protruding from his mouth.[63] It illustrated a growing fascination with medicine, an interest his father initially tried to discourage because it interfered with farm work. A neighbor told of seeing Abram return from town one day to find his sixteen-year-old son sitting by the roadside reading an anatomy text. "Andrew," he shouted," I don't allow any doctor books in my field." The youth merely swiveled his legs back into the road and kept on reading.[64] He was discovering that the human body is made of the familiar mammalian structures and learning "the hard names given to them by the scientific world."[65]

Before licensing laws were introduced in the 1870s and 1880s, apprenticeship to a qualified physician was an accepted route into medicine. When the Stills returned to Macon County, Ed had been understudying his father for four years and, with Abram absent much of the time, largely taken over his practice.[66] Jim was already following in Ed's footsteps. Abram eventually acknowledged where Drew's heart lay and encouraged him to study medicine too.

Drew learned how to diagnose from symptoms and signs, and the art of prescribing the standard pharmacopoeia for purging, puking and sweating: staples such as calomel, quinine, tartar emetic, arsenic compounds, digitalis, opium and whiskey, supplemented by herbs and folk remedies including rhubarb, gamboge, aloes, lobelia and soap pills.[67] He detested taking this "poisonous filth" himself, abhorring the times he was spanked and had his nose held to get down a dose of castor oil, while his father asked God to bless the means used for his recovery.[68] At age fourteen Drew experienced the ravages of calomel, a chloride of mercury administered in reckless quantities for a wide variety of conditions despite severe side-effects: salivation, erosion of gums, loss of teeth, and necrosis of the jaw. "Today I am using part of a set of store teeth," he reflected later, "because I lived in a day and generation when people had no more intelligence than to make cinnabar out of my jawbone."[69]

Andrew's schooldays ended in summer 1848 with a course of mathematics in La Plata. His formal education had been sparse, but he would later come to regard his backwoods upbringing as far superior to that of children raised in the "civilized" Eastern states. Pure air, plain natural diet, outdoor exercise; these he believed essential for balanced physical and mental development.[70] Raised in nature, free from constraints and pressures towards conformity, he learned early to think for himself and make his own decisions, and entered adulthood fearless, courageous and resourceful.

Most importantly, and crucial to his future development of osteopathy, he had unconsciously acquired a way of thinking uncommon in American society. "He thought not in words, as the 'educated' mind would do," one of his later students wrote, "but in terms of pictures, events, forces, wholes."[71] Andrew learned about plants and animals not from books or from specimens in a laboratory, but from the thing itself in its natural environment. Nature to him was not an object to analyze but a subject to experience, one vast protean whole, and he a participant in its ever-changing pattern.[72]

On 29 January 1849, aged twenty and a slim five feet eleven and three quarters, he married Mary Margaret Vaughn, a young woman of Welsh descent, in a service conducted by his father's colleague Lorenzo Waugh. The newlyweds took an eighty-acre tract a mile from the Still family home and Andrew planted sixty with corn, but the signs were inauspicious for a career in farming. On Independence Day a calamitous hailstorm destroyed the entire crop, killing rabbits, birds, and his livelihood.[73] The following winter, to support Mary Margaret and their first child Marusha, born on 8 December, he found work as a teacher in a log schoolhouse one mile west of Barnesville.[74]

He did not know it, but his future was already being shaped by his father's struggles within the Methodist Church.

2

WAKARUSA MISSION

In 1848 Abram and five antislavery colleagues reorganized a Missouri Conference of the parent Methodist Episcopal Church.[1] For his family's safety Abram, despised in Macon County for his abolitionist preaching, sought a distant position,[2] and was appointed presiding elder of the Grand River and Platte District in northwest Missouri. Under his charge came an area bordering the Missouri River and a section on its opposite bank in Nebraska Territory, now Kansas, where twenty-seven reservations had been created to accommodate mainly Eastern tribes displaced by President Jackson's Indian Removal Act.

White settlement was not authorized west of the river, the vast plains stretching towards the Rocky Mountains thought to be a "Great Desert" fit only for nomadic Indian tribes, and the only Europeans permitted to remain on the reservations were a detachment of troops stationed at Fort Leavenworth and a handful of Christian missionaries who vied for Indian converts.

The Methodist Church had established the territory's first mission in 1831 on the Shawnee reservation, a long strip extending along the south bank of the Kaw River from its confluence with the Missouri.[3] By 1844 the church's Tahlequah Indian Conference boasted nearly 3000 members, including most of the 900 Shawnee,[4] and after the schism that year all but a few dissenters fell under the jurisdiction of Reverend Thomas Johnson of Shawnee Mission.

Johnson's Mission, as it was known, grew to become a powerful proslavery stronghold, with close ties to political leaders in Missouri. By the terms of the Missouri Compromise slavery was forbidden in Nebraska Territory, but interested parties turned a blind eye as produce from a farm worked by black slaves and a range of goods manufactured by Indian students at the mission's Manual Labor School was sold to travelers on the Oregon and Santa Fe trails, earning fortunes for Johnson and his associates.[5] "What a heterogeneous company compose of those Missions!" Henry Harvey, Quaker missionary to the Shawnee, wrote:

> Rich slave-holding preachers, exhorters, and school teachers; Indian chiefs, preachers and scholars, too, rich in lands and other property – the whites receiving pay for their own labor (and for the blacks too), the Indians receiving the benefit; all members of the same church, eat their bread and drink their wine at the same communion table, and unite in the same family devotion! But then too, there is another class of human beings at the same Mission, but alas for them, they are black! 'These reap down the fields, and their wages are withheld from them.' Such a course as this does not suit me.[6]

Nor did it suit Abram. To establish an antislavery presence among the Indians he journeyed to the Wyandot reservation, a fertile wooded tract on the north bank of the Kaw where it flowed into the Missouri, since many of the tribe remained uncommitted to Johnson. On 29 October 1848 Wyandot principal chief (and Johnson supporter) William Walker entered in his diary, "Went to Church, and to our astonishment found the presiding Elder of the Quasi Northern District, a Mr. Still; the Deacon, as a matter of Grace, asked him to preach, which he attempted to do. . . . The Church was then divided, South from the North."[7] Forty-one sided with Johnson, sixty-nine with Abram.

The northern Church cemented its presence by appointing Reverend James Gurley missionary to the Wyandot and, the following February, directly after Andrew and Mary Margaret's wedding, Abram returned to hold his first quarterly meeting. In bitter cold he crossed the broad Missouri River, "in a skiff, swimming his horse amidst great blocks of ice," to find Gurley gone, expelled by the Indian agent at the insistence of southern members.[8] In August 1849 the Church installed Reverend Thomas Markham as Gurley's replacement, assisted by Pascal Fish, Jr., a forty-five-year-old Shawnee chief ordained as a "native assistant."

INDIAN LANDS
KANSAS 1853

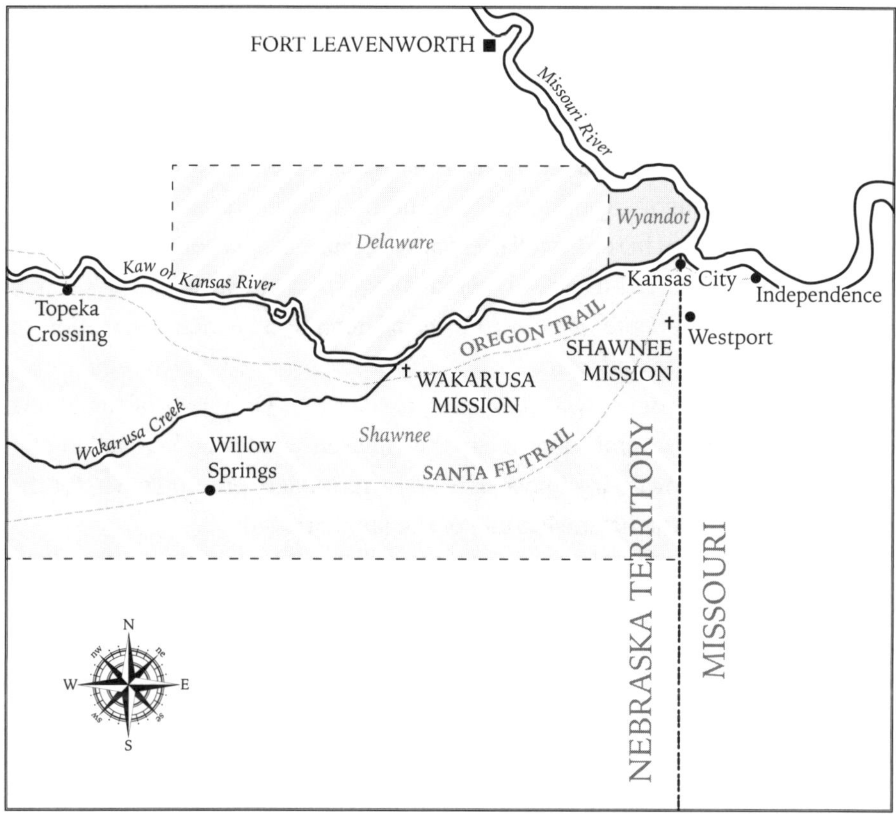

Fish's appointment angered Johnson. The chief's father, Pascal Fish, Sr. (a white man born William Jackson but captured as a child and reared Indian)[9] had been instrumental in the founding of Shawnee Mission, while Fish Jr., a "sober, steady, moral, good man," had been the institution's first interpreter and, since his ordination in 1847,[10] acted as Johnson's missionary to the Kickapoo. In March 1850, as Fish, Jr. suffered persecution for his defection,[11] Indian agent

Luke Lea, undoubtedly at Johnson's behest, forbade Markham from preaching among the Shawnee.[12]

At the following year's annual conference of the northern Church in St. Louis a communication was received from "Bro. Pascal Fish and others" requesting the establishment of a school for antislavery Shawnee. Abram appealed for the project to be supported[13] and, appointed Superintendent of Indian Missions, was charged with establishing a mission school "in the Shawnee Nation."[14]

On his return home Abram broke the news to Martha with great hesitation. She dissolved into tears, reminding him that the Shawnee were the tribe that had captured her father and slaughtered her grandparents. "So they did, over seventy-five years ago," Abram replied. "And now, wife, we are chosen by the Conference to go, and in return tell them about Jesus." It was pointless to object. Ministers were expected to place Church above spouse, and what the Church said, Abram did. In September 1851 he set off for the Shawnee reservation to build a mission house and farm.

His six-month absence was agonizing for Martha. Only two of his letters were delivered and several times a day the children would see her walking far down the road hoping for a glimpse of his return. Anxiety prompted her, for the first time, to relate the harrowing tale of the family tragedy.

Martha's great-grandfather James Moore II emigrated from Northern Ireland "about the year 1726."[15] In 1772, her grandfather James Moore III settled in the remote mountain meadow of Abb's Valley, Virginia, and for defense built a fortified blockhouse cabin, for the valley was a favorite Shawnee and Cherokee hunting ground and location of their summer encampments. When Indians resentful of the white intrusion killed many settlers in the vicinity two of Moore's nearest neighbors abandoned their homes, but he refused to be intimidated even after an entire family with six children was wiped out.

Early on 7 September 1784 Moore sent his fourteen-year-old son James (Martha's father) to fetch a horse from a pasture two miles from their home. James had often gone there alone without fear, but on this occasion had barely lost sight of the house when an unaccountable feeling of dread came over him, "an undefined apprehension of some great calamity that would befall him." He wanted to turn back but, fearing his father's displeasure, continued on, and as he neared the field a Shawnee warrior named Black Wolf and two younger accomplices "sprang from behind a large log, and yelling the terrific war whoop, rushed on him, and laid hold of him." They took the teenager captive to a Shawnee settlement on the Scioto River, Ohio.[16]

Two years later Black Wolf struck again. On 14 July 1786 Mrs. Moore was preparing breakfast when war cries suddenly split the air and forty braves broke from the trees on the Abb's Valley ridge in a headlong charge towards the farm. The field workers scattered into the woods. James's younger sister Mary, who had gone out to call everyone in to eat, barely made it back to the cabin before her mother shut and barred the door, accidentally locking out younger siblings William, Rebecca and Alexander to be butchered and scalped in the yard. Their father, soaking deer skins in the creek, was felled by seven shots as he reached the rail fence. Servant John Simpson, sick in bed upstairs, was killed by a shot in the head as he peered out of the window. As tomahawks splintered the door Mrs. Moore gathered up baby Margaret and knelt to pray with children Mary, Jane, John and neighbor girl Mattie Evans, before opening the door and surrendering to her fate. The warriors ate the food she had prepared, looted the cabin, set it on fire, killed the livestock, and led the survivors away on foot over the mountainous Appalachian terrain.

Their ordeal had only just begun. On the second day John, recovering from fever and struggling to keep up, was taken aside and a Shawnee returned with a scalp hanging from his belt. The following day baby Margaret cried incessantly and, fearing detection, another warrior dashed the infant's head against a tree and threw the lifeless body into the bushes. The twenty-day trek ended in the Shawnee settlement of Chillicothe, Ohio, where the four remaining captives were split into pairs and taken to separate villages. A party of Cherokees, seeking revenge after an unsuccessful raid on white communities in Pennsylvania, entered one village, plied the Shawnee with alcohol and induced them to kill their prisoners.

Jane and Mrs. Moore were tied to a stake, stuck with fine blazing splinters, and burned to death.[17] Mary and Mattie Evans, concealed by Shawnee women in the other village until the danger passed, did not learn what had happened until days later when brought to the scene of the atrocity. Nine-year-old Mary found the charred remains of her sister and mother in the ashes of a fire, gathered the half-burned bones in her hands and, borrowing a hoe from an Indian woman, buried them in a rude grave marked by a stone.

Mary and Mattie were eventually reunited with James who, after two years in Ohio, was bartered for a horse by a French trader and taken to safety in Canada.[18] The three returned to Abb's Valley where, near the ruins of their old cabin, James built the house in which Martha was born.[19]

She need not have feared for Abram's safety. He returned at the beginning of March 1852, saddlebags stuffed with gifts of moccasins and beaded purses for the whole family. A fortnight later all except Andrew, Barbara Jane and Ed, married with young families, set off for Nebraska Territory in two covered wagons, with John and Mary riding horseback driving twenty head of cattle. They crossed a swollen Missouri river by ferry to the small settlement of Kansas City, a handful of houses and stores, a couple of blacksmith shops and a few desultory Indians sitting around on goods boxes.[20] From there they followed the Oregon Trail for another thirty miles, past scattered cabins and Indians dressed in colorful shawls and headgear,[21] until they arrived at a broad prairie dotted with wildflowers upon which stood a four room, two story log structure with a thatched roof.[22] This was the Wakarusa Mission. A mile to the north a ribbon of hickory and oak marked the bottom land where the Kaw River was joined by a tributary, the Wakarusa, a native word meaning *hip-deep*.[23] They were greeted by Pascal Fish and his younger brother Charles who, with a nucleus of antislavery Shawnee, had moved away from the vicinity of Johnson's Mission.

Abram opened a small school and with Pascal's assistance ran Sunday prayer meetings, the Indians singing the Christian songs in their native Algonquin tongue. The Shawnee women were friendly and helpful,[24] and the men dropped in to smoke sumac leaves, their tomahawks doubling as pipes.[25] Pascal visited nearly every day, he and Abram sitting for hours in the shade of the smokehouse relating their experiences.[26] For the first six months the only white person the Stills encountered was William Greiffenstein, a German who had lived for years among the Indians after fleeing his homeland to avoid being drafted into the army. On Saturday evenings "Dutch Billy" closed his small store at Bluejacket Ford on the Wakarusa to spend the weekend at the mission.[27]

Abram's commission was both ecclesiastical and medical.[28] The previous year smallpox and a disease they called "black tongue"[29] had ravaged the reservations, and that winter many more died from cholera, dysentery, pneumonia, typhoid, malaria, and other infections. An inflammatory eye condition blinded an orphaned Indian girl and afflicted the Still family with "dimmed vision, weak eyes, granulated lids &c."[30] Abram was overwhelmed and in spring 1853 sent Andrew a message: could he come and help doctor the Indians that fall?

Twenty-four and the father of two since the birth of a son, Abraham, the previous November, Andrew had spent the last four years farming and pursuing his medical studies at home.[31] In anticipation of his duties he purchased a copy of Robley Dunglison's *The Practice of Medicine* and asserted his ownership with an inscription: *A. T. Still's. Book price $3.00 Ap 15th 1853*.[32] The following month he and his family traveled to the Wakarusa Mission. Over the summer he plowed ninety acres with a team of six oxen while Mary Margaret, with Charles Fish as interpreter, taught thirty pupils up to eighth grade at the mission school.[33]

Andrew soon became on "very friendly terms" with the Indians[34] and earned a reputation among them as a "great talker."[35] He learned their language and as he gained in proficiency began to translate for Abram as he preached.[36]

Many respected Shawnee steeped in the history and traditions of the tribe lived near the mission and assisted with its running.[37] Charles, George and Henry Bluejacket, who ran "a roadhouse or inn" near Dutch Billy's store,[38] were grandsons of the renowned war chief Blue Jacket. Their father Jim Bluejacket was a friend of the celebrated leader and warrior Tecumseh,[39] who was a "cousin" of Pascal and Charles.[40] No Shawnee was more venerated than Tecumseh, a revolutionary thinker, orator and diplomat respected even by the whites. The Fish and Bluejacket brothers had attended mission schools in childhood and spoke good English.

Through a strong oral tradition the Indians recalled significant events affecting their tribe and others for generations. Some even remembered the story of how Martha's grandmother was burned at the stake.[41]

A century and a half earlier the Shawnee had roamed the Atlantic coast south to the Carolinas and Georgia, and west beyond the Appalachians to Kentucky, Tennessee and neighboring states. In the early nineteenth century, driven back by military force and relentless white settlement into an ever-shrinking area of Ohio close to Lake Erie, Tecumseh summarized their predicament:

> Once, there was not a white man in all this country. Then, it all belonged to the red men; children of the same parents – placed on it by the Great

> Spirit, to keep it, to travel over it, to eat its fruits, and fill it with the same race. Once a happy people, but now made miserable by the white people, who are never satisfied, but always encroaching on our land. They have driven us from the great salt water, forced us over the mountains, and would shortly push us into the lakes, but we will go no further. The only way to stop this evil, is for all the red men to unite in claiming a common right in the soil, as it was at first, and should be now, for it was never divided, but belonged to all. No tribe has a right to sell even to each other, much less to strangers, who demand all, and will take no less.[42]

Tecumseh tried to galvanize all Indian tribes in a single alliance to defend their lands, but with limited success, and after his death in 1813 at the Battle of the Thames the vision of coordinated resistance collapsed. Now all that remained of this once powerful tribe were those on the Kansas reservation and an "Absentee Band" in present-day Oklahoma.

Andrew was absorbing more than history. If he had harbored any preconceptions of the native American from his Methodist upbringing they were soon dispelled. John Wesley had characterized the Indian race as morally, culturally and spiritually deficient: "Religion they have none; no public worship of any kind. God is not in all their thoughts. And most of them have no civil government at all – no laws, no magistrates – but every man does what is right in his own eyes; therefore they are decreasing daily. And very probably in a century or two there will not be one of them left."[43] Those who penetrated deeper than stereotypical prejudice, though, commonly discovered admirable traits often lacking in the white race. The Shawnee's Quaker missionary Henry Harvey wrote of regularly finding himself in the humbling position of being asked for counsel by men, "vastly my superior in years, in experience, in public affairs, in intellect and in power of speech, as well as in fine feelings."[44] Qualities not instilled by acculturation, for contrary to Wesley's view Shawnee behavior was guided by an all-pervasive spirituality interwoven with an almost universally observed moral code.

The cardinal virtues, the basis of character and of relationships with others, were self-control and absolute honesty. Each person was his own judge, responsible not only for his own behavior but for the behavior of all.

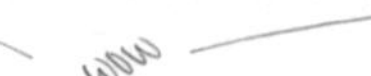

Elders were respected, even those moderately advanced in years.[45] Children were taught that the Creator loves all equally, therefore to injure, wrong or even hate another person was to injure one's self, and to do good to another person and make him happy was to make oneself happy. The Indians had no concept of rich and poor until they saw it in the white population. The love of possessions was a weakness to overcome; those with more than they needed gave to those in want, generosity and gratitude bonding all in a cycle of mutual support. This principle they extended to the Stills, whom they showered with gifts of buffalo jerky, hickory nuts and hominy.[46]

On the reservation Andrew found a notion of God that resonated with his own emerging spirituality. The Shawnee believed in an impersonal Supreme Being who created and ruled the universe and whose ubiquitous power, the Great Mystery of creation, permeated every part and brought everything, material and spiritual, into interrelationship. God and nature were inseparable;[47] nature the embodiment of sacred wisdom and the source of arcane knowledge. Central to their belief system was the principle that the earth and the water must not be harmed, for upon them depend the health of all and the perpetuation of nature's endless cycle.

The colonists showed scant regard for what the Indians held sacred. "Be fruitful and multiply," their Holy scripture urged, "and replenish the earth, and subdue it; and have dominion over the fish of the sea, and over the fowl of the air, and over every living thing that moveth on the earth."[48] Indians the continent over had looked upon these restless intruders with bemusement; their dominant emotion seemed to be fear, their overriding objective the accumulation of riches. The Europeans regarded the earth as "land," a commodity to be parceled for individual ownership or exploited for material gain. They killed the animals, cut down the forests and polluted the waterways. "The white man seeks to conquer nature," Tecumseh's elder brother Chiksika observed, "to bend it to his will and to use it wastefully until it is all gone and then he simply moves on, leaving the waste behind him and looking for new places to take."[49] To the Indians the Earth did not belong to man; man belonged to the Earth.

From an early age Shawnee children learned to observe trees, plants, fruits, and the habits of animals. They kept dates by the waxing and waning of the moon and regulated all work by its stages. They watched closely the position of the sun, particularly at its significant phases around dawn, sunrise, midday, sunset and dusk, and learned to recognize signs for judging the weather and foretelling the seasons.[50] To Andrew these were familiar ideas; his half-Cherokee grandmother had relied upon signs to set hens, kill chickens and butcher hogs.[52] "Who can say how much of this is superstition and how much pure wisdom?" Tecumseh's great-grandson Thomas Wildcat Alford remarked. "To all who listen and look, nature reveals the most astounding secrets."[51]

In the fall, among the Shawnee, Andrew began his career as a medical doctor. Using "such drugs as white men used" he treated fevers, dysentery, pneumonia, the skin infection erysipelas, and other illnesses – while, ever inquisitive, he observed the methods the Indians employed. For fever they wrapped the patient in a wet blanket, left him to sweat it out, and to invoke spiritual aid, "maybe they would dance some hokum to help out a bit."[53] He wrote down the roots and herbs they concocted into medicinal teas – "black-root, lady's thumb, sagatee, muckquaw and chenee olachee" – and noted that their treatment of cholera, pandemic at the time, "was not much more ridiculous" than "some of the treatments used by some of the so-called scientific doctors of medicine." He detailed, "The Indians dug two holes in the ground, about twenty inches apart. The patient lay stretched over the two, vomiting in one hole and purging in the other, and died stretched out in this manner with a blanket thrown over him. Thus they doctored and died, and went to Illinoywa Tapamalaqua, the house of God."[54] He witnessed the appalling cramps caused by the disease. Sometimes the hip muscles were so contracted that he needed to force the legs straight to get the corpse into the coffin.

The Shawnee gave Andrew his first idea of bone-setting, as he observed their crude method of reducing a dislocation. "If a hip came out of joint," he chronicled, "they put that man on his back astride of a small tree trunk and hitched a horse to his ankle and put whips to the horse. Mebby-so the leg got set, mebby-so it came off."[55]

At the end of the year, his medical duties fulfilled, he took his family back to Macon County.[56]

3

BLEEDING KANSAS

On 4 January 1854, Senator Stephen A. Douglas of Illinois reported a bill to Congress to organize the territories of Kansas and Nebraska.

For a decade the idea of a transcontinental railroad had been discussed and, although the route was yet to be established, public consensus favored a scheme financed by public land grants and built by private interests. The success of the venture depended upon sufficient customers and with tens of millions of acres of farmland available in Nebraska Territory the government was keen to open the region to white settlement, but the debate had become mired in Missouri politics and the issue of slavery.

Missouri senator David Atchison supported a route through Nebraska Territory provided that slaveholding was allowed. President Franklin Pierce and other Southern politicians recommended extending slavery into Nebraska Territory, but the Missouri Compromise prohibited the practice in all Louisiana Purchase territories except Missouri north of the parallel 36° 30' north (the state's southern border with Arkansas), and four congressional bills to repeal the agreement had already been defeated. To resolve the deadlock Congress finally agreed upon the principle of "popular sovereignty," proposed by Douglas, whereby settlers could decide the matter themselves in a later ballot.

White settlement demanded extinguishing Indian "title" to the reservations. The government sent a commissioner to negotiate the purchase of surplus land and, in April, invited representatives of all twenty-seven tribes to Washington D.C. for talks. A Shawnee delegation that included Pascal and Charles Fish, with Charles Bluejacket as interpreter, returned having signed a treaty ceding seven-eighths of their land, with each tribal member entitled to 200 acres of the residue.[1] For Abram it signaled the end of the Wakarusa Mission. "The treaties seemed to have been framed upon a scale of favor," his colleague William H. Goode complained, "graduated in accordance with the positions occupied by the several missions upon the question of slavery." Thomas Johnson's Shawnee Mission received rich land grants and generous financial backing; Abram received nothing.[2]

The Kansas-Nebraska Act was ratified on May 30. Passed with an amendment lifting the legal barrier to slaveholding, it effectively invalidated the old Missouri Compromise line and generated a storm of protest in the North. In Douglas's home state, Illinois, former U.S. Representative Abraham Lincoln condemned the Act as a "great moral wrong and injustice," reviled the governing of one man by another as despotism, and warned that the partisan struggle for popular sovereignty would lead to disaster.[3]

He was soon proved correct. A slave was a valuable property, worth up to $3,000 or 500 acres of prime land, and with an estimated 25,000 held in the Missouri counties bordering Kansas their owners, fearing escapes or liberation, felt threatened by the prospect of free territory so close by. To preempt the contest for popular sovereignty Missourians poured into Kansas, staked land claims, established the towns of Atchison and Leavenworth, and organized defensively against an expected influx of abolitionist settlers. In New England, meanwhile, entrepreneur Eli Thayer, supported by *New York Tribune* editor Horace Greeley, set up the Massachusetts Emigrant Aid Company to colonize the territory with abolitionists. Antislavery settlements soon sprang up at Topeka, Manhattan, and at Lawrence, eight miles west of the Wakarusa Mission.

Abram was forced to close the institution that October, and the land reverted to Pascal Fish. The Stills remained there over the winter, and on 10 March 1855 moved to a new cabin that Abram had erected near Blue Mound a few miles southwest along the Wakarusa.[4]

On the same day in Missouri, Andrew and Mary Margaret lost a one-day-old baby, George, and buried his remains in a small private cemetery next to the graves of three of Ed's infant children.[5]

Macon County, with its slave-run tobacco factories and plantations, was becoming increasingly uncomfortable for abolitionists. With the future of

Kansas hanging in the balance, and politicians in Washington debating whether the United States Constitution provided for the rights of blacks as well as whites, Andrew arrived at a decision: "I chose the side of freedom. I could not do otherwise, for no man can have delegated to him by statute a just right to any man's liberty, either on account of race or color."[6] In May, a few weeks after his sister Barbara Jane did the same, Andrew and family left for Kansas.[7]

They arrived in the midst of a deepening crisis. Elections to the Territorial Legislature, held on March 30, had been a fiasco. Of almost 6000 ballot papers counted only 1410 were marked by legitimate settlers, the rest by armed companies of Missourians who crossed the border to systematically cast illegal votes. Elected by this fraud, a proslavery legislature set up temporary headquarters at Shawnee Mission.

Tents and log shanties dotted the prairies as home hunters staked claims, cleared land, killed snakes and poisoned wolves with strychnine. Andrew erected a cabin near that of his parents, resumed a medical practice and, in June, joined a dozen men who formed the Palmyra Town Company to survey and lay out a 320-acre site on a ridge of high ground along the Santa Fe Trail, the trade route linking Independence, Missouri, with Mexico.[8]

At breakfast time one morning a Town Company man, Henry Saunders, galloped up to Andrew's cabin panic stricken, imploring him to make haste. Saunders' wife had awoken at four that morning thinking she had been bitten by a spider, but on lighting a candle and drawing back the covers they found a rattlesnake in the bed. The woman was delirious, striking out at anything that came near. Her eyes were puffed shut, and her face, neck, mouth and tongue so swollen that she "scarcely looked like a human being." Two puncture wounds marked her lower lip.

Innovation was already a feature of Dr. Andrew Still's practice. He seemed to treat medical conditions like everything else on the frontier, as practical problems to be solved by skill and ingenuity – and sometimes by little more than plain experiment. As a child he had once caught a rattlesnake, held its jaws open with a stick, and into its mouth poured hartshorn (spirits of ammonia) to see if it would "cut a caper." It simply died on the spot.[9] Now he took a razor and made seven shallow incisions the length of his patient's neck to drain out the accumulated fluid and, aiming to neutralize the poison, applied hartshorn to the gashes. Mrs. Saunders survived, though her recovery was long and incomplete.[10]

That June, Still improvised another risky treatment. While riding west along the Santa Fe Trail to make a house call, he noticed in the distance a commotion surrounding a convoy of Mexican freight wagons and on arriving at the scene saw a stockman lying on the ground, apparently paralyzed, his head twisted at an odd angle. Onlookers said he had been thrown from his horse at a full gallop and broken his neck. Still introduced himself as a doctor and offered to try and straighten the vaquero's neck, though he warned that the attempt might prove fatal. "Go on," the foreman told him, "he is worse than a dead man now."

Still drove two picket pins into the ground to stabilize his patient's shoulders and, sitting with his feet braced against them, grasped the Mexican's long black hair. Pulling steadily but carefully in line with the spine, he managed to reduce what turned out to be merely a dislocation. As sensation and motion began to return, the man lay quietly for a few minutes before uttering simply, "Muchas gracias, Señor." Relief was mutual. "I was very muchas gracias myself that I had not killed him," Still admitted. Within an hour the Mexican was back on his feet and the foreman rewarded the young doctor, for what was perhaps his first manual treatment, with a $20 gold piece.[11]

On the fourth of July the Stills joined a horseback procession across the prairie to Lawrence, wagons draped in flags and garlanded with flowers, for a grand Independence Day celebration. Settlers mingled with Indians in traditional costume and toasts to the Shawnee were reciprocated in kind by Pascal Fish,[12] but with skirmishes and assassinations on the increase the harmony belied an atmosphere of impending civil war among the white race. Speeches urged vigilance and companies of militia, formed for self-defense, paraded before the crowd. At the end of the month Still joined the Wakarusa Liberty Guards, an eighty-man outfit commanded by Henry Saunders and Connecticut emigrant James B. Abbott, and was assigned the rank of lieutenant.[13] The territory was descending into a conflict known as the Border War or "Bleeding Kansas."[14]

Over the summer the partisan struggle grew entrenched. Territorial governor Andrew Reeder, who had declared the March elections illegal, was removed from office and replaced by Wilson Shannon, a man more sympathetic to the proslavery cause. The legislature ousted all Free-State members and passed a code of "black laws," with slave codes and sedition measures to prohibit criticism of slavery.[15] Representatives of the legal settlers, refusing to recognize the authority of the bogus legislature, convened in Topeka on September 19 to frame a rival constitution and name their own territorial delegate for Congress.

On November 21 an incident sparked a crisis that became known as the "Wakarusa War." A proslavery man, Franklin Coleman, shot dead his abolitionist neighbor Charles Dow in a boundary dispute over adjoining land claims, and fled to Westport, Missouri, into the protective custody of Douglas County sheriff Samuel Jones. Five days later, as abolitionists pressed for the killer to be brought to justice, the sheriff rode out with an armed posse and arrested sixty-five-year-old Jacob Branson, who had shared a cabin with the murdered man, alleging that he had threatened the life of another proslavery supporter, Harrison Buckley. Branson, the only reliable witness to the crime, had merely retrieved Dow's body and carted it home, and to all appearances was being arrested to prevent him testifying against Coleman.

Believing that Branson would likely be hanged, Still's commanding officer James Abbott organized a rescue party. In the early hours, as Jones's posse returned with their prisoner towards Abbott's home at Blanton's Bridge, they ran into ten men lined across the road with rifles and pistols leveled. After a tense standoff, during which Abbott accidentally discharged his revolver, Branson was released.

Retribution was swift. Jones had Governor Shannon issue warrants for the arrest of the "insurrectionists," whose names included Andrew Still, to be tried for violation of Kansas Territory law at the new proslavery capital Lecompton. Briefed that the outlaws were hiding in Lawrence, on December 1 Shannon deployed 1000 troops to surround the town.[16]

The wanted men had already fled. Still, accompanied by James Abbott, went into hiding in a secluded thicket of timber and brush on the banks of the Kaw River, and in this unlikely place was held a conversation that the twenty-seven year old physician would later credit as his inspiration for seeking a better method of practicing medicine.

Ten years Still's senior, cultured, progressive and independent, Abbott had entered the territory with the third group of New England emigrants and quickly established himself as a leader in the abolitionist cause. As the pair

BLEEDING KANSAS 1854 - 57

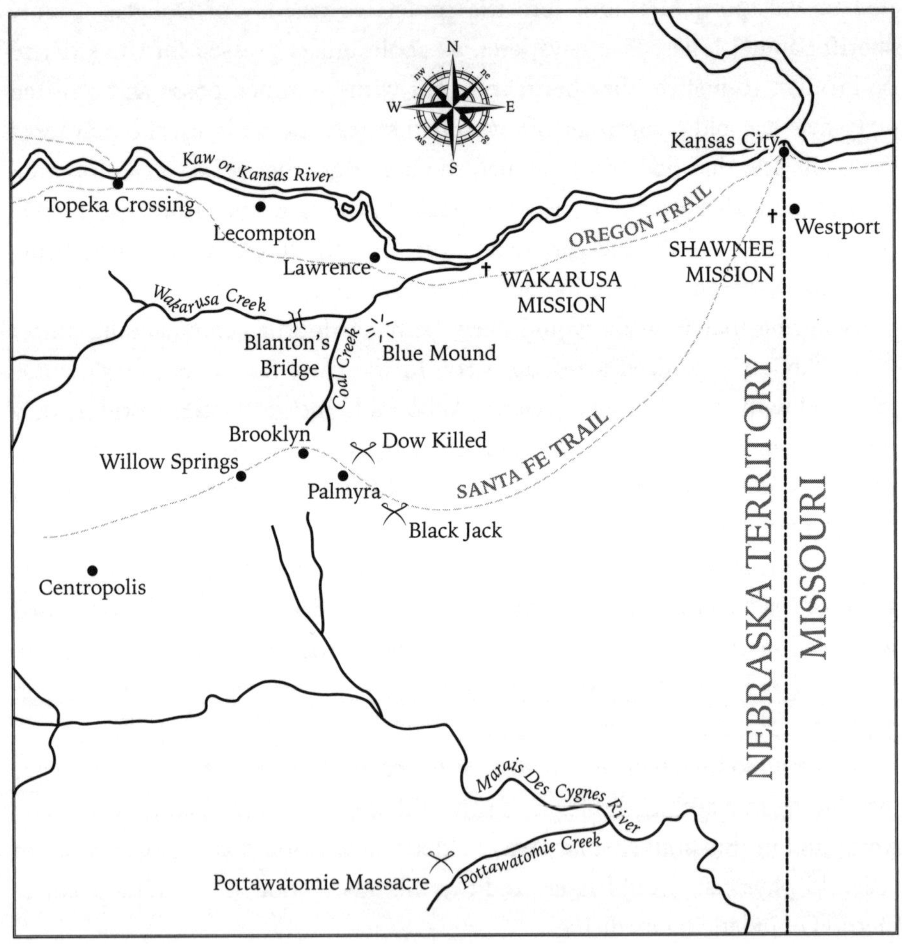

discussed their predicament and the struggle to free Kansas, Still found himself respecting the opinions of this energetic, earnest and public-spirited man.[17]

Abbott spoke of new political reform movements and religious orders that had sprung up in New England over the previous decade, and confided a personal involvement with Spiritualism, a new religion sweeping the country and arousing widespread fascination with intriguing tales of séances and mediums who communicated with the spirits of the dead. He spoke of clairvoyance, describing it as "a curiosity of the day," though to Still the faculty was already familiar. Methodists called it intuition, a working of Divine providence, and Andrew's father always heeded its promptings. While circuit riding in remote areas Abram was known to have returned fifty or seventy miles because of an intuition. Once it was a worry about his horse and he returned home to find old Jim dead. Another time he stopped abruptly in the middle of a sermon, announced he was needed elsewhere, and brought the proceedings to an immediate close. He took up his saddle-bags containing his medical kit and, riding directly to neighbor Jim Bozarth's house, arrived to find him waiting at the door to say his son Ed had broken his thigh.[18]

The conversation turned to the healing arts. "Do you know I have lost all faith in medicine?" Abbott declared. "I am satisfied that it is all wrong, and that the system of drugs, as curative agents, will someday be practically overturned, and some other system or method of curing the sick without drugs will take its place."[19] Still had never before heard his profession criticized and looked at Abbott "in astonishment to hear him talk so wildly."[20] But a seed had been planted.

On December 8 Governor Shannon signed a peace treaty with Free-State leaders and the siege of Lawrence ended. The army withdrew to Missouri and the fugitives emerged from hiding.

A severe winter followed. Three days of snow began on 22 December, the thermometer dipping to -30°F on Christmas day, and the freeze continued until 22 February.

The truce did not last. On January 15 abolitionist settlers held a clandestine election of officers to a rival Free-State legislature, inflaming Sheriff Jones, who reacted by voicing his intent to "wipe out Lawrence and drive every Free-State man out of the Territory, or force them to openly recognize the validity of the Territorial laws." The abolitionist leaders hastily dispatched a letter to President

Pierce requesting he intervene to prevent the invasion. Pierce responded by declaring the Free-State organization "insurrectionary, revolutionary and treasonable," and upheld Sheriff Jones as the only "constituted authority."[21]

The cold weather effectively prevented Jones from pursuing his campaign, and on 4 March 1856, as the Kaw River finally thawed, Free-State men reconvened at Topeka to establish their own provisional government, electing Charles Robinson governor, James Lane senator and James Abbott state representative.

Where Still spent this period is unclear. Mary Margaret was pregnant and on April 11 bore a child they named Susan. At some point she had returned to Missouri, for and the birth was registered in Macon County.

One week later, April 18, a Congressional Investigation Committee entered Lawrence accompanied by Sheriff Jones who, bent upon a policy of intimidation, arrested a number of respectable citizens on trumped up charges. On 23 April, under cover of darkness, an unknown gunman shot the sheriff in the back, but the bullet lodged between his shoulder blades and he survived the attempted assassination.

On May 21 Jones exacted his revenge. His men entered Lawrence, gutted the offices of the *Herald of Freedom* and the *Kansas Free State* newspapers, smashed the presses, threw the types in the Kaw River, and set fire to the nearly completed Free State Hotel, leaving it a smoldering roofless ruin.[22] Wild with drink they plundered houses, destroyed what they could not carry and, as evening approached, looted and burned Governor Robinson's house on Mount Oread, lighting the darkening sky with flames. In retaliation the abolitionist guerrilla John Brown and his four sons massacred five proslavery men on Pottawatomie Creek and mutilated the corpses.

Kansas was plunged into a four-month reign of terror. An atmosphere of fear shrouded the border counties as marauding bands of Missourian "border ruffians" scoured the countryside burning buildings, destroying crops, rustling horses and livestock, and targeting prominent abolitionists. Abram's in-law William Sellers was tarred and feathered and, for preaching against slavery, his colleague Anthony Bewley was hanged by a lynch mob.[23] Colonel Henry Pate, who had participated in the sacking of Lawrence, set out to capture Brown and seized two of his sons, John, Jr. and Jason.

That spring Abram had sold the Blue Mound property to Frederick and Barbara

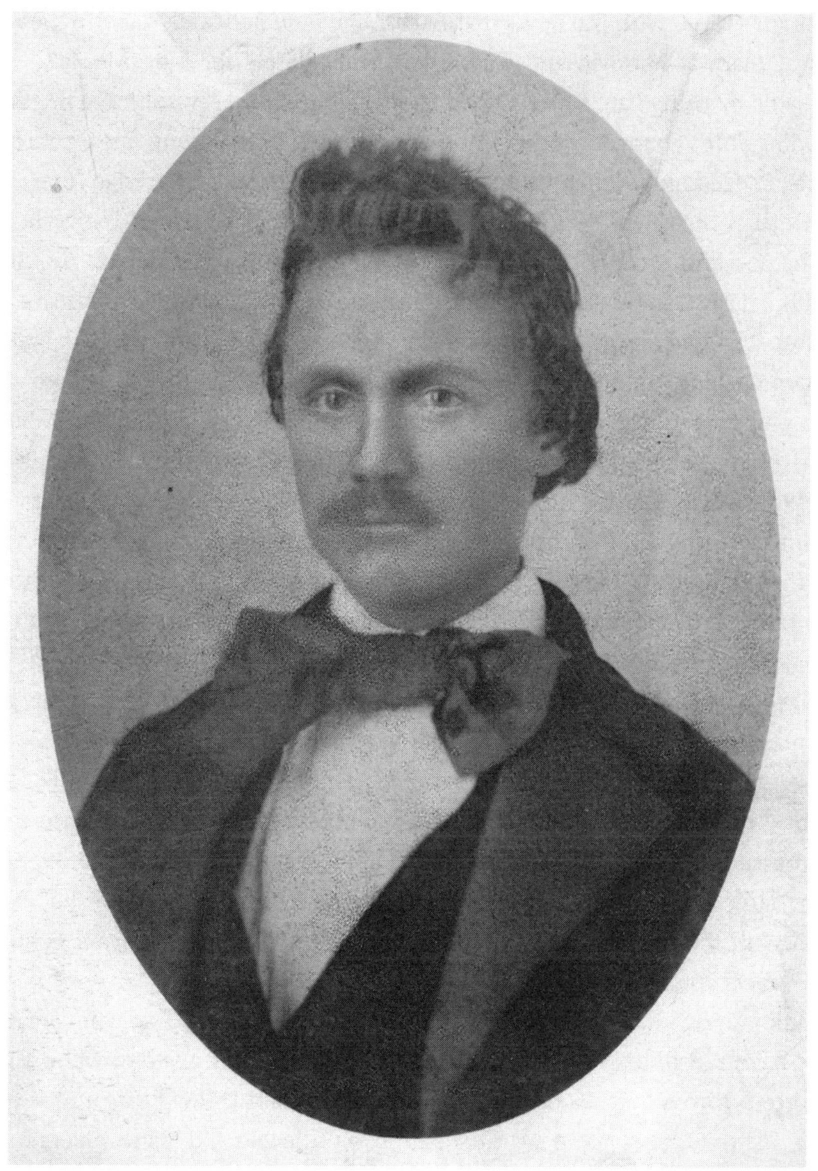

Still aged about twenty-eight, c. 1857.

Jane, and Abram and Andrew staked off claims on the southern boundary of Palmyra to erect shacks of native timber.[24] On Sunday, June 1, a messenger called at Abram's cabin with the news that Barbara Jane was critically ill with measles. Abram, Martha, Marovia and Cassie left immediately for Blue Mound, while that same morning Pate's men raided Palmyra and seized several more prisoners including Still's younger brother Thomas, returning from driving cattle out to the prairie, and led him to their camp beside a small creek called Black Jack five miles southeast of the town. By good fortune one of the proslavery men knew Thomas and helped him escape, but warned that they would take it out on the Stills' neighbor Jake Cantrel instead. Tom remained at the cabin overnight to warn Cantrel, who had agreed to look after the property, that his life was in danger.[25]

Barbara Jane's illness proved providential. Next day, June 2, Brown with twenty-nine men defeated Pate in the Battle of Black Jack and in an exchange of prisoners had his sons released. Later that day a party of Missourians, drunk on whiskey and with blackened faces, rode out to Palmyra in search of Abram, accusing him of "running off niggers on the underground railroad" and threatening to "hang him higher than Haman."[26] Finding no one home, they ransacked and looted the cabin, and scattered the livestock.[27] Cantrel, a Missourian by birth, was not so fortunate. On June 5 he was seized by a proslavery company, and the following day was tried by a mock court, convicted of "treason to Missouri," and shot dead in a ravine.[28]

Neither Abram's nor Andrew's families slept in their cabins again. For self-defense the Still men, Abbott, Saunders and others formed a home guard called the Poker Moonshine Party and at night neighbors for miles around congregated at the large one-roomed house at Blue Mound, the men sleeping out in the brush with their rifles, the women taking turns to keep watch from behind a tent cloth draped over the porch.[29]

Maintaining a medical practice of house calls in this climate, as a marked man, was perilous. Still usually took roads he believed safe, but one day, while taking a shortcut through a wood, his mule slacked up and threw her ears forward, indicating that men were near. He unslung his rifle and slid his revolvers to the front of his belt, but despite his caution blundered into a clearing where fifty or more proslavery men were practicing drill. "What in the devil are you fellows up to?" he yelled, hoping that assertiveness might help defuse the situation.

"Where in the hell are you going?" the surprised commander shouted back, before realizing he knew the intruder. "Attention company," he addressed the platoon, "this is Dr. Still, the damnedest abolitionist out of hell, who is not afraid of hell or high water. When you are sick go for him, he saved my wife's life from an attack of cholera. In politics he is our enemy; in sickness he has proven to be our friend." Captain Owens personally escorted Still to his patient, invited him to dinner, and after that the company allowed him to pass unmolested.[30]

Guerilla warfare presented new medical challenges: penetrating wounds from sabers, knives and gunshot.[31] A surgeon's skill in exploring for bullets or stanching internal bleeding could mean life or death to the patient, and Still was concerned that his anatomical knowledge was insufficient to be sure of avoiding important nerves and blood vessels, so he had Pascal Fish take him along the Santa Fe Trail to the burial grounds of the Shawnee and Delaware Indians. There, by removing a few flat stones from the shallow graves, they uncovered Indian skeletons and freshly buried corpses. Under moonlight and sometimes during daylight Still returned with shovel and scalpel to disinter, dissect and preserve bodies in salt, and remove bones for further study at home.[32] "Someone says the end justifies the means," he wrote in mitigation:

> and I adopted this theory to satisfy the qualms of conscience. The dead Indians never objected to being object-lessons for the development of science. Their relatives knew nothing about it; and as 'where ignorance is bliss it is folly to be wise,' and as the knowledge which I gained by this research has aided me to relieve countless thousands of suffering human beings, and snatch many from the grave, I shall not allow my equanimity of mind to be disturbed by the thoughts that I once sought knowledge from Indian bones.[33]

What he learned was soon put to effect. A Free-State man named Barnes was shot twice through the same thigh, first from the back and then from the front after he fell. Seventeen pieces of coarse buckshot splintered his femur and lacerated the flesh, but the femoral artery (the leg's main blood supply) remained intact so Still decided to try and save the shattered limb from amputation. He cast the leg, knee flexed, in a home-made wooden box and, to cool the limb and reduce inflammation, through this contraption ran water tapped from a six-gallon keg suspended above the bed. He checked regularly for infection or gangrene, removed bits of lead and bone as they pushed to the surface and, after four months, removed the cast. The following summer Barnes was well enough to walk and look after his farm. The case taught Still a fundamental lesson: with appropriate hygiene, even in such an extreme case, an unimpeded supply of arterial blood has an extraordinary power to repair broken bones and heal mutilated tissue.[34]

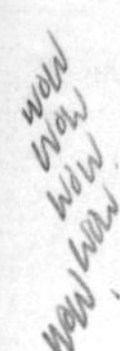

In September 1856 the territory's third governor, John W. Geary, disbanded all armed forces including the proslavery militia, released all Free-State prisoners, and hostilities effectively ceased. A month later, in Lawrence, Bishop Osmon C. Baker presided over the parent Methodist Church's first Kansas-Nebraska Conference,[35] and the following March they reconvened to discuss the establishment of a university, which they agreed to build in Palmyra.

Abram, Andrew, and his younger brothers Tom and John donated their claims – a total of 480 acres – towards a new 640-acre town site on Palmyra's southern border, where Baker University, named by Abram in the Bishop's honor, was to be founded. Andrew, Tom, and James Abbott were appointed ground agents for the three-story limestone structure, and Andrew entered into partnership with brothers Henry and William Barricklow to purchase a forty-horsepower steam sawmill to provide lumber for the building.[36] Abram and Tom staked new claims a few miles south at Centropolis, and Andrew moved to a cabin at Willow Springs, five miles west of Palmyra on the Santa Fe Trail.

Summer 1857 came without organized violence. A wave of new, mainly abolitionist, settlers descended upon the territory, and in October 5 elections to the Territorial Legislature the Free State Party swept to victory in all but two precincts. Still put himself forward as a candidate and was elected Representative of Douglas County.[37] On 2 August 1858 Kansans voted overwhelmingly against a draft constitution to admit Kansas to the Union as a slave state and peace was finally established.

Still practiced medicine and sawed lumber for Baker University and the timber-framed houses that sprang up in the new town which absorbed Palmyra and was renamed Baldwin City. He took a course in milling machinery, attended sessions of the legislature[38] and, on 29 July 1859, voted for the adoption of the

Wyandotte Constitution under which Kansas would eventually join the Union as a free state.

On the same day as the vote Mary Margaret gave birth to a boy they named Lorenzo Waugh after the minister who conducted their wedding. Tragedy followed. Lorenzo lived only six days, and two months later, on 29 September, Mary Margaret also died. The cause of her death is unrecorded and Still left only a brief eulogy: "She was to me beautiful, kind, active, and abounded in love and good sense. She loved God and all His ways."[39] He was thirty-one and a widower with three children.

4

SERIOUS QUESTIONS

Three months after Mary Margaret's passing, Still was summoned by courier to Edgerton, Kansas, to visit two sick girls. Their twenty-five-year-old schoolmistress Mary Elvira Turner, whom the parents had called for advice, thought the children had scarlet fever and suggested they call Dr. Andrew Still, though she knew of him only by reputation.

A physician's daughter from Newfield, New York, Elvira graduated from Poughkeepsie Female Seminary in 1856 and, after working in her father's drugstore for two years, traveled to Kansas in summer 1858 to visit her sister Louise and husband Orson Hulett, who had settled near Edgerton at the end of the Border War. With her father's blessing Elvira decided to remain in Kansas and found work as a teacher at a new schoolhouse in nearby McCamish.[1] As she and a girlfriend waited for the recently widowed doctor to arrive they discussed him with interest.

Still made a poor first impression. Chilled to the bone after a fifteen-mile ride across the prairie, his gruff manner immediately repelled Elvira. "If you want to set your cap for him go ahead," she said to her friend. "He does not suit me." He confirmed her diagnosis and stayed for twenty-four hours to care for the girls, intriguing all by administering no drugs, and left the following morning saying he would be glad to return if they needed him.

The girls made uneventful recoveries, but Still came back anyway – to see Elvira.[2] Despite vowing that she would never marry a doctor, preacher or widower, on 15 November 1860, nine days after Abraham Lincoln was elected president, they were wed. Still had previously known an Elvira he disliked and insisted on calling her Mary; in turn she made him promise to quit chewing tobacco.[3] Mrs. Turner warned Andrew that her daughter was frail, unable to stand hard work, and he would always have to "keep help" for her,[4] but as he visited patients and sawed lumber she milked the cows, did the farm chores and looked after Marusha, Abraham and Susan, aged nine, six and three. And with her knowledge of drug preparation she soon became an integral part of his medical practice.

Meanwhile the country was sliding into chaos. Anticipating that Lincoln would seek to abolish slavery, South Carolina seceded from the Union in December, followed by six more Southern states early in the New Year. On 4 February 1861, less than a week after Kansas was admitted to the Union as a free state, representatives of the seven secessionist states met in Montgomery, Alabama, to formally organize the Confederate States of America. Lincoln, inaugurated on March 4, declared the Union perpetual, secession constitutionally illegal, and violent resistance to federal authority insurrectionary and revolutionary.

The first shots of the Civil War were fired on April 12 as Confederate forces bombarded the Union post of Fort Sumter in Charleston harbor, South Carolina. Three days later Lincoln called for seventy-five thousand volunteers to "stand by the flag" and suppress the rebellion. "You could hear the drums beating in every direction," Still's sister Marovia wrote, "everywhere you were groups were gathered not only men but women & boys & girls singing patriotic songs . . . men & boys were enlisting, women were weeping & the excitement was intense."[5]

Still did not join up immediately. Mary was pregnant and he was busy pursuing a growing obsession. The words spoken by James Abbott six years earlier on the banks of the Kaw, that a system of drugless medicine would someday be found, had made a lasting impression, and the more Still mused upon the subject the stronger the idea grew that he might be the agent of its discovery.[6]

He began some preliminary experiments. On the basis that living nature depends for its survival upon the light and heat of the sun, he planted some corn shoots, measured their height morning and evening, and concluded that growth occurred primarily during the hours of darkness. Reasoning that vegetation must store energy from sunlight during the day and release it for growth during the night, he wondered if the sun's rays might similarly stimulate the growth of animal tissues, perhaps to help promote wound healing, and tested the hypothesis on a patient with a badly gashed knee.

The man had been cutting a stick with a drawing knife when his hand slipped, driving the blade deeply into the knee, partially severing the patellar tendon and slicing into both femoral condyles. Still cleaned the wound and exposed it to "the curative powers of the white solar rays." When the surfaces had dried and a gelatinous fluid appeared he pressed the parts together and bandaged the knee with the leg bound straight. Ten days later his patient was able to begin walking again and the following year enlisted in the Union army, serving until the end of the conflict.

In further researches with sunlight he took two biconvex lenses, two and eight inches in diameter, and focused the rays to cauterize warts and other skin growths. He conducted risky experiments, directing the beam into his own and others' eyes and adjusting the focus. Up to the "cross line or burning point" this had little effect, he noted, but focusing beyond it caused substances to precipitate in the eye "even when it was shut." He employed the lenses "to dissolve opaque bodies such as cataract and floating specks or bodies before the eyes," and found them "valuable in reducing indolent ulcers and assisting in the cure of paralysis and rheumatism." He substituted blue, red and amber glass, but concluded that the sun's power was "complete in the plain white beam."[7]

The war interrupted his studies. By summer eleven Southern states had seceded from the Union and Kansans followed events in neighboring Missouri with growing anxiety. In June, Union commander Nathaniel Lyon declared war on the proslavery Missouri Home Guard under ex-Governor Sterling Price, captured the state capital Jefferson City, and established a garrison at Lexington, thirty miles east of Kansas City. Price retreated southwest with Lyon in pursuit, the two sides skirmishing repeatedly before engaging on August 10 in one of the bloodiest clashes of the Civil War. In the Battle of Wilson's Creek near Springfield, Missouri, Lyon was killed, his army defeated, and an emboldened Price struck north towards Lexington, gathering Southern sympathizers along the way. Union general John C. Fremont, commander of the Western Department, hastily declared martial law and called for reinforcements.

Still reported to Fort Leavenworth on September 6 and enlisted as a regular soldier in the Cass County Home Guards, Company F. The detachment, composed mainly of Kansans involved in the Border War, joined forces with the 9th Kansas Cavalry and marched under orders to Kansas City.[8]

On September 12 Price surrounded Lexington and besieged the garrison for six days before opening fire. The three-day engagement cost the lives of 1774 Union troops and the victorious Price, who lost only 100, fled south into Arkansas chased by 20,000 men including the 9th Kansas Cavalry. The pursuers amassed at Springfield on November 1, and from there Still's battalion was posted to a succession of points along the Missouri border before setting up winter quarters in Harrisonville. In December he was joined by a grieving Mary who, on October 30, lost their first child Dudley Turner, born the day Lexington was besieged. She secured an appointment as a matron in the camp hospital.[9]

Over the winter the men were plagued by ambushes and sniper fire, and Still, appointed hospital steward and scout surgeon, helped care for the wounded[10] – no easy task with a standard issue medical kit that "was complete when it contained calomel, quinine, whiskey, opium, rags and a knife."[11] Among his patients was a young private, six foot and two hundred pounds, shot through the thigh with a two-inch slug of lead while on scout duty, shattering the femur for a distance of about four inches. Two doctors favored amputation, but Still believed that conditions in the camp were too unsanitary to care for an amputee. (With good reason – statistics show that sixty percent of Civil War amputees died of hemorrhage and those that survived stood a high risk of dying from septicemia, gangrene or tetanus.) The soldier's femoral artery was intact so he persuaded his colleagues to let him box the leg as with his previous case. Six months later the man was able to walk with a crutch.

Enemy fire was by no means the only threat. Twice as many Kansan soldiers died of disease than from battle injuries. The camps were rife with dysentery, malaria, typhoid, smallpox, cholera, pneumonia and tuberculosis, and drugs were often ineffective when given to men weakened by stress and poor diet. Still harbored concerns about the safety of the medicines themselves, believing that liquor, opium and other compounds added poison to a body already enfeebled by disease,[12] and he questioned the eagerness of his colleagues to prescribe these substances. "If a patient had one foot in the grave and a half-pint of whiskey in a bottle," he observed, "the doctor would work as hard to get the whiskey out of the bottle as he would to keep the foot out of the grave."[13] Faced with the choice of administering potentially harmful remedies or doing nothing and watching the patient die, he experimented with practical measures of his own.

To relieve the excruciating backache that accompanied cholera he positioned the patient face down, placed a pillow over the lumbar region and kneaded the area over the kidneys with his knees. To his surprise this not only helped ease the pain but within a short time caused the sufferer to pass a large volume of urine. Though cholera was frequently fatal, under this regime his patients generally recovered. Only years later would he understand why.[14]

In March 1862 Confederate forces suffered a heavy defeat at Pea Ridge, Arkansas, and Missouri finally came under Union control. Still's battalion was disbanded and, after a six-month tour of duty, he returned home. In May he was commissioned Captain and instructed to organize Company D, 18th Kansas Militia, with orders to patrol the Santa Fe Trail the breadth of Douglas County to protect the wagon trains bringing gold and silver from western mines. On 13 January 1863 Mary gave birth to a girl, Marcia, and later that year Still's siblings Tom, John and Cassie (the youngest, aged sixteen) left for California with an ox team.[15] Their parents never saw them again.

Sporadic fighting continued in the border counties as pro-confederate "bushwhackers" raided from Missouri before indulging in one final orgy of violence. At dawn on 21 August 1863 the notorious William Quantrill entered Lawrence with a force of 450 guerillas, slaughtered 150 unarmed men and boys, looted indiscriminately, robbed the bank and set ablaze most of the buildings. After a buggy tour of the burning settlement Quantrill turned south towards his next target, Baldwin City.

The morning was bright and clear. Still climbed onto the roof of the barn and, seeing houses on fire in nearby Brooklyn, snatched his rifle and rode off to join a two-hundred strong defense force, while Mary and Abraham hid their valuables in the cornfield. Quantrill however, pursued by federal troops, turned aside and withdrew towards Missouri, burning houses along the way. Still's home, situated in the middle of a field, was spared, but he returned to find it filled with people who had been less fortunate. "The wicked fleeth when no man pursueth," Marovia wrote of the Lawrence massacre. "I hope that the memory of that awful deed haunted them till their dying day."[16] To prevent further atrocities thousands of Missourians were evicted from the counties bordering Kansas.

The raids ended, but Still's world was about to be shattered. A disease known as spine, brain, or spotted fever was sweeping the country. An old Irishman in Baldwin, feigning inability to pronounce its medical name, cerebrospinal meningitis, said it sounded like "finally come and get us."[17] In February 1864 it came to Still's home.

When Abraham and Susan, aged eleven and seven, and a nine-year-old "adopted girl" came down with headache, fever and tell-tale spots, Still called for the assistance of his father, brother James (who had graduated with an MD degree from Rush Medical College, Chicago, two years earlier),[18] and another doctor. But medicine knew neither the cause nor the cure of the disease. The three doctors administered opiates and purgatives, adjusted doses, tried other remedies, and kept vigil day and night. Abram prayed at the bedside,[19] but to no avail. As muscular twitching progressed to painful contractions that convulsed the children's forms, they lapsed through delirium into unconsciousness.

Susan succumbed on the seventh, Abraham on the eighth and the adopted girl a day later. Tragedy was heaped upon tragedy when, on the twenty-third, thirteen-month-old Marcia died of the same deadly disease.[20] Shortly afterwards Still found the decomposing remains of a chicken in the well and, clinging to the ancient theory of miasmas, blamed it for his loss. The dead children had always drunk water straight from the well, while he, Mary and the only surviving child, fourteen-year-old Marusha, preferring coffee, had always boiled it.[21]

Marusha went to live with her grandparents in nearby Centropolis. Mary found the empty house unendurable and went to stay with her sister Louise in Edgerton.[22] Still, "torn and lacerated with grief and affliction," nailed boards across the south window of the house, unable to bear the memory of the children's faces greeting him from it when he returned from his calls. As he languished in heartbreak and disillusionment the words spoken by James Abbott nine years earlier – that he had "lost all faith in medicine" – returned with new vigor.[23] Only now did Still "fully realize the inefficacy of drugs" and he blamed his loss on the "gross ignorance" of the medical profession.[24] He refused appeals to attend other sick children, convinced he had nothing to offer and that "the coffin was a certainty for them."

His crisis transcended medicine. It cut to the core of his doubts about Methodism. "This was brought about by the mysterious providence of God,"

Abram had prayed over the lifeless bodies, "and it pleased Him to take these dear little children."[25] Still could not accept such nonsense; a God who gave life simply to destroy it so young would be "nothing short of a murderer."[26] Nor could he abide the platitude, "the Lord loveth whom He chasteneth," that neighbors trotted out in trying to offer comfort. He could not resign himself to the belief that life was a vale of tears and disease a manifestation of divine intervention.

Troubling him most, though, was the statement, continually repeated by preachers, "all of God's work is perfect" – with great emphasis on the word *perfect*. "Do they believe what they say?" he railed. "If the minister really believes it, why does he send a man loaded with poison into the sick chamber of his family, and drink the deadly bitters himself?" If man – supposedly the epitome of God's work – was perfect, surely he should be capable of recovering from illness without the assistance of drugs. Still questioned how – and this was directed at Abram – "a doctor of divinity could blend his teachings with the foolish teachings of medicine."[27] Suddenly, in the midst of emotional turmoil, there emerged a calm clarity:

> It was when I stood gazing upon three members of my family, all dead from the disease, spinal meningitis, that I propounded to myself the serious questions: 'In sickness has God left man in a world of guessing? Guess what is the matter? What to give, and guess the result? And when dead, guess where he goes?' I decided then that God was not a guessing God but a God of truth. And all His works, spiritual and material, are harmonious. His law of animal life is absolute. So wise a God had certainly placed the remedy within the material house in which the spirit of life dwells.[28]

This assertion was supported by two common-sense observations: few, if any, diseases were invariably fatal; and people were capable of recovering from most diseases without a doctor's help. The human body, he intuited, contains "every sort of drug that the wisdom of God thought necessary for human ›ppiness and health."[29] This momentous insight presaged the existence of as yet undiscovered immune system.

Still's refusal to practice eventually yielded to the tearful entreaties of a young woman whose brother was critically ill with meningitis. He found John Studebaker semi-conscious, neck and jaw set solid by muscle contraction, breathing through his nose and "throwing off what I called the deadly froth from the nostrils."

Still poured out a half pint of whiskey, intending to let his patient take a sip, but Studebaker grasped the cup convulsively with both hands and gulped it all down. Still did not stop him, thinking the young man would be dead in a few hours anyway, but thirty minutes later Studebaker relaxed and opened his eyes. On seeing this Still administered another, slightly smaller, tumbler of whiskey. Within two hours his patient voided a full bladder and after two further hours regained consciousness, with no signs of intoxication. The following morning, to Still's astonishment, Studebaker was up and out of danger.

Shortly afterwards a desperate neighbor implored Still to attend his eight-year-old daughter, sick with brain fever. The two men had harbored "some hard feelings" towards each other, and when Still hesitated the man broke down in tears, saying, "Let bygones go and come with me and help me save my child." At this Still broke down too, and "went off with him, crying also, because his many kind words were not endurable."

Again Still administered whiskey and again it worked; in two or three days the girl was heading towards a full recovery. "I have given the history of these cases of cerebrospinal meningitis and the results that I obtained," he chronicled, "not as a prescription to go by, but because this fact was the pointer which led me to philosophize as a mechanic and find the cause of death." [30] The most significant factor, he later realized, was the spasmodic contraction of the neck muscles.

For the next ten years a multitude of questions troubled his mind. What made a healthy person become sick? What made one person more susceptible than another to a particular disease? Why did some remain well during an epidemic? Why did one person die and another live when given the same remedies? Did the drugs save the first or help kill the second?[31] To account for these individual variations medicine appealed to such factors as mental states, environmental conditions, and heredity – but was there yet another reason?

In summer 1864 Confederate armies suffered a string of defeats. On September 19, in an attempt to relieve the pressure in the East, Sterling Price led a mounted force of twelve thousand men into Missouri, and as they pushed west to Jefferson City and beyond, all Kansan men between sixteen and sixty were hastily summoned into service. Still reported to Fort Leavenworth on the twenty-third and was commissioned Major in the 21st Regiment, Kansas State Militia. The 500-strong unit marched to Kansas City led by the Lawrence brass band, and on October 9 amassed at the Missouri border under Major General Samuel S. Curtis, commander of the Federal Department of Kansas. During the march Still suffered a left inguinal hernia from carrying heavy weapons and ammunition, an injury that would remain lastingly troublesome.[32]

On October 23 his regiment engaged in the Battle of Westport, the largest Civil War battle fought west of the Mississippi River. To halt Price's westward advance Curtis formed his army into a ten-mile north-south defensive line, with the Kansas State Militia stationed at Little Blue Creek, eight miles south of Kansas City. The five-hour engagement cost the lives of 1500 men on each side, among them fifty-six of Still's battalion, many of them his friends. He himself only narrowly escaped death. "During the hottest part of the fight," he recorded, "a musket-ball passed through the lapels of my vest, carrying away a pair of gloves I had stuck in the bosom of it. Another minie-ball passed through the back of my coat just above the buttons, making an entry and exit about six inches apart."[33]

The following day the Confederate rearguard collapsed and Price retreated south. The 21st Kansas Militia joined in the pursuit, skirmishing for ninety miles before giving up the chase near Fort Scott. They returned to De Soto, Kansas, where, on the twenty-ninth, Still received orders to disband the regiment. His Civil War service was over. He made his way back to their desolate home, slumped into a rocking chair and sat in silence with Mary for almost an hour.[34] She was seven months pregnant, and on 2 January 1865 gave birth to a boy they named Charles after her father.

In the East the war dragged on until April 2, when the Confederate capital, Richmond, Virginia, fell to Union forces. At the end of the year slavery was abolished outright, but not before the death of the man who had made it possible.

On Easter Sunday, April 16, as Abram conducted a prayer meeting in Centropolis, news came that Abraham Lincoln had been assassinated. On

Good Friday, while watching the play *Our American Cousin* at Ford's Theater, Washington D.C., the president was shot in the head at point blank range by actor and militant Southern sympathizer John Wilkes Booth, and died the following morning. Abram had greatly admired Lincoln and, in place of the sermon he had prepared, delivered a deep-felt eulogy of the president.

After the service it rained all afternoon and the family sat around the fireplace scarcely speaking a word, "for we felt," Marovia wrote, "that a pall of such impenetrable darkness had settled over us that we would never see the light again."[35]

In truth it was a new beginning.

5

THE SECRET, IMPERCEPTIBLE CHAIN

"The sweet assuring smile of peace fell on Kansas for the first time in her existence when the war of the rebellion ended," William G. Cutler wrote in his 1883 *History of the State of Kansas*.[1] A restless energy born of a decade of turmoil, bloodshed and danger was channeled into intense activity, ushering in an era of progress and prosperity that saw farms thrive, railroads, mines and factories open, and homes, schools, churches, villages and cities appear.

Andrew and Mary abandoned the log cabin and its painful memories for a fresh start in Baldwin City.[2] They took a house four blocks east of Baker University[3] and Still settled back uneasily into medical practice, his shattered faith in drugs compounded by two disturbing observations: a widespread problem among ex-soldiers of alcoholism and addiction to substances initially taken as medicines,[4] and, during the war, a perceptibly lower incidence of infant mortality in the parts of Kansas and Missouri lacking doctors due to army conscription.[5] He told a neighbor that "if there was nothing more in the healing system of drugs than to let children die like hogs with the cholera," he would "take a solemn oath to never give another dose of medicine."[6]

To test his concerns about the safety and efficacy of drugs he conducted a private survey, noting what he prescribed and how his patients fared. The results pointed to a dismal conclusion: dissatisfaction "to the degree of disgust."[7] His conscience told him to stop administering medicines altogether, but in practice this was impractical. Patients expected drugs – they were virtually synonymous with medical practice – so he continued to prescribe those he considered least dangerous.

To further his medical knowledge he enrolled as a student at the College of Physicians and Surgeons in Kansas City.[8] It proved a disappointing experience. The curriculum covered no more than he already knew: a meager outline of anatomy,[9] a smattering of physiology, and a course in *materia medica,* the science, preparation and uses of drugs. Some have questioned his attendance of this college and even if the establishment ever existed. Evidence is inconclusive, but forty years later a conversation between Still and his brother Ed was overheard:

> You really had several years of schooling, didn't you Drew?
> Well, I had six months of anatomy, six months of physiology, six months of pharmacy, six months of chemistry, six months of dissection – how much does that make?
> About thirty months, I make it.

The listener "forbore to ask if these were the same six months." They were – the equivalent of one school year.[10]

What Still wanted to know was the rationale behind medical practice. What was disease? What caused it? What lay behind the almost universally accepted notion that when a person is sick some substance must be given to vanquish the disease? Did the different patterns of illness represent internal changes in the state of the human system, or were diseases, as some theorized, distinct objective realities – *entities* – that invaded the body from the outside? The stark truth was that medicine did not know. "I learned," he lamented, "that a king was just as ignorant of the nature of disease as his coachman, and the coachman no wiser than his dog."[11] Medicine knew equally little about the drugs it employed for curing. Knowledge of their physiological effects was at best rudimentary, with explanation lacking on the mechanisms by which even the most familiar remedies acted against specific diseases.

Still fell back on his own resources. He immersed himself in texts on anatomy, physiology and surgery;[12] perused tomes on physics, geology, astronomy and other natural sciences; and became an "ardent student" of philosophy, ancient and modern.[13] The subject, he was coming to realize, was of crucial importance to medicine.

Philosophy – literally "the love of wisdom" – was concerned with the nature of ultimate reality and man's place in the universal scheme. Nothing was set in stone. As ideas changed so did concepts of man and his relationship to nature and God, leading to different theories about the workings of the human organism and the role of the doctor in trying to restore lost health.

Since antiquity medicine had oscillated between two fundamentally different approaches: reliance upon measures to assist the *vis medicatrix naturae,* the healing power of nature; or reliance upon the skill of the physician to apply the correct remedy or procedure.

In the time of Hippocrates man was regarded as part of nature, and nature as part of God, the relationship of man to God one of microcosm to macrocosm. Medicine was guided by the humoral doctrine; the four humors or body fluids (blood, phlegm, choler, black bile) analogous to the four natural elements (air, water, fire, earth). Health was the natural state of body and mind, to be maintained by living in harmony with one's environment through a sensible regimen of diet, work and lifestyle. When harmony prevailed within, right thought and action followed, leading to harmony with nature. Disease represented an upset in the humoral balance, to be remedied by the removal of adverse factors. Medicines, if prescribed at all, played no decisive role in curing, but simply aided the healing power of nature.

After the Christianization of the Roman Empire medicine became closely associated with the Church, and from the second to the seventeenth centuries the Greek physician Galen, whose writings were endorsed by the Church and found in every monastic school, reigned as the supreme and virtually unchallenged medical authority. The new religious philosophy, hierarchical and anthropocentric, promoted the idea that God created man as lord of the earth with dominion over nature. Guided by this thinking, medicine came to rely less upon the body's innate healing tendency and more upon the knowledge and skill of the physician to control the humoral balance. Galen saw disease as an unnatural accumulation of humors, to be relieved by a variety of measures including copious bloodletting.

The Christian philosophy profoundly influenced Western concepts of knowledge, truth and reality. "The prevailing world-view of the period was marked by a deep and persistent assurance that man, with his hopes and ideals, was the all-important, even controlling fact in the universe," Edwin Arthur Burtt wrote in his 1924 *The Metaphysical Foundations of Modern Science*:

> This view underlay medieval physics. The entire world of nature was held not only to exist for man's sake, but to be likewise immediately present and fully intelligible to his mind. Hence the categories in terms of which it was interpreted were not those of time, space, mass, energy, and the like; but substance, essence, matter, form, quality, quantity – categories developed in the attempt to throw into scientific form the facts and relations observed in man's unaided sense-experience of the world.[14]

Thoughts and emotions were the measures of reality, with "the crowning scientific fact" the religious experience, "that transitory but inexpressibly ravishing vision of God . . . in which the whole realm of man's knowledge gained full significance."[15] The testimony of the senses was considered unshakable. From man's perspective the Earth was a fixed center of the turning astronomical realm, and time a fixed present moment drawing the future towards it.

Science changed everything. In the early 1600s Galileo Galilei proved, through mathematics, that the Earth is not a fixed center of the universe but a planet that revolves on its axis and circles the sun, and through studies of velocity and acceleration demonstrated that time can not only be measured but has a mathematical relationship to motion and space. Time, represented as a straight line and divided into regular intervals, became an irreversible fourth dimension progressing at a regular cadence from past to future.

Beguiled by science's ability to explain previously inexplicable phenomena, Galileo became convinced that God had made the world a mathematical system, simple and orderly. Nature's book was inscribed in the symbols of geometry – number, figure, magnitude, position, motion – and mathematics was the key to deciphering her immutable laws.[16] To accommodate the objection that personal experiences and feelings could not be resolved into geometrical representations, Galileo distinguished between "primary" and "secondary" qualities. Only the primary, *objective*, qualities gave the true picture; the secondary qualities were merely subordinate effects on the sense organs. The senses could deceive, and he deprecated the partial and possibly distorted knowledge they revealed as *subjective*.

In the 1630s the French physiologist and philosopher René Descartes carried the idea further. Descartes insisted that the "certain principles of material things" must be derived not by "the inconsiderate judgments of childhood" – the deceitful senses – but by "the dictates of mature reason."[17] But reason generated theory, and if a theory's initial premise was incorrect so too was everything deduced from it. To obtain true knowledge, he asserted, science should therefore purge itself of all speculative assumptions and include only "self-evident truths" that require no experimental verification. To Descartes nature was self-evidently geometrical and mathematics the key to unlocking her secrets; there was "absolutely no other way of discovering the truth."[18]

Descartes theorized a universe composed entirely of an absolute uncreated substance – God – that brought into being the "created substances" of matter and mind.[19] These substances, equivalent to Galileo's primary and secondary qualities, occupied two mutually exclusive realms: the *res extensa*, the physical world of matter and motions (including the movements and physiological workings of animal bodies); and the *res cogitans*, the non-physical world of the thinking, sensing rational soul. To explain the undoubted interaction of body and mind, Descartes hypothesized that they communicate through the mediation of the conarium (the pineal gland), a small pine-cone shaped organ in the middle of the brain, from where, he maintained, the mind "radiates forth through all the remainder of the body by means of the animal spirits, nerves, and even the blood."[20] But to all intents and purposes the mind could be ignored. So too could God, reduced to the status of a great mechanical inventor accountable for the first appearance of the world's fundamental particles.

Thus liberated from the awkward questions of ultimate causation, Descartes could treat the universe as a vast machine of geometrically predictable motion. "If anyone could know perfectly what are the small parts composing all bodies," he proclaimed, "he would know perfectly the whole of nature."[21]

In the late seventeenth century Isaac Newton provided the definitive formulation of the modern worldview. Newton regarded the mind as a unique but nevertheless relatively insignificant substance, and located it in an undefined part of the brain he called the "sensorium."[22] Later materialists took the marginalization of the mind to its logical end point. The philosopher Thomas Hobbes described the mental faculty as an *epiphenomenon*, a spontaneous outgrowth of matter; the naturalist Thomas Huxley (who pictured the mind as an "aura" of matter) declared that, "we shall, sooner or later, arrive at a mechanical equivalent of consciousness, just as we have arrived at a mechanical equivalent of heat."[23]

As the realm of matter came to overshadow all others, there came a profound shift in the nature of inquiry from the ultimate *why* of events to their immediate *how*. Knowledge was no longer the qualitative possession of the individual, but something external, quantitative and exact.

The mind made unimportant, science could order the incomprehensible chaos of the universe into the mathematical constructs of matter, motion and force, within an independent frame of immovable space and uniformly flowing time. The new scientists believed that plants and animals differed from man-made machines only in level of complexity, and were therefore subject to the same inorganic laws. "Man was a machine, inhabited and ruled by a rational soul, which touched the body only at one small point, the pineal gland in the center of the brain," wrote Ralph M. Eaton, editor of the 1927 book *Descartes Selections*:

> The actions of the human organism were for the most part automatic, while animals, having no rational souls, were nothing but automata. Like the solar system, the living body was a mechanism, at bottom to be explained on the same principles. This was the idea in physiology that fascinated Descartes, and if we put aside the question of the rational soul, it was the same idea that the physiologists of the next three centuries worked out, with more and more careful descriptions of the mechanisms within mechanisms which make up a living organism.[24]

Descartes had been inspired by William Harvey's 1628 demonstration that the blood circulates around the body, propelled by the mechanically pumping heart. Harvey's astonishing discovery disproved the old Galenic theory that blood, cardinal of the four humors, is "concocted" in the liver and washes out towards the periphery to be "consumed" by the various parts of the system.[25]

This not only discredited the old humoral doctrine but also, by association, eroded the authority of the Church. Medicine thereafter turned to science for knowledge.

Chemists analyzed body fluids for acidity or alkalinity; physicists applied hydraulic models to the circulatory system; mathematicians counted, measured and weighed to establish physiological norms. New forms of humoralism appeared as a profusion of speculative theories were propounded to explain the genesis of disease, upon which a plethora of rival and often conflicting systems of practice were elaborated.

In Germany, Friedrich Hoffman described medicine as "the art of properly utilizing physico-mechanical principles" to maintain or restore health.[26] In Holland, Herman Boerhaave held that health demanded a free movement of fluids in the vascular system, with disease caused by blockages, constriction or stagnation. In England, John Hunter attributed all structural changes of disease to perversions of "nutrition," with deficiency to be restored by diet and excess to be removed by bloodletting or drugs to induce purging or sweating.

When the Swiss physician Albrecht von Haller demonstrated the "irritability" (contractility) of muscles and the "sensibility" (responsiveness) of nerves, the new humoralism lost favor to "solidism." Solidists maintained that the body's physiological balance depended ultimately not upon the circulatory but upon the nervous system.

In Edinburgh, William Cullen, building on Haller's work, proposed that the body is maintained in a normal state by "nervous energy," with health dependent upon an appropriate equilibrium between the stimulation of living tissue and its innate "excitability." Cullen believed that all pathology was initiated by external influences that adversely stimulated irritable tissues to produce a disordered action or "spasm" of the nervous system (a theory that earned him the nickname "Old Spasm"). Too little stimulation led to weakness, requiring tonics and supportive treatment; too much – by foods, climatic conditions, noxious substances, contagions, emotions – led to fever and "debility," requiring sedatives or bloodletting. For half a century Cullen's 1778 *First Lines of the Practice of Physic* remained Europe's principal text on the classification and treatment of disease, and made the Scottish capital the preeminent center of medical thought, drawing students from all over the Western world.

The system Still learned from his father was that of the influential Philadelphia physician Benjamin Rush, a 1768 Edinburgh graduate and student of Cullen. Rush regarded debility not as a consequence but as a predisposing cause of disease. Theorizing that adverse stimuli cause hyperactivity of the blood vessels (a state he called "hypertension") and ultimately exhaustion, he declared that there was "only one disease in the world" – namely "morbid excitement."

Rush disagreed with Cullen about the role of drugs. Cullen had followed the Hippocratic teaching that medicines do not conquer disease directly but merely assist nature to restore health; Rush, favoring the Galenic approach, advocated extensive bloodletting and massive doses of purgatives and laxatives to counteract his hypothetical hypertension, measures that earned his system the name "heroic medicine."

Rush's followers prescribed prodigious doses of quinine for all febrile conditions; large amounts of drugs regarded as "blood purifiers" for all kinds of skin eruptions; and reckless quantities of the mercury compound calomel ("a safe and nearly a universal medicine")[27] for a wide variety of intestinal and other maladies. Under the dubious logic that children could tolerate higher fevers, they were commonly administered higher doses of calomel than adults, despite (as Still had experienced as a teenager) the drug's harsh side-effects.[28]

Rush dominated American medicine, but even before Still served his apprenticeship the speculative foundation of all the medical systems was being challenged, even by an American president. "The adventurous physician," Thomas Jefferson wrote in 1807:

> establishes for his guide some fanciful theory . . . of mechanical powers, of chemical agency, of stimuli, of irritability . . . or some other ingenious dream, which lets him into all nature's secrets at short hand. . . . I have lived myself to see the disciples of Hoffman, Boerhaave, Stahl, Cullen, and Brown succeed one another like the shifting figures of a magic lantern. The patient, treated on the fashionable theory, sometimes gets well in spite of the medicine.[29]

Jefferson might have added Rush to the list, but Rush was a personal friend and cosignatory of the Declaration of Independence.

In Europe, meanwhile, scientists were pursuing a promising new avenue of inquiry. Since ancient times concepts of disease had been rooted in abnormal physiology, with anatomy largely ignored. Human dissection had been forbidden in ancient Greece and, since the soul's salvation depended upon an intact body, tabooed by the Church. With the rise of science this taboo was lifted, opening the way for the study of pathological anatomy.

In 1761 Giambattista Morgagni, professor of anatomy at Padua, published his landmark *On the Sites and Causes of Disease*, a correlation of pathological findings at autopsy with patients' symptoms and signs before death. At the beginning of the nineteenth century, hospital doctors in Paris, inspired by Morgagni, conducted the first systematic medical research with the routine performance of autopsies. They hoped that the study of pathological anatomy in the corpse might enable them to make more accurate diagnoses in the living.

As dissection revealed tumors, inflammation, gangrene and other pathologies – *lesions* – in specific organs, the Parisian doctors concluded that disease processes were localized anatomical problems rather than diffuse disturbances of the body's fluids or forces. Humoralist and solidist systems were pushed aside in a new scramble to discover which organs harbored the "seat of disease." When Xavier Bichat further discovered that organs are composed of different tissues, each tissue, distinguished by appearance and function, became a possible seat of disease.

The new focus on morbid anatomy drew attention away from the person and his generalized responses and towards specific diseases. Under the assumption that each disease obeys laws of its own and affects all people alike, doctors came to rely upon objective signs to interpret the pathological changes that might be occurring within the patient's body, and to regard symptoms – subjective and variable – as confusing and unreliable. New instruments like the stethoscope and thermometer, and procedures like percussion, enabled diseases to be more precisely named and classified, so that previously vague diagnoses such as inflammation of the chest could be more accurately identified – *defined* – as pneumonia, pleurisy, bronchitis, tuberculosis.

Detailed classification made it possible to test the effectiveness of various modes of treatment against named diseases. In 1835 Pierre Louis developed a "numerical method" to evaluate the efficacy of bloodletting for pneumonia, comparing one group who were bled with another who were not. The results were startling: the treatment provided no benefit. Further experiments revealed that bloodletting was equally ineffective for the skin infection erysipelas, and the drugs used for purging fared no better. Statistical analysis soon became the standard test for methods of treatment, and systems that failed it were labeled "quackery."

Unsubstantiated theories and large doses of drugs were all discredited. Paris criticized Edinburgh and to a new generation of Americans the French capital became the enlightened place to study. Parisian graduates like Elisha Bartlett and Oliver Wendell Holmes then returned to challenge the old heroic practices. "In the whole compass of medical literature," Bartlett wrote in 1844 of Rush's essays, "there cannot be found an equal number of pages containing a greater amount and variety of utter nonsense and unqualified absurdity." Bartlett reminded his colleagues that the cause of disease remained unknown and warned against systems founded on unproven speculations.[30] Holmes, in an 1860 address to the Massachusetts Medical Society, cautioned that medication "should always be presumed to be hurtful. It always is directly hurtful; it may sometimes be indirectly beneficial. Throw out opium, throw out a few specifics, throw out wine, which is a food, and the vapors which produce the miracle of anesthesia, and I believe that if the whole materia medica as now used could be sunk to the bottom of the sea, it would be all the better for mankind, and all the worse for the fishes."[31]

Most American doctors continued to prescribe drugs nonetheless. Some carried Rush's measures to the extreme, others turned to less debilitating alternatives founded upon further unsubstantiated speculations. Samuel Thomson's botanical medicine rested upon the notion that illness is caused by cold and cured by remedies to restore body heat – steam baths, cayenne pepper – and the natural emetic lobelia to induce vomiting; Samuel Hahnemann's homeopathy relied upon the theory that a minute dose of a substance that produces a set of symptoms in a healthy person will cure a sick person suffering from similar symptoms; Wooster Beach's eclecticism employed a mix of herbal and any other remedies considered efficacious. Still investigated homeopathy and eclecticism, only to conclude that both were "a conglomerate mess of conjectures and experiments on the ignorant sick man."[32]

Alongside the problems of disease and cure, medicine was also grappling with an ancient and perennially tantalizing riddle: the nature of the body's mysterious animating power.

In the Middle Ages the alchemist physician Paracelsus promoted the idea that life was a special indwelling spirit, a force different from matter and separable from it, and that the ultimate goal of all future research should be to discover its essence. A succession of vitalist schools employing mysticism and "contemplation" followed, but none found the answer. At the cusp of the scientific revolution the German physician Georg Ernst Stahl, believing that all purposive actions of living organisms – consciousness, physiological regulation, healing – required the guiding power of an immaterial soul, replaced the spirit with the psyche or *anima*.

Science demanded more concrete explanations. Vitalism and animism were swept aside as materialists sought to account for the extraordinary properties of organic nature not in some vague spirit or psyche, but in some special property of the body itself.

Humoralists found new meaning in the old Mosaic dictum *the life of the flesh is in the blood* and propounded a congeries of hypotheses. Some envisioned the animating power as a kind of amorphous fluid substance, and located it variously in blood, in lymph, in other body fluids, and even in the clotting substance fibrin; others theorized that blood contains a living substance called "plasma," responsible not only for growth and nutrition but also the exudations blamed for all pathological conditions. Solidists, meanwhile, maintained that life originated in the brain, the nervous system, or elsewhere. William Cullen identified life with the ethereal fluid thought to be the basis of light, heat, magnetism and electricity, and postulated that it signified no more than a state of nervous excitement induced by environmental stimuli.

Chemists and physicists influenced the argument. In 1828 Friedrich Wöhler heated ammonium cyanate in the laboratory and produced urea, undermining the belief that organic compounds could only be synthesized by living organisms under the influence of a vital force. Justus Liebig contended that just as the organization of elements in some chemical compounds can generate a characteristic chemical force, the organization of elementary particles of matter in the tissues can generate a characteristic vital force. In his 1847 essay *On the*

Conservation of Force, Hermann von Helmholtz wondered whether vital forces might transmute into physical forces, or "energies" as they came to be known. When Luigi Galvani discovered that an electric current passed through the legs of a dead frog produced reflex movement, life became equated with electricity and magnetism.[33]

But despite the development of better scientific instruments the body's animating power remained stubbornly elusive, and the series of metamorphoses it passed through – from spirit to principle to substance to force – clarified little. Medicine, deeming as questionable anything not proven by scientific methods, thereafter restricted itself to investigating life's manifestations: the body's movements and physiological processes – its "actions." The word *life* slipped quietly from the medical lexicon.

The Church abhorred the new scientific gospel. Genesis taught that "the Lord God formed man of the dust of the ground, and breathed into his nostrils the breath of life; and man became a living soul."[34] The body was not the man. Man was "not only a house of clay," John Wesley insisted, "but an immortal spirit; a spirit made in the image of God."[35] Behind the body's seemingly mechanistic operation lay occult truths known only to the Creator. "Do not we know ourselves?" he asked:

> Our bodies and our souls? What is a *soul*? It is a spirit, we know. But what is a spirit? Here we are at a full stop. And where is the soul lodged? In the pineal gland? In the whole brain? In the heart? In the blood? In any single part of the body? Or (if anyone can understand those terms) 'all in all, and all in every part?' How is the soul *united* to the body? A spirit to a clod? What is the secret, imperceptible chain that couples them together?[36]

Again,

> When and how was the immortal spirit superadded to the senseless clay? 'Tis mystery all. And we can only say, 'I am fearfully and wonderfully made.'[37]

The biblical teaching was, “We know in part.”[38] Better to admit limited knowledge than hubristically assume that life somehow emanates from matter. “It behooves us to humble ourselves before God,” Wesley admonished, “and to acknowledge our ignorance.”[39] This was also Shawnee teaching and there was a story Still liked to tell.

At the Wakarusa Mission he was called to see a patient, the “daughter of an Indian chief.” The chief kept firing question after question about the intricacies of the girl’s illness until Still was eventually forced to admit he did not possess all the answers. The chief took a stick and drew a circle in the sandy earth. “Indian know so much,” he said. Taking the stick again, he drew a larger circle circumscribing the first. “Pale face know so much,” he continued. Then, with a wave of his hand, he concluded, “Outside this, Indian know as much as pale face.”[40]

6

VITAL UNITIES

On 15 May 1867, Mary gave birth to twins, Harry and Herman. The day after Christmas that year Abram fell ill from exposure while conducting a funeral[1] and contracted pneumonia. On December 30, his condition deteriorating, he asked Andrew his chances of recovery. Still replied honestly that they were slim. "Well I have lived all my life for this day," Abram said, and Andrew seized his opportunity to raise a subject increasingly preoccupying him. "Father," he said, "I want to ask you a question now; a serious question. What do you know of tomorrow after the body is dead?"

Methodism had indoctrinated Still with the notion of the soul's continuity after death. Church dogma enshrined the immortality of the soul as an article of faith, but faith did not satisfy this enquiring mind – he craved firsthand proof, and had long wondered if those nearing death might be able to provide it. As early as 1858 he had asked family friend Abraham Rothrock, dying from intestinal gangrene, if he could glimpse anything of the life beyond, and during the Civil War had ventured the same question to a number of dying soldiers, but none had been able to offer illumination.

Still hoped that fifty-two years of devoted service to the Church would afford his devout father a clearer view, but Abram's reply was profoundly disappointing. "Andrew, my son," he said simply, "I hope and feel that I am in the hands of a merciful God, but I know nothing beyond. It is all a leap in the dark."[2] Abram died on New Year's Eve.

Six weeks later Still joined the Freemasons, a brotherhood for whom the immortality of the soul was a key tenet. On 12 February 1868 he was initiated into the Palmyra Masonic Lodge and on the first of July completed the sequence of degrees to become a Master Mason.[3] Sometime during this period he also became involved with Spiritualism, presumably through his old comrade James Abbott. Spiritualists believed not only in the soul's immortality but also that direct communication could be established with the spirits of the dead.

Still and Abbott had maintained a close friendship since the Border War. They shared many ideals and interests, from the welfare of the Indians to politics, from mechanics to books. Throughout the Civil War Abbott had acted as government agent to the Shawnee, and in 1866 re-entered politics to serve a two year term as a Kansas state senator. He possessed an impressive library, collected art and specimens of nature, and in a home workshop invented and repaired a wide range of objects for neighbors – "cabins, dug-outs, shakes, tables, shoes, bedsteads, culverts and bridges" – and devised curious tools to fashion them.[4]

Still, too, was pouring his energies into invention. He designed a safety pin sprung with wire and a wooden model for a railway switch identical to the one later adopted. Both had the potential to make him a fortune, but he patented neither.[5] Nor did he patent his next contrivance, a labor-saving modification to a reaping machine. On the existing model the cut grain was deposited on a platform on top of the machine and when enough for a bundle had collected it was pushed off by a man with a rake. To dispense with the rake man Still designed two steel forks to catch the grain and a lever to drop the bunch to the ground ready for binding. He naïvely demonstrated the device to a traveling representative of the Walter A. Wood Mowing and Reaping Machine Company of Hoosick Falls, New York, only to find the following summer the company selling reapers with forks of his design. "Wood had the benefit of my idea in dollars and cents," he commented wryly, "and I had the experience."[6]

He made sure to patent his next invention, a churn to speed up the laborious chore of butter-making. Studying the chemistry of milk and cream, he learned that the milk fat was encased in a membrane of the phosphoprotein casein which needed breaking to release the fat globules and allow them to coalesce as a single mass. Reasoning that more force would hasten the process he constructed a device similar to an old-fashioned ice-cream maker, with gears to turn it at 500 rpm and tapering tubes to dash the milk at high velocity against the inside of the drum. The machine completed the task in an impressive three to ten minutes and,[7] in September 1871, won him a prize from the Douglas County Agricultural and Mechanical Association for the best butter churn. He had the product manufactured in Dayton, Ohio, and marketed it for the next three years.

Meanwhile, in fall 1870, his medical quest took an unexpected turn. A Scottish physician and naturalist "sent by the British government on a research study in Africa," and visiting America on a "special mission" before returning home, found his way to Baldwin City where he heard of a local doctor who prescribed very few drugs and sought him out. Dr. John M. Neal disliked medication and disapproved of his profession's business values. Drugs were "bait for fools," he told Still, and the practice of medicine no science but "a trade, followed by the doctor for the money that could be obtained by it from the ignorant sick." It was not drugs that cured, he said, but nature.

Still invited him to stay. Neal remained for "several months," the two doctors studying together all winter.[8] During this period, on 6 December, Still's daughter Marusha (now almost twenty-one and a Baker University student) married wealthy physician's son John William Cowgill, a nephew of author Robert Louis Stevenson.[9]

Neal introduced Still to a trove of knowledge that would prove crucial to the development of osteopathy: the latest literature on natural history, evolutionary biology and medicine, including the works of Herbert Spencer, Charles Darwin, Thomas Huxley, Ernst Haeckel, Alfred Russel Wallace, and the German physician Rudolf Virchow.

Virchow's *Cellular Pathology, as Based upon Physiological and Pathological Histology*, a transcription of twenty lecture-demonstrations at the Pathological Institute of the University of Berlin in 1858, was the most influential book on disease to appear in the nineteenth century.[10] Still held the work in "high regard."[11] It provided him, for the first time, with a solid basis for reasoning on health and disease.

When Morgagni had traced the "seat of disease" to organs and Bichat to tissues, they had labored under the prevailing belief that the smallest unit of living structure was the "fiber," with organisms formed by their agglomeration in a process the organic equivalent of crystallization. But in the late 1830s botanist Matthias Schleiden and embryologist Theodor Schwann, peering through the newly invented compound microscope, saw that the basis of all living matter is not the fiber but the nucleated cell. Or nearly all. Schwann remained uncertain about connective tissues – bone, ligament, tendon, cartilage, fascia and the ubiquitous intercellular substance – believing they contained cells in early embryological development which changed into fibers upon maturation.

Virchow disproved this. In a seven year study from 1848-55, examining human tissues under the microscope, he established that mature connective tissues are composed of cells that lack individual cell walls, with nuclei embedded in communal ground substance.

The cell theory was complete. The human organism begins as a fertilized ovum, a single cell that divides and differentiates to become bone, muscle, brain and all else; each cell type possessing its own specialized physiology, each individual cell a separate living being contributing an essential function towards the common expression of the whole. The human body is composed entirely of cells and all arise from preexisting cells, a concept expressed in Virchow's aphorism *omnis cellula a cellula*.

Humoralist and solidist theories were both wrong (or, perhaps more accurately, both partially right); the body's animating power does not reside exclusively in the vascular or nervous systems, but in every single cell. Virchow asserted that the nerves could no longer be considered as "so many wholes, as a simple, indivisible apparatus," or the blood "as a merely fluid material," because both nerves and blood teem with an "enormous mass of minute centers of action."[12] And, he pointed out, life is present in the egg long before the heart and brain develop, while plants and many animals possess neither organ.[13]

Though a person looks and acts like a single living being, his life is actually the coordinated lives of uncountable separate beings, a "democratic group of individual creatures with equal standing, although not equally endowed,"[14] as the German put it. *"The organism is not a single unit,"* he italicized, *"but a social system."*[15] Virchow presented a new concept of the living being:

> Every animal presents itself as a sum of vital unities, every one of which manifests all the characteristics of life. The characteristics and unity of life cannot be limited to any one particular spot in a highly developed organism (for example to the brain of man), but are to be found only in the definite, constantly recurring structure, which every individual

> element displays. Hence it follows that the structural composition of a body of considerable size, a so-called individual, always represents a kind of social arrangement of parts . . . in which a number of individual existences are mutually dependent.[16]

Medicine, accustomed now to the scientific method, abhorred Virchow's terminology: cells as *vital unities* and his philosophy *new vitalism* – words that raised the unwelcome specter of vital spirits or animating forces. In his defense Virchow insisted he was not arguing for the existence of the soul, but added that he found it impossible to reconcile his observations with the accepted paradigm. "Does this new kind of vitalism not stand in irreconcilable opposition to the dominant tendencies of modern science?" he asked. "Should it be possible to present life as a whole in terms of a mechanical result of known molecular forces – and this has admittedly not been done up to the present – it would remain impossible to avoid designating with a special name the peculiarity of form in which the molecular forces manifest themselves, thus differentiating them from other expressions of these forces. Life will always remain something apart, even if we find that it is mechanically aroused and propagated down to the minutest detail." [17] He added, "It is high time that we give up the scientific prudery of regarding living processes as nothing more than the mechanical resultant of molecular forces inherent in the constituent particles."[18] Despite abundant scrutiny, nature's animating power remained stubbornly elusive. "Millennia have passed over the heads of mankind, but no one has yet grasped the secret of life," Virchow lamented. "All have turned to dust before solving the great riddle."[19]

The cell theory brought the mystery of life no closer, but it revolutionized the understanding of disease.

The pathological anatomy inspired by Morgagni and Bichat had enabled a wealth of new diseases to be localized, described and named: Addison's disease of the adrenal glands, Graves' disease of the thyroid, Bright's disease of the kidneys, to name a few. The objective, analytical search for morbid lesions pioneered in Paris led to the idea that what killed were underlying pathologies – tumors, inflammation, gangrene, and so on – but what autopsy could not reveal was what these anatomical changes represented.

Did disease arise from within or from without? Was each disease a discreet entity with its own laws of growth, development and decline, like the life history of a plant? Did pathology indicate the presence of some parasitic life form that sucked the strength out of its host? What was the process by which the first seed of disease grew into a visible abnormality? Until these questions were answered methods of treatment would remain speculative. "We know only in a very fragmentary fashion the conditions which determine the appearance of abnormal phenomena in the living organism," Virchow stated on the eve of his cell studies, "and even when we do know these conditions, often enough we do not, to our regret, know the means to eliminate them."[20]

Taking that as his starting point, the German examined normal and abnormal tissues. The microscope revealed that diseased tissues exhibited a variety of changes ranging from potentially reversible fatty accumulations within cells to inflammatory conditions that resulted in cell death, tissue destruction and atrophy of the part. It revealed that one cell could die while its neighbor remained healthy, and that pathology could be confined to a single cell without adjacent cells being affected. And, crucially, it showed that disease in all its variety and diversity was never accompanied by new cell types. Even tumors turned out to be modifications of existing cells. He concluded that all pathology manifests as disturbances of living cells, and that all abnormalities are degenerations, transformations or repetitions of normal cellular structure.[21]

Virchow had traced both the awkward concept of life and the elusive "seat of disease" to the same fundamental unit – the cell. Disease was not an entity, not a parasite (with the possible exception of microorganisms, but they were yet to be implicated). Health and disease were not two mutually exclusive states, but two ends of a continuum from normal to abnormal physiology. "What Virchow accomplished in *Cellular Pathology* was nothing less than to enunciate the principles upon which medical research would be based for the next hundred years and more," historian Sherwin B. Nuland wrote:

> In one sweeping declaration, he cleared the medical air of all residue of humors and humbug. . . . He discovered that even the finite structure of disordered anatomy is only a clue – the real cause of disease is to be found not in disorders of form but in disorders of function. It is not

> the way the cell *looks* that is the problem, but the way it *acts*; the key is therefore not the cell itself, but what goes on inside of it; it is not to pathological anatomy but to pathologic physiology that physicians must look to solve the fundamental riddles of sickness.[22]

Research laboratories sprang up as scientists probed the physiological and biochemical minutiae of living cells to establish the normal range of various chemicals in the blood and urine (and similarly of body temperature, blood pressure, heart rate, and other aspects of function) relative to a person's age, sex or physique. They hoped that once the changes associated with specific diseases were known, new drugs could be found to counteract the abnormalities.

Still read *Cellular Pathology* critically. Having intuited that all the remedies needed to cure disease exist naturally within the body, he did not favor a search for new drugs. Virchow himself had recognized that the body exhibits a constant drive towards health, noting that even in a disease as devastating as tuberculosis the microscope showed numerous and extensive foci of healing. "But what is done," he asked, "to investigate the conditions of spontaneous healing?"[23]

This was precisely what Still set out to explore. He began by applying what he learned from his surgical work on the battlefield: with a normal blood supply the body possesses remarkable powers of healing, regeneration and, with appropriate hygiene, resistance to infection. Upon this foundation he formulated the "first postulate" of his new medicine: *An unobstructed, healthy flow of arterial blood is life.*

Medicine had long recognized that an occluded vessel led to the death of the parts supplied, but Still was thinking (similarly to the old humoral pathologists, who reasoned that disease results from blockages, constriction or stagnation of the vascular system) about the effects of a partial obstruction to blood flow. "I reasoned that disease, which is really a fractional death," he wrote, "must be due to a partial cessation of the blood stream from some mechanical obstruction to the artery or vein of the organ primarily affected."

Still returned to the Indian burial grounds in search of corroborating evidence. "Studying hundreds of post-mortem specimens," he reported (with frustrating lack of detail), "I found this to be true in every case, that is, there was some derangement of the blood supply, either causing or accompanying all disease processes." On his patients he experimented with manipulations to invigorate the circulation to the liver, the bowel and other organs within easy reach. "I got some results," he related, "but realized that I was only on the first round of the ladder. I had not yet found the real underlying cause of disease."[24]

Cellular Pathology provided further valuable clues. The book presented a new vision of the body and its inner workings: an impossibly complex world of cells and connective tissues and nutritive channels, of fluids and secretions and exudations; a colony of tiny living beings coexisting in cooperation and mutual dependence, every cell dependent upon its immediate environment – a fluid-filled connective tissue labyrinth – to supply nutrients and carry off wastes; and disease in any one part affecting the whole by polluting the circulating juices. "As a continuous ingestion of injurious articles of food is capable of producing a permanently faulty composition of the blood," Virchow lectured, "in like manner persistent disease in a definite organ is able to furnish the blood with a continual supply of morbid materials."[25]

Still employed the metaphor of the body as a self-sufficient community; the organs and tissues workshops for manufacturing products indispensable for the health and comfort of its citizens, the cells a brotherhood of laborers each performing skilled work, and disease the failure of one section to perform its task correctly. "Just as a filthy sewer will produce disease in the whole city," he paraphrased Virchow, "so the failure of one organ will produce disease in the whole body."[26]

This was a plausible account of how disease developed, but it failed to explain what initiated the morbid changes. Again Still drew upon Virchow, who indicated that cellular health relies not only upon the quality of blood but also upon its quantity.

In 1840 the German anatomist Jacob Henle had established that blood vessels contain a muscular layer whose constriction and dilatation – as seen in the veins of the hands – decreases or increases the supply of blood, an arrangement his fellow countryman Benedict Stilling termed a "vasomotor system."[27] Eleven years later the French physiologist Claude Bernard demonstrated which nerves were involved when he severed a *sympathetic* nerve in a rabbit's neck. Virchow described the effects: "a state of hyperæmia ensues in the whole half of the head; the ears become dark red, the vessels greatly dilated, the conjunctiva and nasal mucus membrane turgidly injected."[28]

Charles-Édouard Brown-Séquard further found that electrically stimulating the cut end of the nerve caused the same blood vessels to constrict, and the stronger the stimulus the greater the contraction. "When an artery is acted upon by any influence which causes a contraction of its muscular tissue," Virchow elaborated, "it must of course become narrower, inasmuch as the contractile cells lie in rings around the vessel; this contraction may under certain circumstances proceed until the canal is almost entirely obliterated, and the natural consequence then is that less blood penetrates into the corresponding part of the body."[29]

Medicine had probed no further. "Very little was known of the vasomotor nerves, sympathetic ganglia, or the brain and spinal centers for the different viscera and organs and special centers for special functions," Still wrote. "Nerves were supposed to carry motor impulses to the muscles and to carry back sensations from the periphery, and beyond this little had been worked out."[30]

Even the origin of the sympathetic nerves remained in dispute. Early investigators, seeing them emerge from the jugular openings in the base of the skull and pass down the neck as chains of *ganglia* on either side of the spine, concluded that the body possesses two separate nervous systems that function independently of one another. Since the ganglia, like the brain, are composed of nerve cell bodies, some believed they were a chain of little brains. The influential Bichat even assumed a separation into *animal* and *organic* life: the former, centered in the brain, the life of the intellect; the latter, centered in the sympathetic ganglia, the life of the internal organs, concerned with the "passions."

Virchow, though, had observed in the brain and spinal cord, cells "perfectly analogous" to those of the sympathetic ganglia and, since the ganglia communicate with the cord via branches from the spinal nerves, believed the sympathetic nerves emerged not from the skull but from the spinal cord.[31] He was correct, but not until 1885 was it conclusively proven that the sympathetic nerves emerge from the cord, *ascend* via the ganglionic chain, and pass through the jugular openings to supply the head.

Still, crucially, adopted Virchow's position. He studied the anatomy of the nervous system: thirty-one pairs of spinal nerves emerging from apertures – *foramina* – between adjacent vertebrae: eight cervical, twelve thoracic, five lumbar, five sacral and one coccygeal. Only spinal nerves from the first thoracic (T1) to the second lumbar (L2) give off branches to the sympathetic ganglia. The T1 ganglion supplies the head (the nerve severed by Bernard), T2 the neck, T3-6 the thorax, T7-11 the abdomen, and T12-L2 the legs. Still marveled at how the spinal nerves, "joined with the gangliated cord or sympathetic nervous system lying in front of the spinal column, and then penetrated every organ and tissue of the body, whether there was any apparent need for it or not."[32] (He also recognized, profoundly, that arteries and veins passed through the foramina to and from the spinal cord: "Thru these tiny openings, then, went all the vital impulses between the cord and viscera, and also the gross nourishment of the cord.")[33]

Still reasoned that since pressure on motor or sensory nerves by tumors, dislocated bones, contracted muscles and other factors frequently gave rise to neurological symptoms, similar interference with sympathetic nerves should give rise to symptoms peculiar to that division – and he identified the intervertebral foramen as a prime site for such irritation. He theorized that a strained spinal joint, by altering the relationship between adjacent vertebrae, would narrow the foramen, irritate the exiting spinal nerve, and produce motor, sensory or sympathetic symptoms depending on which fibers within the nerve were compressed. Two experiences supported this hypothesis.

On a reconnaissance mission near the end of the Border War he crested a hill on his mule and was spotted by a band of Missourians below, who set off in pursuit. His life in danger, Still took a risky short cut, edging his mule carefully over a foot log spanning a swollen creek. They had almost reached the far bank, and fortunately cleared the water, when the bark suddenly detached, the mule stumbled, and Still was thrown to the ground, striking his sternum on the pommel of the saddle as he fell. He made good his escape but the injury, although minor, resulted in the immediate onset of heart palpitations.

These persisted for nearly a decade. During the Civil War, at winter quarters in Harrisonville, he asked the camp's twenty-five doctors to examine him. By consensus they diagnosed valvular disease of the heart and prescribed rock candy and whiskey. Then, one day after the war, he accidentally cured himself. Suffering from an ache in his upper back while watching a game of croquet, to try and ease it he placed one of the wooden balls close to a tree, lay down with the ball between his shoulders and his feet up the trunk, and twisted around. He felt something slip and, after initially worrying that he might have broken a rib, soon realized that his backache had disappeared – and so too had his palpitations. They never returned.[34]

The second experience was even more dramatic. One cold winter's day a boy rode up to the house in haste, announced that his mother needed urgent attention, and without further elaboration galloped off. Assuming that a birth was imminent, Still grabbed his obstetrical kit and followed on, twenty-five miles, to a farm. When they got there he found the woman not pregnant but sick, and a chest examination revealed pneumonia. A blizzard had meantime blown in, making it impossible to return for his medicines.

As he sat on the bed wondering what to do, absentmindedly continuing his examination, Still suddenly became aware of his fingers unconsciously following the lower border of a rib. Something about its contour seemed wrong and the woman found it painful to touch. She told him that the previous day the family had been slaughtering hogs, hanging the carcasses to be cleaned from a tree limb by their hind feet, and one finished carcass tied against the trunk had swung free to hit her firmly, snout first, in the chest. A small bruise marked the spot. Still surmised that the impact had strained a rib at its attachment to the spine, altering its alignment, and managed to work the joint free. This resulted in an immediate diminution of pain, and soon no pain at all. To his astonishment, within an hour the woman's fever broke and her labored respiration ceased. He remained overnight waiting for the storm to pass and in the morning found his patient well enough to be up and about.[35]

The woman's dramatic recovery led Still to formulate a tentative hypothesis: "A rib, slipped from a transverse process of the spine, would cause pressure on the structures of the intervertebral foramen, derange blood and nerve action to intercostal spaces, resulting in venous congestion and inflammation of pleura, followed by pneumonia in some division of the lung, or of the whole pulmonary system."[36] He wondered if his palpitations had a similar cause; the displaced rib perhaps irritating a sympathetic nerve supplying the heart or its vessels, to confound the organ's action and generate an irregular beat.

"The history of medicine teaches us, if we will only take a somewhat comprehensive survey of it," Virchow had stated, "that at all times permanent advances have been marked by anatomical innovations, and that every more important epoch has been directly ushered in by a series of important discoveries concerning the structure of the body."[37] Still's anatomical innovation was to look at the body structure from a radically new perspective.

As a mechanic he knew that the efficient operation of a machine depended upon the correct adjustment of its parts. In the sawmill, when the circular blade was properly aligned it made a harmonious hum, but with any deviation the hum became a warble, the blade wobbled and buckled, become hot with friction, and cut inefficiently.[38] The cardinal principle for adjusting or repairing any mechanical device was *cause and effect*: trace back from the fault to its underlying source.

Did similar mechanical principles apply to the human body? Would structural derangements produced by strains, injuries, postural stresses or other factors irritate nerves, alter circulation, disturb physiology and therefore, by definition, cause disease? And – the corollary – would correcting deranged structure free nerves, normalize circulation, and restore normal physiology, with recovery dependent on the extent of cell death and the regenerative capacity of the part?[39] It was a revolutionary theory, but if correct it had profound implications for medicine: to cure disease, treatment should be addressed not to physiology but to anatomy.

Johannes Müller's *Elements of Physiology* lent support to this idea. On page 596 of his copy Still underlined, "the division of the vagus in the neck is followed by the effusion of bloody fluid in the lungs, and although the chemical process of respiration is at first not essentially disturbed, yet the animals die a few days after the operation."[40] The vagus was a *parasympathetic* nerve, responsible for a host of involuntary functions including the slowing of heart rate and the orchestration of digestion. Would irritation of the vagus anywhere along its course from the jugular foramen to the abdomen produce physiological discord in the organs supplied? Might irritation of any nerve, artery, vein or lymphatic vessel anywhere in the body predispose to disease? Had Still found a universal principle applicable to all medical conditions?

He began to look at his patients from a different perspective. Instead of employing symptoms and signs as guides for naming diseases and prescribing drugs, he started employing them as guides for seeking and correcting structural derangements.

A pattern soon emerged: a consistent and reliable correlation between anatomical causes and physiological effects, conforming accurately to the pattern of the nervous system. And, as he had surmised, the spinal nerves were especially vulnerable at the intervertebral foramen.[41]

By 1872 Still was applying his new method to every chronic case,[42] falling back on drugs only if it failed to help. If a patient agreed to try the new treatment but still expected drugs he would send one of his sons to deliver the remedy with strict instructions on dosage. "Little did these people think," Harry wrote, "[that] all the time father was quietly getting away from the poisonous drugs, and at the same time some of these people were taking the drugless treatment without their knowledge." Even the boys were unaware that some of the "medicines" they were delivering were only dough pills and colored water. Still merely told Harry, "You will see the day when the doctor will give very little medicine, if any, and this is one of the principles I am striving for."[43]

In February 1873 the U.S. Government passed the Fourth Coinage Act, replacing a bimetallic (gold and silver) standard with a gold standard. With the supply of money tied to the amount of available gold (less plentiful than silver) the quantity of dollars in circulation was reduced, making them more valuable. For Kansan farmers, already burdened by debts from the boom years and plagued by a drought that summer, the "Crime of '73" proved catastrophic. Interest rates rose, agricultural prices declined, banks folded, and farms collapsed.

Still lost nearly all he had. The family "nearly starved to death" in the famine that followed, though they fared better than some. "We were lucky," Charley related. "We had a cow that was fresh, a little corn, and some pigs, and that was the only thing we could live on. No money was being exchanged by anyone."[44] To make ends meet they took in three Baker University students as lodgers.[45]

Mary was expecting another baby, Fred, born on 15 January 1874. She wrote her physician father that Andrew now prescribed very few drugs, and in some cases none at all. Intrigued, Dr. Charles Turner paid them a three month visit that winter. While there he said little about Still's practice, but on returning home wrote Mary that although he did not fully understand what her husband was doing, he thought him honest and sincere, and undoubtedly achieving startling results. He closed by saying he hoped she would give Andrew her support and encouragement.[46]

He would soon need it.

7

PERFECTION

Andrew Taylor Still "discovered" osteopathy at 10 a.m. on 22 June 1874. So he always maintained, though this was neither the moment he propounded his radically new theory of disease nor when he first applied it to his patients, for he had been doing so for two years already (and another fifteen years would pass before he employed the word "osteopathy"). At this hour he experienced a life-changing epiphany, a dramatic moment of illumination when, he wrote, "like a burst of sunshine the whole truth dawned on my mind, that I was gradually approaching a science by study, research, and observation that would be a great benefit to the world."[1]

One flash of inspiration did not bring him here. "It seems to have been not one but quite a series of discoveries," his later student Ernest Tucker elaborated, "some by accident, some by intuition, some by sheer backwoods mental habit of looking facts straight in the face and talking straight back at them. But these eventually grouped themselves into a great concept."[2] It was on that June morning that the great concept suddenly coalesced, its disparate elements united by a profound insight that hinged upon the word *perfection*.

Ten years had passed since Still's children died of meningitis and his doubts about medicine and Methodism remained unresolved. Troubling him most was the apparent contradiction between the doctrine of original sin and the phrase, continually repeated by ministers, "All of God's work is perfect."

Genesis taught that God created Adam and Eve perfect, immortal beings, knowing neither sin nor sickness. "But since man rebelled against the Sovereign of heaven and earth, how entirely is the scene changed!" John Wesley preached.

"The incorruptible frame hath put on corruption; the immortal has put on mortality. The seeds of weakness and pain, of sickness and death, are now lodged in our inmost substance."[3] Fallen man was forever tainted. "The highest perfection which man can attain while the soul dwells in the body does not exclude ignorance and error, and a thousand other infirmities."[4] Why then, Still questioned, did ministers preach that "God's works prove His perfection"? If man – supposedly the crowning glory of "God's work" – was imperfect, surely that would prove His *imperfection*.[5]

In raising this objection he was in good company. Wesley himself had agonized over the same quandary – in fact it was over the concept of Christian perfection that he broke with the Church of England to establish his own nonconformist order. Anglicans traditionally regarded perfection, or perfect love, as a gift bestowed upon the righteous at or after death, but Wesley could not reconcile this teaching with the words of St. John: "God is love; and he that dwelleth in love dwelleth in God, and God in him. Herein is our love made perfect, that we may have boldness in the Day of Judgment: because as He is so are we in this world."[6] Wesley finally settled on the compromise embodied in his doctrine of perfection: man's judgment is clouded, but at the ground of his being the knowledge of truth and goodness remains. Vigilance is required to hear its promptings, but through "holy living" – dwelling in a state of perfect love of God and neighbor – a believer can attain perfection during life.

Still had encountered the same word, perfection, in the evolutionary literature provided by James Neal. Biologists regarded "higher" organisms – those with a greater degree of organic complexity – as being more "developed." Erasmus Darwin and Jean Baptiste Lamarck had proposed that "lower" forms transmuted into higher forms over historical time. To explain the mechanism of this process Charles Darwin (grandson of Erasmus) and Alfred Russel Wallace independently proposed a theory of "natural selection," whereby random mutations confer superior or inferior characteristics and competition weeds out the weak. The new discipline of sociology assumed that the mind obeyed the same evolutionary laws, with happiness increasing as social structures became more developed. "As natural selection works solely by and for the good of each being," Charles Darwin concluded in his *Origin of Species*, "all corporeal and mental environments will tend to progress towards perfection."[7]

The English philosopher Herbert Spencer – the man who coined the phrase *the survival of the fittest* and gave the word *evolution* its modern connotation – took the idea further, suggesting that natural selection described only a particular instance of a general Law of Evolution applicable to absolutely everything in the universe. In his prodigious ten-volume *System of Synthetic Philosophy* Spencer applied evolutionary ideas to biology, sociology, psychology and ethics. He envisaged the creation as "a single metamorphosis universally progressing,"[8] one vast protean whole advancing in one glorious direction: "always towards perfection is the mighty movement."[9] He imagined man climbing ever upwards and society rising to ever increasing happiness, the whole journeying inexorably towards "the highest conceivable state of humanity."[10]

Spencer was immensely popular in nineteenth century America, his idealistic, anthropocentric arguments matching the aspirations of the age of "progress" where scientific, technological, economic and social advances all seemed to confirm the belief that by enhancing man's control over nature the attainments of each successive generation could be built upon to ever greater, and therefore better, levels.

Not all shared Spencer's unfettered optimism. The Church abhorred the theory of evolution. Christian dogma depended upon the fixity of species and man's special creation as lord of the earth, not some lineal descendent of lowly forms by the serendipity of natural selection. God was the reason why things happened, all events in the world directed by His divine providence.

Still retained a belief in providence, but he also accepted the paleontological evidence for the transmutation of species over historical time. He believed in progress, but he disagreed with those who linked natural selection to nebulous visions of utopian societies or man's apotheosis.[11]

At ten in the morning on Monday, 22 June 1874, he engaged his brother James, now practicing medicine in Eudora, in a theological discussion. Still pressed Jim, a Methodist minister from 1849 to 1852,[12] on a specific doctrinal issue: "the extent of the laws of God of which man, a miniature representation of the universe, was the result."[13]

For Methodists the *law of God* held a precise meaning: "the law engraven on the heart by the finger of God, the conscience also bearing witness."[14] "What is the law," John Wesley explained, "but the original ideas of truth and good, which were lodged in the uncreated mind from eternity? It is God made manifest in our flesh, and bringing with him eternal life." This was the law "originally given to angels in heaven and man in paradise, and which God has so mercifully promised to write afresh in the hearts of all true believers."[15]

During the conversation Still was suddenly struck by a profound, almost overwhelming, insight. He wrote twenty-two years later:

> I was shot in the dome of reason by an arrow charged with the principles of philosophy. Since that eventful day I have sacredly remembered and kept its anniversary . . . sometimes withdrawing from the presence of man to meditate upon the event of that day wherein I saw that the word 'God' signified perfection in all things and in all places.[16]

He saw that both God *and* man are perfect – a revolutionary, even heretical, idea for the time and place, for it not only contradicted the doctrine of original sin but also undermined the very foundations of the Methodist faith. This was the same difficulty that Wesley had encountered, but unlike the Church founder Still would entertain no semantic fudges to get around the problem; he simply took the statement "all of God's work is perfect" at face value. "In all time past," he now wrote sarcastically, "man has felt and acted as though the Creator had provided all things for him that he could ask or desire but one, and that was what to do or take when sick. We have lived under the tradition that man is made sick as a punishment for a few apples that Grandma Eve took, and that he has never been well since."[17] Having dispensed with original sin he further dismissed the doctrine of perfection as an artifice of Wesley's invention, and with it disappeared the need for salvation by faith.

Even more radically, Still's insight challenged the Christian concept of God: an anthropomorphic Father in Heaven, omnipotent, omnipresent and omniscient, merciful and compassionate in one guise, wrathful and vengeful in another, ruling over but separate from the natural world below. Still favored a Deity similar to St. John's "as He is so are we in this world." Similar, but not the same. He was veering towards a concept of the Creator much like that of the Shawnee: a Great Spirit whose sacred and incomprehensible power pervades the entire Creation, imbuing everything, animate and inanimate, with infinite wisdom.

When Still applied this idea to medicine everything fell into place. In a dramatic moment of realization he apprehended, as he put it, "the immutable truth underlying the cause and cure of disease."[18]

He saw that the "laws of God" extend to both mind and body, the great mystery of creation permeating every fiber of man's being; every aspect of anatomy, physiology, biochemistry, emotion and behavior under the fiat of nature's perfection, every living cell constantly striving to express the ineffable quality known as health.

Health and disease could be regarded as the interaction of two opposing forces: spiritual forces generating order; material forces – physical derangements – generating disorder. He now understood why his new medical approach worked: because all living cells constantly strive to express nature's perfection. Echoing St. Paul, who declared in *Romans* that the moral law "hath dominion over a man as long as he liveth,"[19] Still now asserted, "When every part of the machine is correctly adjusted and in perfect harmony, health will hold dominion over the human organism by laws as natural and immutable as the laws of gravity."[20]

He realized he had unconsciously absorbed a worldview that insidiously shaped his thoughts and actions, a belief system that upheld a set of material values – money, power – espoused by not only Western society generally but also by medicine. A way of thinking based upon controlling nature rather than harmonizing with its inherent wisdom. "For twenty years or more I was content to be governed by the opinions and customs of older and more experienced physicians," he wrote. "I gave the disease its proper name. I gave the medicine as taught and practiced, but was not satisfied that the line of procedure was philosophically correct."[21] Materialism had profound limitations when applied to the living being. "Science cannot deal with fundamental questions," Still wrote:

> Only philosophy can do this. Science is only a tool or a key, and it can unlock only certain material problems. It cannot appraise itself. It is not a judge but a witness. Problems of mind, of character, moral, aesthetic, literary, artistic problems are not its sphere. It counts and weighs and measures and analyzes, it traces relations, but it cannot appraise its own

> results. Science and religion come in conflict only when the latter seeks to deal with objective facts, and the former seeks to deal with subjective ideas and emotions. On the question of miracle they clash, because religion is then dealing with natural phenomena and challenges science. Philosophy offends science when it puts its own interpretation on scientific facts. Science displeases literature when it dehumanizes nature and shows us irrefragable laws when we had looked for humanistic divinities.[22]

Within the living human body were mysterious workings, laws unknown to science that enabled trillions of vital unities to cooperate in perfect harmony; laws that coordinated growth, repair and healing; laws that potentiated the incomprehensible association of body, mind and spirit. To accommodate these arcane laws medicine needed a more appropriate philosophy.

Still found the basis for one in Herbert Spencer's 1862 *First Principles*, the introductory treatise of the *Synthetic Philosophy*. The book became one of Still's "most treasured volumes."[23]

Spencer's thesis, a reconciliation of science and religion, centered upon the limitations of man's knowledge. He challenged the idea that science might one day discover everything, arguing that it did not, and could not, know the ultimate genesis of *anything*. Even if physics could resolve all material objects into manifestations of force within a framework of space and time the nature of matter would remain a mystery since, he held, force, space and time "pass all understanding." Science generated only "partially-unified knowledge," Spencer asserted, and he accused it of being "unscientific" for tacitly ascribing life and mind, without proof, to chemical, electrical or other general powers.

In similar vein he accused the Church of being "irreligious" for presuming to know what was unknown, for contradictorily upholding God as a power transcending human knowledge while anthropomorphizing Him as a great Father in Heaven. If God is utterly transcendent, Spencer argued, it is impossible to know His nature, acts or motives, and presumptuous to invest Him with human attributes and qualities.[24] He further charged that moral codes accompanying religions were "supplementary growths," social rather than spiritual. Spencer maintained that "completely-unified knowledge" could only come through a union of science and religion.[25]

"Science and Religion express opposite sides of the same fact," he wrote, "the one its near or visible side, and the other its remote or invisible side."[26] These two sides he termed the *Knowable* and the *Unknowable*. The Knowable represented everything "capable of being perceived by consciousness" – the inorganic, organic and "super-organic" (man's endeavors in science, art, language and literature, the political and industrial organization of society). The Unknowable represented the transcendental cause of the perceived things, manifesting as three mutually dependent attributes: matter, motion and force. For organic nature Spencer adapted this, substituting "mind" for force.

This was the scheme Still adopted. "In this one form," he set down his new philosophy of the human organism, "you will find all that heaven and earth contain, fully represented, mind, matter and motion, blended by the wisdom of Deity."[27] Under Still's philosophy matter represents the body's anatomy and physiology, and behind it the unknown laws governing the creation of form. Mind represents rational thought, memory, imagination and intuition, and the hidden wisdom of the body that orchestrates trillions of cells in one common expression. Motion, a word he used interchangeably with spirit, represents not only movement and all physiological and mental processes but also the body's unseen animating power.

Science and religion – man's attempts to interpret nature – provided only partial truths. To find absolute truth demanded learning from nature itself – its visible and invisible sides – unclouded by assumption or preconception. Still had reached a fork in the road:

> With the iron hand of will I barred the gate of memory, shut out the past with all its old ideas. My soul took on [a] receptive attitude, my ear was tuned to Nature's rhythmic harmony. . . . My spirit was o'erwhelmed with the unmeasurable magnitude of the Divine plan on which the universe is constructed.[28]

From now on he would challenge the veracity of everything, regardless of source or authority.

He would conduct an experiment, not under the rules of scientific materialism, but under his new philosophy, to test the hypothesis that disease is the physiological effect of anatomical disorder. Since every patient would present a unique problem there could be no control group against which to compare results. The instruments used for diagnosis and treatment would not be objective but subjective – his own hands and reasoning faculties – and the remedy under trial not a drug but the healing power of nature.

If correcting deranged structure led to the restoration of normal function it would demonstrate two things: that nature constantly strives to express health, and that the body possesses all the agencies required for healing. If the normalizing of anatomy led to the normalizing of physiology time after time, in condition after condition, it would also, to his mind, prove the Methodist assertion "all of God's work is perfect."[29] And, by implication, it would challenge the appropriateness of a materialist philosophy for medical practice. Still set himself a high standard; if he proved his hypothesis false, even in a single instance, he would be forced to discard the whole idea.

Echoing Lincoln, who had rallied the American people to "stand by the flag" in defense of liberty, Still determined to raise his own flag, the "emblem of truth," in defense of nature's work, and to "stand by that flag as long as life shall last."[30] It was this vow that made 22 June 1874 the "birthday" of osteopathy.

It also marked the beginning of fifteen years of poverty, ostracism and the desertion of most of his patients, family and friends. For something unusual occurred at ten that June morning. Something that charged the moment with overwhelming influence; something that disturbed his brother Jim, who witnessed it; something that Still did not reveal publicly – and then only partially – for another thirty years.

8

APOSTATE OF THE FIRST WATER

Dr. Andrew Still was well respected in the small rural community of Baldwin City. Conscientious and caring, he had helped his patients through epidemics, set fractures, reduced dislocations, and run a "sort of sideline" as a dentist – the only one in the vicinity – pulling, filling and making false teeth.[1] A patriot, popular and public-spirited, he had fought for the freedom of Kansas and served as a representative of Douglas County in the territorial legislature. But his good reputation was about to be shattered.

In summer 1874 he embarked upon a challenging new project: to elaborate a system of medicine based upon mechanical principles.

> This year I began an extended study of the drive-wheels, pinions, cups, arms, and shafts of human life, with their forces, supplies, framework, attachments by ligaments, muscles, their origin and insertion; nerves, their origin and supply; blood supply from and to the heart; how and why the motor nerves received their power and motion; how the sensory nerves acted in their functions, voluntary and involuntary nerves in performing their duties, the source of their supply, and the work done in health, in the obstructing parts, in the places through which they passed to perform their part in the economy of life; all this study awoke a new interest within me.[2]

Fired with enthusiasm over his great discovery he approached the local, county and state medical societies, of whom he was a member, only to find them uninterested and scornful. To suggest that the body is a machine whose derangements can cause disease was a subversion of every current medical belief.[3]

Undeterred, he turned to the laity. On the streets of Baldwin he declared that too many deaths were occurring under the "guesswork" of medication and that God's purpose in making man was not for him to fertilize the earth in the prime of life. He told the people they did not need medicines, for the body already contains "every quality of drug that the wisdom of God thought necessary for human happiness and health." He explained the necessity of unimpeded blood circulation, proclaiming that all who "wished to successfully solve the problem of disease or deformities of any kinds in all cases without exception would find one or more obstructions in some artery, or some of its branches."[4] He said he intended "to revolutionize the old order of things; to free them from the slavery of drugs and restore to them their inalienable right to health."[5] And, most provocatively, he asserted that by applying the law of cause and effect to health and disease he could demonstrate, where ministers could offer only faith, that "all of God's work is perfect."

"Three sows among ten goslings would not have made such a fuss,"[6] he wrote. These were days of strict fundamentalism, when to challenge the authority of the church was no light matter, especially for the son of a prominent churchman; and to question Christian dogma was tantamount to sin, for it raised the suspicion of demonic possession. This was precisely what Jim believed had happened. "My honorable brother honestly believed that I had one foot in hell," Still told, "and he would have to catch me by the coat-tail and jerk me out." When he tried to argue that "God blessed no such things as quinine, morphine, opium, whiskey, or fly-blisters," Jim replied sternly, "You are talking wild. I advise you to quit that right now. There is great danger of your being lost."[7] He refused to speak to Andrew for the next nineteen years.

To reach a wider audience Still applied to deliver a public lecture at Baker University, but the Methodist institution his gift of land helped found turned him down,[8] its president Werder Davis accusing him of trying to imitate Christ by laying on hands to perform miraculous cures. "I have seen my mother also perform miracles then," Still responded sarcastically, "for she put her hands on corn meal and turned it into bread."[9]

His troubles began in earnest when he asked a member of the Baldwin Methodist Church, "George," to interpret some (unspecified) "signs" he had seen. "I believe it is the evil spirit which the devil has set to draw you into his rabbit snare," George responded ominously, saying he would lay the case in front of "Brother D." and report back the next day.

George returned the following morning bearing a written statement from Brother D. Headed *Baldwin, July 7, 1874,* it listed ten charges that Still was adjudged to have committed, the most serious of which were sacrilege and blasphemy (his talk of employing the "divine" law in healing). When George asked Still's opinion of organized religion he answered truthfully:

> I have no use for the churches of the world when I take them as a whole; I think there is good and bad in all of them. I see rivers of blood running from the most of them, and more coming. I look on them as clandestine in effect, and as having fallen far short of the great need of the world. To be a Methodist means to hate a Campbellite; and to be a Campbellite is to hate the Baptist; and all will unite as one to fight the Roman Catholic. I believe the principle given to man is high above all churches, and it is Love to all mankind, with all the soul, body and mind as the law and gift of God to man. My confidence is fully builded and will ever stand upon the goodness and love of God outside of all church organizations.[10]

Still's timing could not have been worse. Kansas was a land of climatic extremes, of winter snows and icy blasts, of spring tornadoes and scorching summers. In only two decades of white settlement its residents had weathered years of partisan conflict, seen young men from the farms leave to fight in the Civil War to never return, enjoyed boom times, and finally suffered financial collapse. Debt hung over nearly every head, and with money scarce the means of exchange had returned to a system of barter. "We should get this condition of affairs firmly fixed in mind," an observer wrote, "because into the center of this picture a man, courageous and resourceful, pushed his way to teach a new doctrine of health to men sullen and maddened by their lot." What the people of Baldwin craved was stability. They had little tolerance for innovation, let alone revolution.[11]

The community closed ranks. Damaging stories began to circulate that Dr. Still had lost interest in his regular medical practice, was neglecting his farm, had stopped marketing his butter churn, and was failing to support his family. It was rumored that he was spending extended periods shut away in his room conducting what he called "research" (scrutinizing books and obsessively examining bones), and that on moonlit nights he had been seen roaming the countryside to plunder Indian graves.[12] Seven-year-old Harry overheard people asking what in the world had gone wrong with his father. Patients petitioned Still to quit being a dreamer and return to being a normal physician.[13]

It was nevertheless acknowledged that his peculiar new brand of medicine was effective. "Yes, he was a queer sort of man," an acquaintance named Webster recalled. "He didn't doctor like the others did, but his patients most usually got well."[14] But even Still's cures were looked upon with mistrust. His uncanny ability to locate and remove pain and disease simply by placing his hands on a person raised fears of supernatural powers, malign forces, or evil spirits. Some blamed his "crazy ideas" on his friend James Abbott and, by implication, Spiritualism.

This suspicion hardened when Still's student lodgers organized a picnic in the country. Two of the three young women had been disabled, but under his ministrations Anna Hagler had discarded her crutches and Viola Duboys was no longer a "cripple." Abbott asked Still to deliver a talk at the picnic and invited a number of people to come for treatment. The seventy-five who attended reportedly witnessed Still cure two "paralyzed" women and restore the sight of a boy "blinded by a fall from a horse."

News of these "miracles" filtered back to Baldwin before he returned home and were immediately seized upon by the Methodist minister as convicting evidence of the devil's work. The cleric dispatched a Mr. Beebe to deliver Still an ultimatum: quit what he was doing or be expelled from the church. Still told Beebe that what he was doing was too important for quitting, church or no church.[15]

That Sunday in the Baldwin Methodist Church, with Mary and two of the boys among the congregation, from the pulpit the preacher castigated Still (who was not present) as "an apostate of the first water" who must change "his tactics or land in hell."[16] The minister prognosticated that their family "would be better off if Dr. Still were removed from the earth, that nothing good could come of

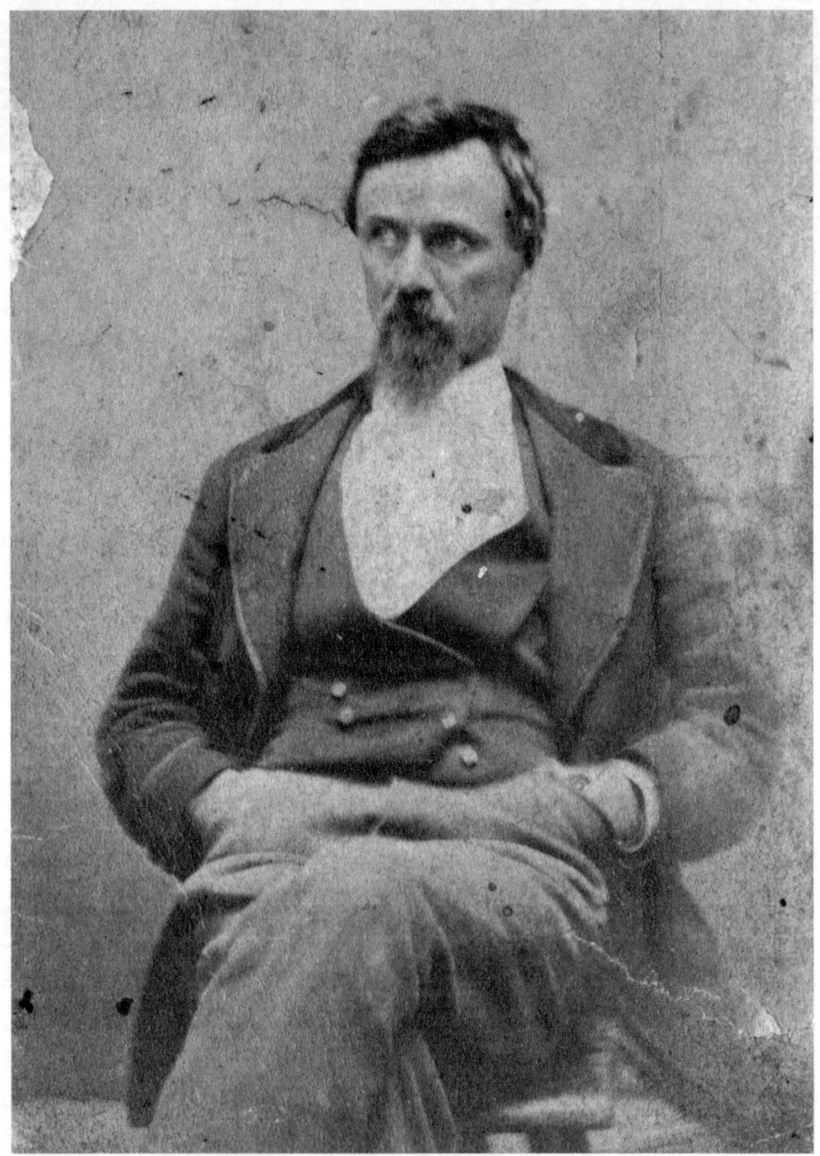

Still purportedly in Civil War uniform, c. 1874.

them, and that with such a husband and father they would become harlots and gamblers and even murderers."[17] "He raved," Still related, "so that those whom he could influence thought me demented."[18] And they did. As he walked down the street the following Tuesday, "more than two hundred children" fled from his path as though he were "an unclean leper, a huge serpent, or a wild boar from Russia."[19] People who had previously respected him turned their backs.[20] The Palmyra Masonic Lodge reconsidered his membership. Still escaped expulsion, but only by a single vote.[21]

On August 6, his forty-sixth birthday, a locust swarm of biblical proportions darkened the Kansas sky. Chickens went to their roosts as the "grasshoppers" stripped crops bare, devoured the next year's fruit buds, and reduced Abram's orchard to the surreal sight of one thousand trees denuded of leaves with the unripe apples left untouched.[22] At Atchison a train was left stranded at the station, unable to gain traction for crushed insects.[23] For Kansans already in the grip of a deep depression it proved catastrophic. Famine, contaminated drinking water, disease and debt forced many to abandon their homes, including Still's sister Mary and husband Thomas who, with the motto *In God we trusted, in Kansas we busted,* joined a wagon train for California.[24] Still wrote to old friends in Missouri requesting donations of food and clothing to help families in need, and traveled to Macon County to visit his eldest brother.

Ed had moved to Macon City during Civil War to act as assistant surgeon to the 11th Missouri State Militia, stationed in the town, and would continue to act as an examining surgeon for the army pension business.[25] As the pair toured the district gathering a wagonload of supplies Still related his woeful predicament. Ed had problems of his own. In poor health for a number of years, his self-medication with morphine had become an addiction, leaving him "so reduced he could scarcely walk." Still returned to Baldwin to distribute the gifts and, concerned that "bad could be worse,"[26] went back to Macon to try and wean his brother off the morphine, leaving Mary and the children behind for the time being.[27] On August 29 he had his name entered on the Macon County Roll of Physicians and Surgeons, entitling him to practice medicine in Missouri.[28]

Fall was approaching but Macon City remained hot and humid. One day, while strolling around town, the brothers noticed drips of fresh blood on the sidewalk and on following the trail for about fifty yards caught up with a woman with two children. One, a boy of about four wearing only a calico dress, was sick and his bare legs were covered from top to bottom in blood. Flux – bloody dysentery – was common in the autumn and often fatal for a child.

Still offered to help the woman get her children home. He took the sick boy in his arms and as he walked noted something curious: the back of the child's head, neck, and lumbar region were hot, while his abdomen, face, nose, and forehead were cold. Surmising that the temperature variation reflected a circulatory disturbance, Still pressed and rubbed methodically along the spine from the base of the skull to the pelvis, hoping to stimulate the vasomotor nerves to increase blood flow to the cold parts. In doing so he noted another curious finding: areas of rigidity in the muscles adjacent to the vertebral column, with the lumbar region feeling particularly tight and congested. The standard remedy, Dover's powder (a mixture of opium and the emetic ipecac), often proved ineffective, so he spent a few minutes loosening and softening the stiff areas, and asked the mother to report on her child's condition the next day. Both he and Ed feared the boy would die, but morning brought the surprising news that he was better.[29]

The woman told others about the cure and within a few days Still had treated seventeen cases of dysentery, all without sedatives, astringents or sweating powders, and all made uneventful recoveries. "I felt proud to be able to say to the people that I could throw all the known remedies for flux out of the window," he proclaimed, "and give them a reliable and demonstrative substitute that I had found on a prescription written by the hand of the Infinite." His services were soon in demand for "all kinds of fevers, summer and fall diseases," all of which he treated without drugs, and within a short time he found himself "in possession of a large practice."[30]

His success was short-lived. As in Baldwin, his public assertions that he "did not believe that God was a whisky and opium-drug doctor" alerted the local Methodist preacher, who assembled Ed's wife and children in prayer. "The old theological blank poured out his idiotic soul to the Lord," Still wrote, "telling Him that my father was a good man and a saint in heaven, while he was of the opinion that I was a hopeless sinner. He stirred up a hurrah and hatred in Macon, which ran to such a stage that those whom he could influence believed I was crazy."[31]

Soon afterwards Still was called to attend a young woman, diagnosed with "nervous prostration from fall heat" and given up to die by a council of physicians. Led into the bedroom, he immediately noticed the girl's head lying in a twisted position on the pillow, and on examination "found the atlas or first [bone] of her neck one-half inch too far back [so that] it had shut off the vertebral artery from supplying the brain."[32] Four hours after carefully freeing the offending joint the young woman was back to her normal self, and in gratitude her father pressed fifty dollars into his hand to send to Mary and the children.

This cure further inflamed the Methodist preacher, who now sent up prayers that Dr. Still was possessed of the devil. "I don't think the Lord listened to such howling old fools," Still responded, "who would kill a cow with the carnal sword if she gave a bushel of milk with a drop of progress in it. My father was a preacher, but was no fool seeking popularity among the ignorant."[33] The people of Macon turned on Still, calling him infidel, crank, insane.

At his brother's home Still found a letter from Jim warning Ed to "watch Drew" for he had "gone crazy" and lost his "mind and supply of truth-loving manhood." "I read it," Still related, "and thought, as the eagle stirreth up her nest, so stir away, Jim, till your head lets down some of the milk of reason to the starved lobes of your brain." By the onset of winter Still had managed to wean his brother off the morphine and, restored to health, Ed mailed Jim a reply: "I have watched Drew closely now for three months. I think it would be well if some more of the Stills went crazy."[34]

But for Andrew, with the community of Macon set against him, it was time to move on.

9
KIRKSVILLE

Still did not return to Baldwin. Instead he boarded a train for the rural community of Kirksville, Missouri, population eighteen hundred, thirty miles north of Macon. Situated on a divide between fertile agricultural land to the east and prairie scarred by deep wooded valleys as the country fell westwards to the Chariton River, the early settlement had been on Abram's circuit and he had preached its first sermon.[1] Selected as the seat of justice for newly organized Adair County in 1841 and incorporated as a town in 1873, it had earned a degree of renown as the site of a minor Civil War battle.

Still alighted at the St. Louis, Kansas City and Northern Railroad depot on 1 December 1874 and walked the short distance to Court House Square. The rectangle of timber frame stores interspersed with vacant lots actually lacked a courthouse, destroyed by fire in 1865, the two-story brick structure replaced by an open space known as the "park," a grassy area planted with a geometric pattern of trees.[2] He called at Ivie's Hotel on the square's northeast corner and to its Baptist proprietor Julia Ivie explained his straitened circumstances. She told him her creed was "feed my lambs" and offered him room and board for a month without charge.

The town was decidedly rustic, with rough sidewalks and unpaved thoroughfares of dust or mud depending on the weather. An ordinance forbidding hogs was generally ignored. They roamed freely, rooted in gardens, and after a rain wallowed in prodigious mires in the streets. Merchants fed them potatoes and rotten apples emptied into the mud holes on the square.[3] Outside his grocery on the square's north side Joe Ivie kept a cow tethered to a post, fed from a slop bucket, a convenience that afforded his customers fresh milk in their coffee, sometimes expressed directly into the cup. Loose horses and stray dogs created nuisances, and that spring a spate of dog poisonings left canine carcasses putrefying by the sidewalks. Offsetting these "repulsive features," local newspaper *The Tattler* reported, were the town's pleasing churches, the State Normal School and "numerous representatives of the angelic gender, who are noted for their beauty, mental development &c."[4]

Pleasing, too, for the teetotal Still, Kirksville was a temperance town. Nominally, at least, for a prohibition on selling alcohol did not stop it being freely available.[5] At the Pool Hotel customers could pay a dime to see a bear and return to find a glass of whiskey waiting on the counter. In Sam Furrow's restaurant and ice cream saloon a dime placed in a tin cup granted unlimited whiskey from a barrel mounted on a goods box.[6] The judicial process was equally lax. "The peculiar justice court trials of this county would fill volumes," the compendious *History of Adair County* relates in recounting the verdict of an 1873 trial. "Justice Link in delivering judgment said, 'I find there is not much evidence against the defendant, but if he is not guilty it is the first time of his innocence, and in any case I will fine him a couple of dollars on general principles.'"[7]

Still had some handbills printed and began disseminating his revolutionary ideas to anyone willing to listen. Speaking "as a man whose mouth would not be closed through fear,"[8] he criticized medicine, held forth about Spiritualism, and rapidly attracted "a great deal of attention."[9] Medical doctor and spiritualist Frederick Grove absorbed his ideas with interest.[10] Gunsmith and wagon maker Robert Harris, another spiritualist, readily accepted the concept of man as a machine. "Plant that truth right here," he told Still.[11] Local residents Bill Parsons, Wash Conner, George Cain and Bill Linder received his new medical doctrine with refreshing enthusiasm. Linder encouraged him to locate in town and even promised to help for six months.[12] Still wrote Mary that the initial signs were good – he had met "three or four thinking people" and would stay to fight it out.

Harris's wife claimed to have been Still's first Kirksville patient. Plagued for years by a litany of distressing symptoms – vomiting, cramps, convulsions, fainting, and an inability "to raise her head" – she had been given up as hopeless by the local MDs. "I don't understand Mrs. Harris's case," Dr. Grove advised the woman's husband, "but I understand it as much as any of the others. Try Dr. Still, there is something wonderful about him." Three months later, to general disbelief, all her symptoms had disappeared.[13]

Harris and Grove became Still's firm friends, but most regarded as preposterous the idea that disease could be caused by falls, strains, shocks and even changes in the weather.[14] "People who first heard of the claims of Dr. Still only laughed and sneered," an observer noted. "The idea of anyone claiming to restore the afflicted to health without the use of drugs, pills, plasters or blisters was, in those days, a sure sign of degeneracy. They said he must be crazy."[15]

Attorney John R. Musick listened incredulously to a story about a mysterious new doctor in town who could find and cure pain and disease simply by placing his hands on a person. Soon afterwards someone pointed out a tall, pleasant looking, square-shouldered man and, with a sly chuckle and a gesture towards his forehead indicating he "was wrong in the upper story," said it was "the great Dr. Still."[16] Musick happened to be co-editor of *The Tattler*. On February 6 the paper ran an editorial, "A Town for Humbugs":

> Of all places on earth or in the air, above or below, where mortal man could or ever will live, Kirksville is certainly the grandest for patronizing first-class, downright, shameless humbugs. Let a quack doctor come in town and only put out a few bill posters, and all the old tried physicians are thrown aside, and he has his pockets filled, while they are left in a worse condition than before. Ghost, and witch stories are preferred to reason, science, Bible, or anything else common sense might dictate. Now we don't believe in spirits, except in case of snake bite or in time of measles, and then a quart is amply sufficient for the entire case. But let a traveling imposter come, in the form of a lecturer, and all our own true and tried ministers, who have labored faithfully for us so long, are cast aside and we cannot do too much for the new humbug.[17]

The cures of Mrs. Harris and others prompted retailer Charlie Chinn to rent Still a suite of rooms over his hardware store on the south side of the square,[18]

NORTHEAST MISSOURI

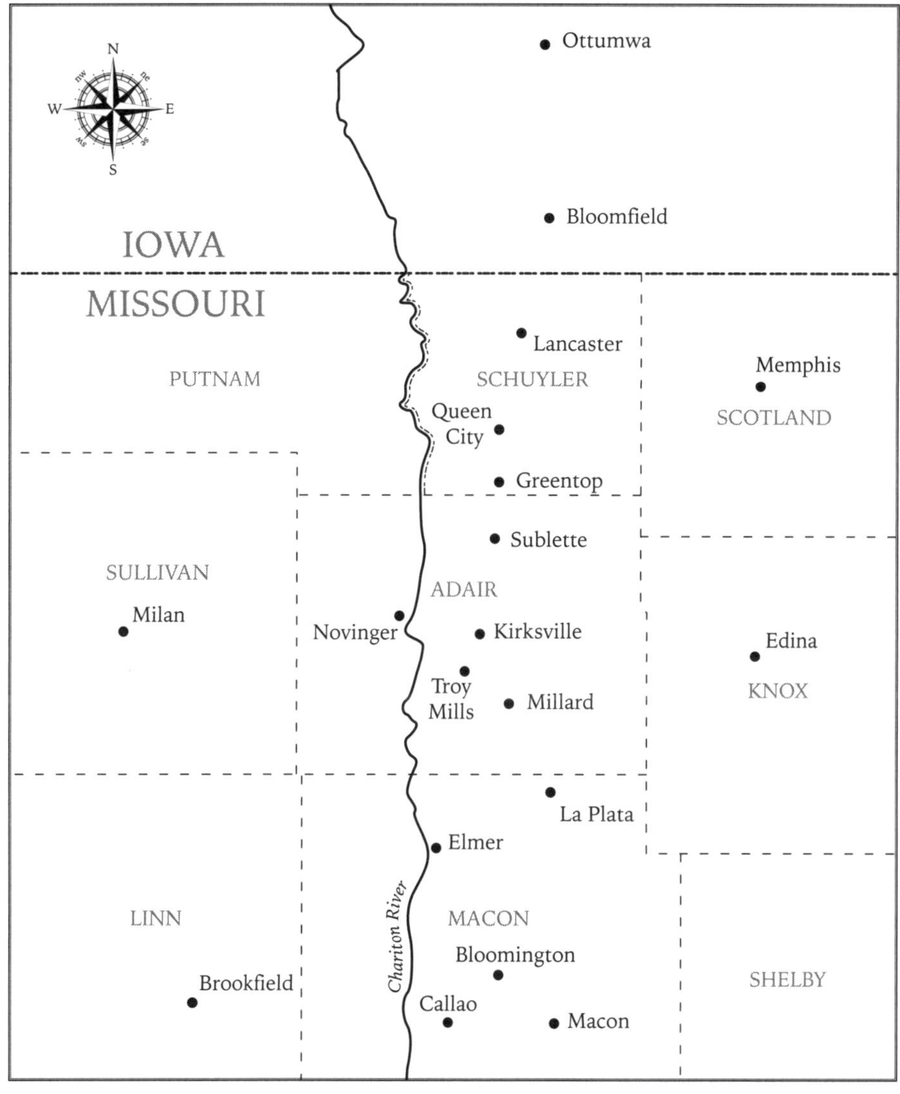

and as Still plied his new trade he also began investigating a controversial fringe medicine called magnetic healing, making train journeys to Ottumwa, Iowa, sixty miles north of Kirksville, to visit the Paul Caster Infirmary.

Caster was six foot ten, illiterate and renowned for spectacular cures. A serious speech impediment and "some mental peculiarities" had denied him a regular school education, throwing him "entirely upon his own resources mentally," but since childhood he had shown a "wonderful magnetic power to heal." It was said that he could divine a person's medical history purely by intuition and that in giving treatment became "charged with a super-abundant amount of nerve vital fluid, which by the force of will and manipulations he imbues and unfuses into the system of his patients."[19] Caster regarded his uncanny healing power as God-given and he believed Still was endowed with a similar gift. "It was soon discovered," the *History of Wapello County, Iowa*, records, "that Dr. Still possessed the same magnetic virtue as Doctor Paul, and the latter advised Doctor Still to start on the practice and shortly thereafter began treating patients according to his preceptor's system."[20]

On March 18 a small box advertisement appeared in Kirksville newspaper *The North Missouri Register*:

> The attention of the readers of the Register is called to the card of Dr. Still, magnetic healer, who has quietly opened up an office for the healing of disease and from the success attending his profession thus far at this place he with others now associated with him expect to build an Infirmary which will be noted for its good works in the healing of the afflicted. They now occupy the two rear rooms over Chinn's store and expect to occupy the whole of the upper story thereof.[21]

The notice, with the title "Dr." conspicuously absent, appeared in a different column from those of the town's half-dozen other physicians. The title "magnetic healer," however, was merely a device to attract attention.[22] The only suggestion that he may have briefly employed Caster's method comes from the testimony of Annie Cavitt, a farm girl who suffered a temporary loss of vision after falling from a horse. While Annie was blind, a friend related, "she could always tell when Dr. Still touched her even though no words were

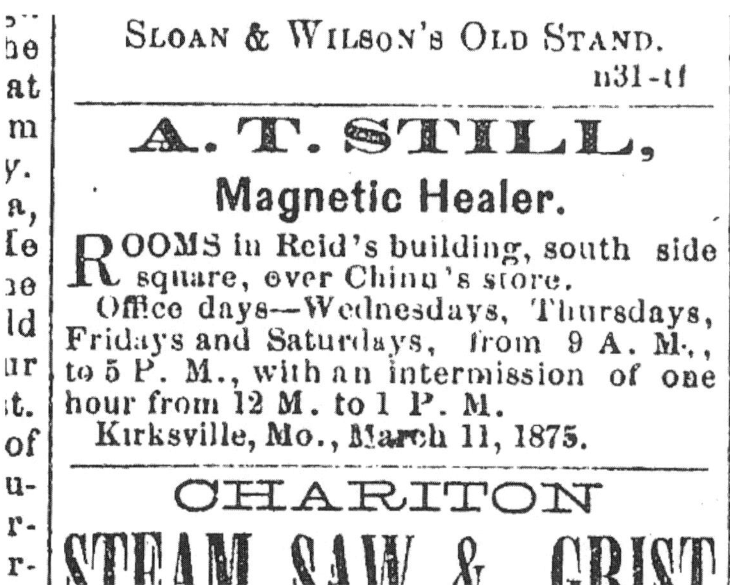

SLOAN & WILSON'S OLD STAND.
n31-tf

A. T. STILL,
Magnetic Healer.

ROOMS in Reid's building, south side square, over Chinn's store.
Office days—Wednesdays, Thursdays, Fridays and Saturdays, from 9 A. M., to 5 P. M., with an intermission of one hour from 12 M. to 1 P. M.
Kirksville, Mo., March 11, 1875.

CHARITON
STEAM SAW & GRIST

spoken. She thought he was charged with some kind of magnetic power that seemed to go through her entire body at his slightest touch." A few weeks later her eyesight returned to normal. "Annie could not tell how it was done. All she could say was like the case in the Bible – 'whereas I was blind now I see.'"[23] Still's grandiose dream of emulating Caster's infirmary collapsed when Judge Jess Linder, who was due to finance the project, left for Arizona to speculate in silver mining.

Still gravitated towards the community's free thinkers. He fraternized with Dr. A. H. John, a "keen and brilliant" physician interested in metaphysics and the philosophy of Spencer, Kant, Leibniz, Plato and Aristotle,[24] and befriended many spiritualists.

The previous fall a "spiritualistic circle" had been founded in Kirksville by the wife of medium Harvey Mott from nearby Memphis, Missouri.[25] At séances in their home Mary Mott tied Harvey to a rocking chair inside a closed pine cabinet, dimmed the lights, and as he entered a trance state the participants viewed the manifestations of spirits through an aperture in the door.

Mott's authenticity was hotly debated. Some alleged that he had once been a saloon keeper and circus performer, and that the "spirits" were generated by trickery using masks and wigs. Newspapers, initially curious and impartial, turned increasingly to ridicule. "There [we] found Mrs. Mott, who is a singular, weird appearing woman, having very much the appearance of a gypsy," one reporter wrote on being denied access to a séance. "There were with her in the house several queer spoonlike looking men, reminding one of the cadaverous, lank, inferior men, found among the clayeaters of the south."[26] Others claimed to have conversed with dead relatives and friends. Robert Harris's brother-in-law Judge John Porter professed to have talked with the apparition of his deceased brother about family and business matters and, after attending three séances, was convinced that Mott was genuine.[27]

In mid-May, Still, stationer Billy Gill and dry goods merchant E. B. Brewington traveled to Memphis to visit Mott.[28] The following month Brewington, Gill, John Porter and Robert Harris formed the Spiritualist Society of Kirksville. Still held no official position, but the group met at 3 p.m. every Sunday "in one of the rooms over Chinn & Bro's store" – the location of his office.[29] The society invited a number of noted traveling lecturers and aroused the bitter opposition of many in the community.[30]

In Kansas, meanwhile, Christian Aid societies had distributed supplies to families left destitute by the grasshopper invasion, but deliberately ignored those like Still's deemed spiritualist or liberalist.[31] Neighbors heaped scorn and pity upon Mary, some telling her bluntly that her husband, absent and contributing no income, would amount to nothing, while others suggested she raise money herself by selling subscriptions to *Harper's Magazine* and *Godey's Lady's Book*. "Evidently people liked her and sympathized with her," Charley wrote, "for she won two cash prizes of twenty five dollars each." She sent half the money to Andrew to enable him to remain in Kirksville.[32] In spring he wrote telling Mary to sell everything and join him, though he warned that things would not be easy. "I will stand by you," she wrote back, "we'll be cussed together; maybe we can get it done cheaper."[33]

Mary and the children arrived in May. Still rented a house on the east side of town and as they unloaded their belongings seven-year-old Herbert Bernard peered through the fence across the street to size up the new neighbors, hoping they would be an improvement on the last tenant, a minister with the irritating habit of giving "good advice promiscuously." When everything had been carried inside Herbert leaped over the fence and threw his new baseball to a boy about his own age. Charley caught it and pelted it back. Things were looking up, Herbert thought, but then a tall man, straight as an arrow with long black hair and keen eyes, came out and ordered his new friend to "go and help Ma straighten up." Without saying another word the man looked Herbert over, grabbed hold of him and, mumbling in a foreign tongue (a mixture of Shawnee and anatomy) ran his fingers up and down the boy's spine. "Scared? I was scared stiff and you bet I wriggled loose," Herbert related, "doing a hotfoot through that yard and over the fence faster than any boy ever got out of a watermelon patch in front of a dog."

Herbert "kept rather shy" of the strange man after that. Then one day, as he was playing with Charley's brother Herm, Still began telling an interesting tale of the plains and the Indians. Herbert maintained a safe distance at first, but with a few more stories was won over and after that let Still examine any bone of his body, though did not know what he was doing or why he kept repeating the phrase "man is a machine." In time he came to understand that Still was scanning his surface anatomy like a blind man reads raised letters.

Still was always talking about bones, even to the boys. They often found him out in the Kellogg woods, sitting on a stump or a fallen tree with a gunny sack containing a disarticulated human skeleton. He might have in his hands a humerus, radius and ulna, or the wrist and hand bones, diligently uncoupling and recoupling them with rubber bands, so engrossed that he rarely heard them approach. But when they interrupted he would lay down the bones and with patience and enthusiasm answer their questions at length.

He taught them a range of practical skills: how to make snares and dead fall traps, stuff birds, cure hides, and build a fire correctly. He showed them how to scout, make bows and arrows, read the stars the Shawnee way, and he instructed them to report their doings Indian fashion, with the sacred pipe "pointed just right for a council of grave importance." One day he showed them how to build a tipi in the traditional manner. They cut the poles, with two extra for the smoke vent, and around the framework fastened bed sheets he had cut and sewed to the right shape.

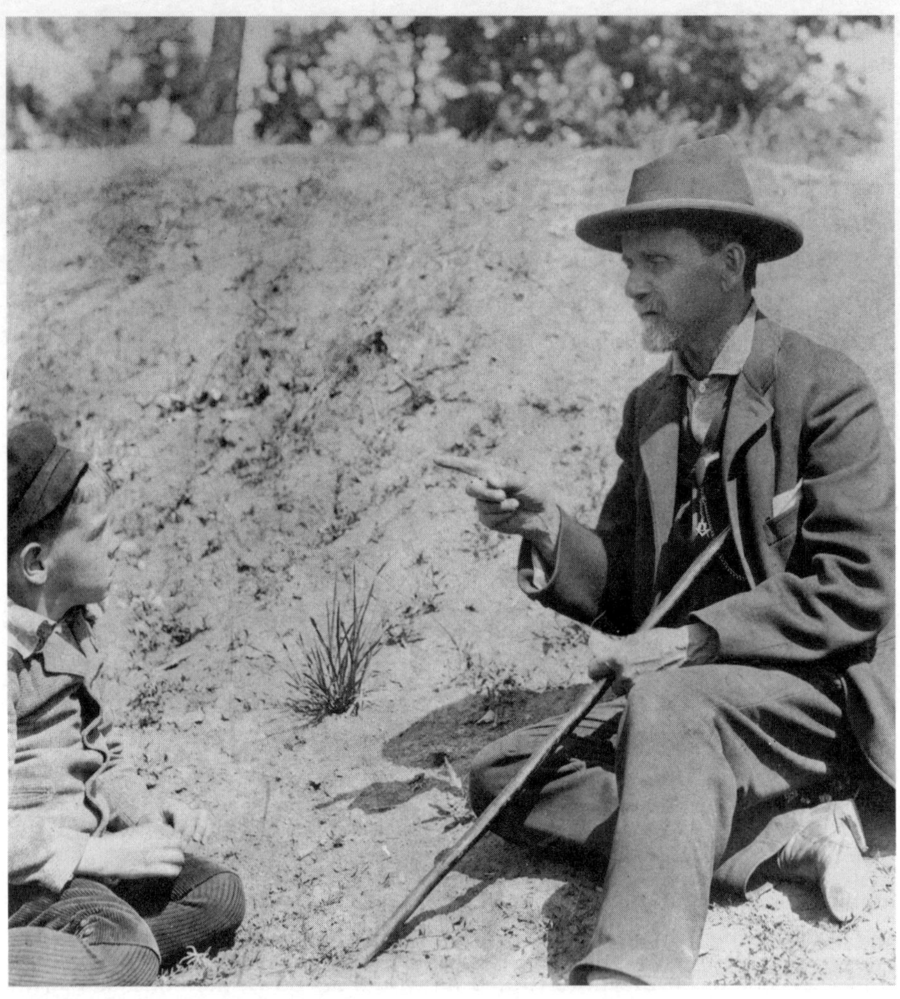

Still speaking to an unknown boy.

They learned of his deep respect for the Shawnee. "He knew all the Indian ways having lived among them," Herbert related, "and he was their defender always, especially of their beautiful faith, their just laws and their bravery. He told us boys that an Indian hated fear above all other things, as it would make a coward of him, and the next thing he hated was a liar."[34] Still told them the Shawnee believed in a Great Spirit, present everywhere, who could be reached by prayer and sacrifice – and they learned that he shared similar spiritual beliefs. "His religion was something akin to the North American Indian, something like their Great Spirit," Herbert wrote. "[The] shrine at which he worshipped and prayed was a shag-bark hickory tree. His prayer never in any way asked for anything for himself nor his friends, it was that everything was all right – akin to the Indian religion. He taught us to reverence our bodies as the sacred temple of our spirit and he told us how to perfect the body so that our earthly record might be the better. Old Doctor Still believed in beautifying all things in this life."[35] A curious phrase, one seemingly derived from the Shawnee orator Tecumseh, who said:

> So live your life that the fear of death cannot enter your heart. Trouble no one about their religion, respect others in their view, and demand that they respect yours. Love your life, perfect your life, beautify all things in your life. Seek to make your life long and its purpose in the service of your people. Prepare a noble death song for the day you go over the great divide. Always give a good word or a sign of salute when meeting or passing a friend, even a stranger, when in a lonely place. Show respect to all people and grovel to none.
>
> When you arise in the morning give thanks for the food and for the joy of living. If you see no reason for giving thanks, the fault lies only in yourself. Abuse no one and nothing, for abuse turns the wise ones to fools and robs the spirit of its vision. When it comes your time to die, be not like those whose hearts are filled with the fear of death, so that when their time comes they weep and pray for a little more time to live their lives over again in a different way. Sing your death song and die like a hero going home.[36]

Still applied a remarkably similar code to his life – and perhaps his essentially American Indian spirituality generated more prejudice than his spiritualist leanings. "The good people of Kirksville called him an infidel," Herbert told, because "he truly believed that God and his Creation was one and the same thing."[37]

One day Still was sitting on a log in the yard with two bones in his hands when he saw a doctor leave the Bernard house. Herbert told him his mother was in bed with one of the frequent headaches she had suffered for years since being thrown from a carriage. "Come on, boy," Still said, "Let's go over and see if we can't make big medicine for her." He examined Mrs. Bernard's neck and made a correction that resulted in a popping sound – and no further headaches. The medical doctors made capital of this; the ludicrous suggestion that a displaced bone in the neck could cause headaches was sure proof of Dr. Still's insanity.[38]

While adults belittled, the young generally beheld Still in a positive light. "He was a man who inspired fear and awe," his nephew M. F. Hulett wrote, "yet there was something attractive in his kindly face that drew the interest of children. While rather gruff in his behavior, we followed his every movement as does a faithful dog its master."[39]

Charley's friend Edwin Pickler initially thought Still a "strange, silent man" whose "eyes, when he looked at me, always gave me the impression of knowing just what I was thinking about" – and even stranger when he produced some bones from his pockets and said they were "the upper end of an Injun."[40] But with familiarity Ed grew to like Charley's father.

Still took the boy on rock hunting forays down a little creek west of town, rewarding him with praise and perhaps a small coin for his finds. At home Still kept in boxes a "magnificent collection" of pebbles and crystals, among them a clear blue-tinted agate shaped like a sheep's head that Ed coveted, thinking it would make a beautiful scarf pin. Still's sons encouraged him to take it, but warned to say nothing to their father. The next time Ed ran into Still the agate was in his pocket. To his excruciating guilt, Still looked at him steadily and thoughtfully. "Ed," he said, "have you been trading rocks with the boys?" Ed denied it, fully expecting to have his pockets searched, but instead Still reached into his own pocket and handed over a dime. "I would not like to lose any of them," he said kindly. The agate was replaced at the first opportunity.[41]

The boy remained skeptical of the doctor's odd medical theories, though, until one cure made a deep impression. Ed's friend Ellsworth "Ec" Hawkins gashed his knee with a knife and was confined to bed, unable to bend the joint or bear weight on the leg. After the regular physicians failed to help the parents finally called Still, who approached the bed and asked the child what was wrong. "I don't know Doc," Ec replied, "but I guess the devil's in my knee." "All right," Still said, "let's knock the devil out of it." The following day Ec was on crutches and in a short time was well.[42]

Still was a man possessed by a great idea. In an old flour sack he kept the 206 bones of a complete Indian skeleton. Removing one bone at a time he familiarized himself with their contours: the bumps and rough areas where ligaments and muscles attached, the smooth joint surfaces, the small holes where blood vessels and nerves entered and exited. To help memorize these intimate details he took a penknife and whittled soft pieces of wood or plaster of Paris into the exact shape of each bone, and covered the walls of the house with home-made anatomical charts and diagrams.

He explored the relationships between the osseous elements and the soft tissues: the bones acting like levers, the muscles moving the bones around the fulcrum of the joint, the ligaments fastening the bones together to stabilize the joints and check excess movement, the joint capsules enclosing the thin film of synovial fluid that lubricated and protected the articular cartilage at the ends of the bones. To sharpen his tactile sense he devised a demanding exercise. On long strips of cardboard he drew accurate outlines of the bones – the arm, wrist and hand; the leg, ankle and foot – and onto them placed the bones themselves, each labeled with its correct anatomical name. Standing with his back to the table, he had an assistant hand him one bone at a time and tried to identify it solely by touch. After mastering the limbs he progressed to the head, pelvis and spine. The vertebrae were a close study; no two were alike and he learned to distinguish each by such subtle details as differences in rib attachment.

Through repeated practice he developed a detailed mental picture of the vertebrae and their relationships to the spinal centers and vasomotor nerves that controlled the circulation of the various parts. "Dr. Still studied and experimented for many months that he might learn by personal observation the location of these centers," one of his students wrote later:

> With this knowledge as a guide, he literally 'felt his way' along the spines of his patients, comparing the abnormal with the normal, the pathological with the physiological. And – mark this, for it is the gist of the whole subject – there was impaction of tissues upon a given nerve or derangement of structures at a given spinal center whenever

> the function controlled by that nerve or center was impaired. In other words if an organ or part was not in proper working order, the structures surrounding the nerve or spinal center that controlled the functioning of that organ or part were found to be out of their normal relations.[43]

Systematically correlating anatomical derangements with physiological effects (changes in the digestion and assimilation of food, detoxification and elimination of wastes, and every other function), Still concluded that "no human body was normal in disease." So engrossed did he become with this mechanical approach to medicine that he entered his occupation in the 1875 Kansas census not as a physician but as a "Machinist."

For many years he carried in his pockets perhaps the bones of a hand or foot, an arm or leg, or a portion of the backbone. When giving treatment he might draw from his coat a column of neck vertebrae strung together with a rubber cord and, mimicking what he found in his patient, bend it into different positions to help decide how to make the correction.[44]

For every condition he applied the same principle: trace from physiological effect to anatomical cause, trust in nature's ability to heal, and await results. In these early days, though, working out the intricate relationship between structure and function could be a complex and occasionally lengthy process.

A youth working in a Kirksville cooper shop gashed his knee with an adz. The cut became infected, the leg inflamed, and when the first signs of septicemia appeared his parents called in a council of three physicians. Two advised immediate amputation; the third, Dr. Grove, favored calling Still first. Still called at the house that evening, and the boy's parents watched anxiously as he examined the knee for a few minutes. Then he drew up a chair to the bedside, sat with his feet upon another chair, and pulled his hat down over his eyes. He remained motionless in this position for so long that they feared he would do nothing, but then he suddenly stood up, worked on the pelvis and thigh, and gently rotated and stretched the injured leg to relax the inflamed and contracted tissues. By morning the swelling had subsided and the boy was out of danger.[45]

Such incidents fueled endless gossip and rumor. Businessman F. D. Parker expressed the typical sentiment:

> Not knowing him at this time personally, any too well, I could not look upon him other than a poor, misguided man whose mind was a little 'off' as compared with the average citizen. Imagine one going about town, or strolling in the woods, dropping down perhaps upon a curb stone, taking a bone from among many hidden about his person, wholly oblivious of his surroundings, and studying it as if his whole future depended upon the exact origin or attachment of a muscle, perhaps mumbling to himself; and you will see Dr. Still. His neighbors did not know exactly what he was doing, but thought his actions the singular notions of an unbalanced man, penning himself up, or wandering in the country, apparently dreaming his life away, often trying to induce some colored, or poor white person, to come under his treatment.[46]

Still's last newspaper advertisement appeared on August 5 and with it his final mention of magnetic healing. By now most called him the Bone Doctor anyway.

To help keep the family solvent Mary continued to sell magazine subscriptions, and they took in a string of patients as lodgers: Martha Bunch, the invalid daughter of an old friend from Macon County; Valie Chapman, bedridden for five years after a fall from a haystack; and Blanche Meeks, the eighteen-year-old daughter of a Bonaparte, Iowa, jeans manufacturer, who Still cured of "granulated eyelids," a fungal condition that frequently led to blindness.[47] On 5 January 1876 Mary gave birth to their last child, a girl they named Blanche after their houseguest.[48]

Lacking money and patients, mocked and maligned for his seemingly bizarre preoccupation with bones, Still began to suffer spells of self-doubt and despondency.[49] Convinced his brother was suffering a form of insanity, Jim wrote Mary that Andrew was unworthy, unfit to raise a family, and she had no business living with him.[50] On a visit to Kansas Still confided in his sister-in-law Louise how hard he had tried to convince others that what he had to offer was really worthwhile, but they were set against him and it seemed as if he might as well quit. Louise looked him in the eye. "Dr. Still I believe in you, and in your work," she said, "and someday the world will look upon your discovery as one of the greatest, and that will not be many years hence."[51]

A handful of others offered needful encouragement. "Dr. Drew, you are on the right track," Hez Prudom said after Still cured his wife of an unspecified eleven-year illness. "Keep on investigating and no one can horoscope the possibilities."[52] Charlie Chinn, too, foresaw a brighter future for his tenant, and was always ready with uplifting words to cheer him in his gloomiest hours. "Shout on brother," he would utter with a reassuring pat on the back, "some day you will outride the storm."[53]

The greatest comfort came from a philosophical insight of Robert Harris. During a walk in the woods Still told the gunsmith he might have to quit his idea to provide an income for his family. "No, stick to it," Harris said, "and you will come out all right."[54] But why, Still asked, were people so reluctant to accept a truth? "Man naturally dreads to travel a road he has never been over and fears that which he does not understand," Harris replied. "He does not understand life or death therefore he dreads to talk or think on such subjects." He concluded with a phrase that would help Still through many difficult times in the coming years: "Only few men allow themselves to think outside of popular ruts."[55]

10

LIGHTNING BONE SETTER

The people of Kirksville called him the crazy bone crank, impostor, spiritualist and other terms "still more uncomplimentary." They dismissed his cures as the work of the devil, hocus-pocus, fakery. Black people said there was something "funny" about him – he had "power" – and they preferred to submit to his treatment than risk being hoodooed.[2] Preachers denounced him from the pulpit.[1] Physicians besmirched his reputation, belittled his work,[3] and refused to have anything to do with him or any case he had attended.[4] Neighbors feared exchanging visits. Patients dared not summon him, fearing the likely ridicule, abuse and even ostracism of their families. The few who did usually insisted on secrecy, asking him to come after dark or by the back door. Many had second thoughts when he arrived and turned him away.[5]

Lacking patients in town, Still adopted a new strategy, offering evening lecture demonstrations in country schoolhouses throughout the surrounding district. Under a program billed as *Man's Lost Center,*[6] he presented to audiences of perhaps a half-dozen or more his "advanced ideas both of medicine and religion"[7] and after speaking invited sufferers to step forward for free treatment. Charley and Harry acted as assistants, holding a part of the patient's body as their father made the correction, all the while describing what he was doing and why. Occasionally someone might offer them a bed for the night, but usually they had to walk home, up to fifteen miles, often setting off after midnight.[8]

One Saturday evening Still spoke to a small gathering in Troy Mills, three and a half miles south of Kirksville. On this occasion farmers Harvey and Jane Hildreth, who lived a mile from the school, collected him from town and put him up for the night. Jane had worked as a water cure practitioner since before the Civil War, riding horseback to rural communities to treat typhoid, smallpox, scarlet fever and other infections with hot baths, hot packs, hot water bottles and hot ears of corn to induce sweating and eliminate toxins. She had first met Still in summer 1875 when she climbed the rickety flight of stairs outside Chinn's store with her twelve-year-old son to seek advice about a sick neighbor, Mrs. Bush. For the child the visit was memorable both for the generosity of the doctor and for his apparent power of prescience. "Until my dying day I shall never forget the scene nor the impression made upon me, boy though I was," Arthur Hildreth recalled:

> The morning was a bright, beautiful, sunshiny one, the weather was warm, and the west door of his office was open. He was standing just a few feet in front of where we were sitting. After mother's question, he turned and gazed out the door, seeming to be lost in thought for a few minutes. Then turning to us he said, 'Why your friend has a goiter and if you will have her come up here I will remove it.'

Jane protested that the Bush family lived out in the woods near the Chariton River, barely eking a living by felling trees for railroad ties, and could not afford his fee.[9] "Tell them to haul me a load of wood," Still responded, "they can afford to do that can't they?" After a few treatments the swelling on Mrs. Bush's neck grew smaller and finally disappeared.[10]

Still became a frequent visitor to the Hildreth farm. He often carried a copy of *Gray's Anatomy* and, sitting on the porch or with his chair tilted against a tree, read to Arthur and philosophized on the words. The boy regarded Dr. Still as "more than just another human being" and would remember as "one of the real worth-while things" of his childhood the day they strolled together two or three miles along a nearby ravine, the doctor picking up one pebble after another and describing the geology of the rock strata they came from.[11] Arthur Hildreth would grow to become one of the most important figures in the early history of osteopathy.

Just as Still had begun to attract enough patients to pay the rent and put food on the table he suffered a devastating setback. In September 1876 he contracted typhoid and for nine months was too weak to work. Overwhelmed by discouragement he wallowed in uncharacteristic self-pity and began to entertain morbid thoughts:

> Days and years may come and go, seeming to show us trees loaded with ripe fruit and heaven's perfume. But tomorrow comes [and] cyclones of fire pass over the shade trees of hope, tearing them up by their roots and piling them in heaps of ruin, to ever remind us that the road we have traveled only leads to defeat, and that life is a succession of failures. Not even the feeble flash of a firefly tells us that such a thing as light exists. We look for friends in vain. We pray, trust, and cry, but neither bread nor pillow of rest comes. We throw high in the air the rockets of distress, but no mortal friend sees the signs of misery. We feel that death is the only friend left, and would gladly give it an open-armed welcome, but the cries of our children call a halt to the thought of the deadly drug and knife of suicide.

A "vision of the night" broke the downward spiral. In his slumber Mary came to announce that their "ten-year-old son" had gone out in search of work to support the family and found paid employment for a month. Then appeared an image that seemed to indicate hope and joy: a golden banner floating on the breeze and next to it, atop a large stone, a dish containing a human brain – not just any brain but "the brain of a man who had been used to success in all things." Upon the stone was embossed an emblem: *This is of no use to any other man, it is no better than others only in one way, this man had the courage to use his own brain and let all others alone*. Still awoke with the dream still vivid in his mind and in an instant his despondency melted away.

It taught him "one of the most valuable lessons" of his life: the only person he could truly rely upon was himself. He realized that his greatest problem lay not in external circumstances but in his own lack of self-confidence. He had been lecturing that God constructed man to the degree of physical and mental perfection while ignoring his own teaching and languishing in dependent helplessness. No longer would he rely upon the opinions of experts or authorities; no longer would he defer to ministers, politicians, doctors, the rich or the powerful. From now on he would be his own judge, guided not by the laws of man but by the moral law engraved on his heart.[12]

As he convalesced he continued to study. After two years of examining bones by touch he was now able to identify every bone of the body, including each individual vertebra and each tiny phalanx of the fingers and toes, left and right, of any skeleton. He whittled wood, ornamenting the living room window sill with a long row of "small various-sized flat bottom domes" for treating feet.[13] He immersed himself in the works of Huxley, Darwin, Wallace, Béchamp, Spencer and other biologists, sifting truth from theory and evolving new ideas and novel interpretations.

The origin of species concerned him little. "Whether we sprang from monkeys or buzzards," he opined, "does not help us much."[14] He accepted the principle of the survival of the fittest, but disagreed with those who equated developmental complexity with increasing perfection, believing that everything in nature was already perfect regardless of its level of development. He held that all life forms had "reached a state of anatomical and physiological perfection very early," and that natural selection had "accomplished little or nothing except possibly in brain development since the time of Paleolithic man."[15]

To assert nature's perfection dissolved the argument between evolutionists and creationists, for both camps labored under the premise of man's imperfection.[16] "Whichever side of the case, 'Religion vs. Charles Darwin et al.' one wishes to take," Still declared, "whether one believes that man was made from dust in a finitely short time by an infinite being, or whether he was made from protoplasm in an infinitely long time by the action of finite forces, one must admit that the result has been a practically perfect creation."[17] But in the theory of natural selection he identified an important principle that the eminent biologists had overlooked.

The evolutionary literature emphasized the anatomical adaptations made by species in the struggle for survival, but Still recognized that in order to survive they must also have developed physiological adaptations to enable them to resist and recover from disease. "The European naturalists, although some were physicians," his student John Deason wrote, "did not realize that these same principles would apply to the building of resistance to disease. It was Still who first presented this view." Deason added, though, that with the religious furor over evolution Dr. Still was "far too wise to discuss such things for it would have made him even more unpopular than he was at that time."[18]

Since the flux cases in Macon, Still had mulled endlessly over the "diseases of the seasons." The cause of these epidemics remained unknown. Some suspected microorganisms, though so far none had been positively implicated.[19] But while medical researchers were looking for external causes, Still's gaze was turned inward. Since 1864 he had wondered why some people caught a particular disease while others did not, and why sometimes even the most serious cases made spontaneous recoveries. The body patently possessed an inbuilt mechanism for its own defense. Speculating on its possible nature (the immune system remained undiscovered) he formulated a tentative hypothesis: during periods of stress from infectious disease the blood and tissues produce curative or protective "chemico-biological substances" he termed *body ferments*.[20]

The word fermentation had traditionally been employed to represent a variety of spontaneous changes occurring in organic solutions: alcoholic fermentation of beer and wine, acetic acid fermentation of vinegar, lactic acid fermentation of souring milk. Putrefaction, a word given to the spoiling of meat, eggs and other foods, was assumed to be a related process, and both were thought to be catalyzed by chemical agents known generically as ferments. Still's "theory of ferments"[21] drew heavily upon the research of French chemist Louis Pasteur.

In 1855 Pasteur was asked by an alcohol manufacturer to investigate why his product frequently became contaminated. The process involved adding yeast – thought to be a chemical – to beet juice to catalyze the conversion of plant sugars into alcohol. Pasteur took samples of the fermenting juice and looked at them under his microscope. To his surprise he saw that the small globules of yeast were not chemical in nature but tiny living organisms, the plant sugars were their food, and alcohol a waste product of their metabolism. The solution also contained some smaller objects. These, too, turned out to be living organisms – bacteria – and the undesirable contaminants were *their* waste products.

Pasteur tested other organic solutions. In his landmark 1857 paper *Mémoire sur la fermentation appelée lactique* he described the souring of milk by the bacterial conversion of milk sugar into lactic acid, and went on to show that other bacterial strains are responsible for the spoiling of beer and wine.

Seeking methods to prevent bacterial ingress, he took contaminated solutions, adjusted various parameters, and monitored the metabolic activity of yeast and bacteria. He altered the pH. Yeast produced more alcohol in an acid solution. He altered the aeration. Yeast grew slowly in conditions of low oxygen but produced a large amount of alcohol; it grew abundantly in conditions of excess oxygen but produced only a small amount of alcohol. The results were consistent and replicable. By knowing the pH and the available oxygen he was able to accurately predict the level of proliferation of either yeast or bacteria.

It had previously been thought that living organisms could only respire by assimilating free oxygen from air, but these experiments showed that yeast can derive energy from food by two separate metabolic pathways: respiration with free oxygen, an efficient process that produces much energy and only a small amount of toxic metabolites; and *fermentation*, "respiration in the absence of air," a more wasteful process that produces little energy and a large amount of toxic metabolites.[22] Pasteur now employed the word *ferments* in a new way to signify a "class of organized beings . . . similar in all particulars to those [that respire with free oxygen], assimilating in the same manner carbon, nitrogen and phosphates, requiring oxygen like them, but differing from them in the ability to use the oxygen from unstable organic combinations instead of free oxygen gas for their respiration."[23] Some bacteria, he found, thrived only when starved of oxygen.

Since the biochemical activity of all living cells is remarkably similar, Pasteur postulated that the level of oxygen should be a factor of universal importance. "The relation between fermentation, respiration and availability of oxygen is not limited to microbial and plant cells," he wrote. "Similarly, in animal economy, oxygen gives to cells an activity from which they derive, when removed from the presence of this gas, the faculty to act in the manner of ferments."[24] The principle is illustrated by muscle cells. In aerobic exercise, when oxygen supply exceeds demand, the cells respire with free oxygen, converting glucose into carbon dioxide and water in an efficient process that liberates a great deal of energy. In anaerobic exercise, when oxygen demand exceeds supply, the cells switch to lactate fermentation, converting glucose into lactic acid and water in a more wasteful process that liberates far less energy.

Pasteur never experimented with animal tissues, but he did speculate on the fundamental importance of oxygen to cellular metabolism. "There lies, certainly, the mystery of all true fermentations," he declared, "and perhaps of many normal and abnormal physiological processes of living beings." Profound though this thought was, he pursued it no further.[25]

Instead Pasteur followed a thread that led to the germ theory of disease. He had early referred to the contamination of beet juice, milk, beer and wine as "diseases of fermentation" and, ruminating on the bacterial breakdown of plant and animal tissues by fermentation and putrefaction, declared that "everything indicates that contagious diseases owe their existence to similar causes."[26]

In the mid-1860s Pasteur was appointed to head a commission to investigate a disease ravaging the French silkworm industry. In a three-year study he found that the worms had two separate diseases, one protozoal, the other bacterial. The protozoal disease was controlled relatively easily by breeding methods to avoid contamination, but the bacterial disease demanded deeper investigation. Applying what he had learned from his fermentation experiments, he exposed infected worms to different parameters. The bacteria thrived when the worms were kept in conditions of poor nutrition, excessive heat and humidity, inadequate aeration and even during stormy weather.[27] These experiments showed that the prevailing environmental conditions – what Pasteur termed the "terrain" – formed the single most important factor for the health of the worms, the presence of microorganisms being less the *cause* of disease than the *effect* of lowered resistance.[28] Measures to raise the worms in conditions of optimum hygiene and nutrition saved the industry from ruin.

Still took Pasteur's conclusions, blended them with Virchow's teaching that normal physiology demands unimpeded blood circulation, added his own principle of cause and effect, and applied this assemblage of ideas to his understanding of human infections. "It is only reasonable to look for fermentation of fluids if delayed too long in the cellular system," Still declared. "A closing of cells with their fluids holds their contents, and this is followed by fermentation. . . . A collapse of cells comes with fermentation."[29] A sluggish circulation, from any cause, would result in poor oxygenation and, beyond a certain point, cellular respiration by the inefficient process of fermentation. But what would cause a delay of fluids in the first place?

Pasteur had suggested that circulation might be altered by atmospheric changes and extremes of temperature, and even that mental states might affect the course of many diseases. Still speculated that since dysentery usually struck around harvest time, overexposure to sun or overexertion of spinal muscles might irritate sensory nerves and, by reflex stimulation of motor and vasomotor nerves,[30] cause circulatory stasis and poor oxygenation of intestinal cells. "I defy the oldest sages of philosophy to show me the difference between flux and no flux; to show me the time when flux was not there," he wrote:

> [They] must take the number of hours in which this milk soured and began to curdle. It first commenced by being in a stationary position and under a curdling temperature: then the milk sours, in a common pan, and it would sour just the same in pans of the bowels or the mesentery arteries, veins or muscles. Therefore you simply have an effect, and you call that effect a disease, a particular disease, just as you call your brother Jim and your sister Sarah Ann.[31]

Flux, he concluded, was simply "an abortive effort of the artery to feed the vein,"[32] an effect traceable to "a cause in the spinal cord or its branches."[33] He believed that relaxing muscles and freeing joints calmed the sympathetic nerves, normalized the circulation (and therefore oxygenation, nutrition and acidity at the cellular level), and enabled the body's endogenous "body ferments" to overcome the infection. "I took the position," he set down a prototype theory of immunity, "that the living blood swarmed with health corpuscles, which were carried to all parts of the body. Interfere with that current of blood, and you stream down the river of life and land in the ocean of death."[34]

By June 1877 Still felt strong enough to resume working and, maligned in town, turned again to the outlying district.[35] Among the farming community he found a refreshing openness to his revolutionary ideas and people interested in helping develop them. They allowed him to test his theory on their ailments and experiment with different methods of treatment.[36]

He usually took Harry on his rural calls, as helper and companion – and to keep an eye on him. Ten and big for his age, Harry was by his own admission the bad boy of the family. He was always getting into fights, usually provoked by some taunt about his "crazy Pa." If he heard another boy make fun of his father "it was like shaking a red rag at a bull, or touching off the fuse of a charge of dynamite." Either the boy apologized or one or the other of them took a thrashing. Another source of trouble was a youthful enthusiasm for the art of spitting. For added mastery he took a pin and worked a hole between his front teeth, but one day his technique faltered and he accidentally sprayed his mother. To escape her wrath he ran off to hide under the barn, pursued by his father, crawling after him with a big stick. "What's the matter Pa," Harry blurted out, "did you spit on Ma too?" Still dissolved into laughter and on this occasion the beating was averted.[37]

In late 1878 father and son traveled to Baldwin in response to an urgent telegram from an old patient whose daughter had pneumonia. Regular medical treatment carried a poor prognosis. "In young children and old persons almost always fatal," Still's copy of Dunglison's *The Practice of Medicine* stated. "Double pneumonia generally fatal." The standard prescription was morphine to relieve the pain, but Still believed that by slowing the circulation the drug increased the risk of congestion, fermentation and mortality, so he persuaded the girl's parents to withhold medicines until he tried his treatment first. Employing the same principle as for flux, he placed his hands on either side of the girl's thoracic spine, applied gentle but sustained pressure to relax muscles hardened by reflex contraction, and raised the ribs to restore mobility to the chest, aiming to free blood and lymph to allow the body's own "drugs" to overcome the infection. This simple procedure resulted in an immediate improvement and by morning the crisis had passed.[38]

Pneumonia was epidemic and before returning home he treated further cases in western Missouri.[39] In Pleasant Hill he received a telegram from Captain Sandy Lowe, his former commander in the 21st Kansas State Militia, whose wife was dangerously ill with pneumonia of both lungs.[40] Her speedy recovery prompted Lowe to invite Still to practice from his home in Wadesburg the following year.

From the flux and pneumonia cases Still learned that just as different infectious diseases show characteristic signs and symptoms, they also show characteristic patterns of muscle contraction and joint irritation related to the "spinal centers" connected neurologically to the site of infection. He reasoned that joint restriction and muscle tension initiated "a stoppage of fluids in the body long enough to permit of fermentation usually resulting in fever."[41] He was also learning that pneumonia (and all other infectious diseases) could

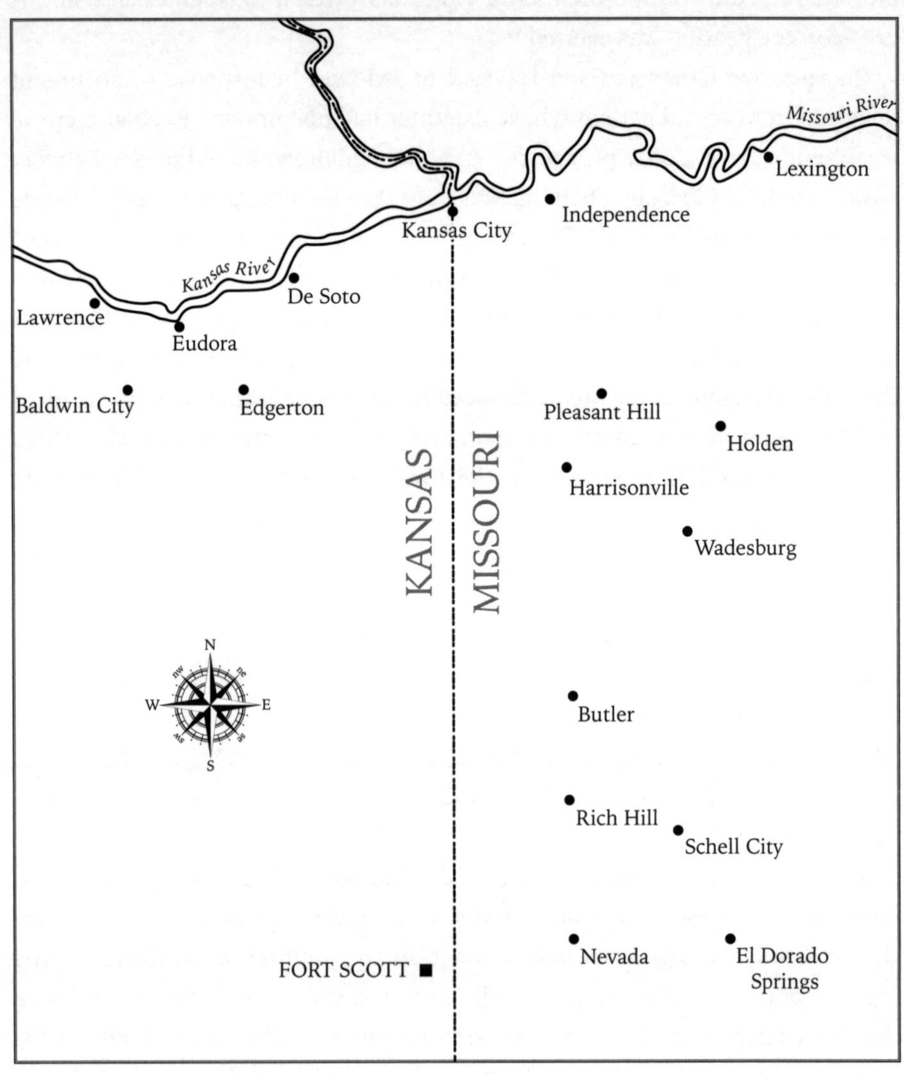
SOUTHWEST MISSOURI
Missouri River
Lexington
Independence
Kansas City
Kansas River
De Soto
Lawrence
Eudora
Baldwin City
Edgerton
Pleasant Hill
Holden
Harrisonville
Wadesburg
KANSAS
MISSOURI
N
W
E
S
Butler
Rich Hill
Schell City
Nevada
El Dorado Springs
FORT SCOTT

have *predisposing* or *exciting* causes. In the woman hit in the chest by the hog's snout a displaced rib had predisposed to nerve irritation, circulatory stasis and lowered resistance. The cases in Baldwin and western Missouri were different, the characteristic pattern of lung congestion, heat, and muscular rigidity being the secondary effects of an exciting cause later found to be microorganisms and their toxins. And, pondering the similarities of the body's response to different infectious diseases (generalized aching, chills, malaise and fever), he further concluded that fever is a powerful natural remedy.

The following summer, at Lowe's and in nearby Holden, Still experimented on a variety of new conditions. He cured (with two months of treatment) a woman with erysipelas, another with "running sores" from shoulder to wrist caused by a displaced acromioclavicular joint, and a man rendered almost blind by corneal ulceration from a purulent eye infection. He cured headaches by adjusting cervical vertebrae and upper ribs to normalize cranial blood circulation,[42] and finally came to understand why his childhood headache remedy provided only temporary relief: because it failed to remove the underlying cause.

In the fall he and Harry traveled across the state to Hannibal, the Mississippi river town familiar from Still's childhood corn-milling trips, and rented an office there for the winter.[43]

A pattern was set. For the next ten years Still conducted a peripatetic practice reminiscent of his father's circuits, visiting a dozen or more towns in western Missouri, others in Hannibal and vicinity, while continuing to treat patients in Macon, La Plata and Kirksville.

Announcing his itinerary in newspapers, carrying perhaps a thousand handbills to scatter at his destination,[44] he plied his trade more like a vendor of elixirs and quack medicines than a qualified physician. Perched upon a spring wagon or ox cart on the sidewalk of a public square, a street corner or, in poor weather, a hall, schoolhouse or hotel lobby, he lectured to gaggles of curious bystanders who gathered to listen.[45]

From his old flour sack he produced the bones of an Indian skeleton and in plain language described the wondrous workings of the marvelous machine run by the unseen power of life. He demonstrated how the bones join together, described how injury or illness alters their relationships to irritate nerves and upset circulation, and told his listeners to quit taking drugs and place their confidence in the healing power of nature. After his talk he invited sufferers to come forward for treatment and, as he worked to normalize joints and loosen muscles, described what he was doing as if repairing a machine.

Crowds needed to be won over quickly before he was deemed a failure or a fake.[46] They jeered and scoffed and demanded to be shown results. Sometimes the barracking and name calling upset his sons, but Still seemed to thrive on it. "He rather enjoyed having the finger of scorn pointed at him," Charley related, "and he would do things sometimes that would encourage it."[47] Remaining calm and assured, Still turned the abuse to his advantage. "If you had as much sense as a sheep on this subject," he singled out one heckler, "I would feel hard towards you, but you are perfectly excusable." Since most knew nothing about anatomy he quizzed them on such things as the number of bones in the foot and, after capturing their attention, introduced the relationships of bones to muscles, blood vessels and nerves, and explained how structural derangements marked the beginning of disease.[48]

The affluent generally stayed away from these street performances, but his frankness and common-sense explanations appealed to the common folk. They compared his prognoses with those of their regular doctors,[49] and when they recovered just as he predicted – especially when beyond their expectations – they grew more confident in him and his treatment. "Of course he would be looked upon as some mysterious being, crazy or at least daffy," his printer Homer Bailey told, "but with his intuitive insight he would pick out a cripple, or someone with a severe headache or some disease he could cure quickly. He was always eccentric and did what you least expected him to do; but the impression left was usually a good one. It created talk and interest in the mysterious old doctor."[50]

Rapid cures sometimes generated mistrust. An Irish laundress in Holden suspected trickery. While washing Still's shirt she discovered a hole in the right side and convinced herself it was the exit for a wire connected to a hidden battery. She believed the various ways he pulled people around was a pretense and that the real restorative was electricity. (He had actually made the hole to insert a handkerchief during the sticky summer months to prevent his shirt becoming soiled with sweat.)[51] Others imagined metaphysical forces. Rumors spread that he was a medium, a clairvoyant, a man gifted with spiritualistic and magnetic healing powers – and not entirely without foundation. To engage audiences he often attempted to read people's minds, a practice he eventually discontinued because it generated a belief that his cures relied upon hypnotism or suggestion.[52] Some divined malign influences. A month after correcting another Irish woman's shoulder and two displaced upper ribs she accused him of having "hoodledooed" her, for not only was her shoulder better but her asthma, which she had not even mentioned, had also disappeared.[53]

This outcome surprised Still, too, and proved a valuable lesson. One freezing December day, passing through woods outside Kirksville, he came upon an old woodchopper named Joe Hall sitting astride a chair outside his cabin, stripped to the waist in a biting north wind, fighting for air. "I have asthma and am smothering to death," Hall uttered in panic between gasps. "I can't get my breath." Still examined him, corrected some ribs, and the man's respiration soon calmed. "My God, Doctor, what have you done to me?" he exclaimed, alarmed at his rapid relief. "My lungs are as free as ever they were in my life." Four months later they ran into each other in a Kirksville dining room and Hall reported that his asthma had not returned since being "fumbled." After treating a few more asthmatics Still tentatively announced that the condition was curable, provided the patient did not have tuberculosis or some other cause of lowered vitality.[54]

Real estate agent George Compton of Independence, Missouri, vehemently disbelieved the stories of cures. Certain the whole business was an elaborate confidence trick, he was "very much disgusted" when his daughter, suffering from "a spinal affection which gave rise to a distressing complication of ailments," asked to be taken to the bone doctor. Compton tried to dissuade her, offering to take her to specialists in New York, Philadelphia, Chicago or anywhere, but finally relented when she "womanlike began to cry." To humor the girl he took her to Nevada, Missouri, where Still was due, only to find he had already left, leaving in his wake accounts of marvelous cures. It hardened in Compton an obsessive resolve to track down and expose the quack.

They waited a fortnight in El Dorado Springs, but Still failed to appear. They traveled to neighboring St. Clair County, and there heard tales of a boy cured of fits, a woman relieved of asthma, and many other wonders. On returning to El Dorado Springs they heard a story about a girl he cured in Schell City. They finally tracked him down in Rich Hill, where Compton watched cynically as people entered a room on crutches and exited without them, sure they were hired accomplices. But a seed of doubt was planted when he saw a woman with a hand so swollen it looked as if the skin would burst and a few hours later the swelling had gone. Then he saw a girl with "hip joint disease," pronounced incurable by the celebrated Dr. John C. Gunn (author of *Gunn's New Domestic Physician*), and within a week she was walking around without crutches. "The evidence was too much for me," Compton related. "I had to be convinced." As skepticism gave way to curiosity and finally to enthusiasm, he invited Still to open a temporary office at his home in Independence.

Within a few days up to three hundred people were congregating daily at the house. Still cured Compton's brother-in-law of chronic diarrhea, a Kentuckian of agonizing sciatica, and a jeweler unable to raise his arm for nine months. Some needed only a few treatments, others more, while a few showed improvement only "some time" later. "I cannot begin to tell all the cures the doctor made there," Compton wrote:

> There was a Mrs. Furnish, who had been in a railroad wreck. She had walked with crutches five years and could not stand alone without them. In five minutes after the doctor treated her she walked without her crutches. This was on Wednesday. On the Sunday following she walked four blocks to church without her crutches. As she walked down the aisle everybody in the church was amazed. The preacher looked like one struck dumb. 'Is this sister Furnish,' he asked. 'Yes, I am sister Furnish, and I was cured by Dr. Still,' shouted the happy woman. 'Bless God,' said the minister, 'Let us sing *Praise God from Whom All Blessings Flow*,' and the congregation arose and made the old church ring with joy over the good sister's restoration to health.

Compton's daughter, too, was much improved, though a spinal curvature remained. For the real estate agent it was "a grand lesson" to witness not only the doctor's work but also his philanthropic attitude. Still accepted money only under the greatest protest and not at all if he thought it would hurt someone to pay. He treated the poor for free and, if he had or could borrow it, gave money to those unable to afford travel or lodging.[55] "Those who were able, paid him,"

Compton told, "but those who could not pay were treated just as well, and many a poor creature who came there in misery and without money, went away cured and happy with enough coin to buy bread for several weeks."[56]

Such philanthropy meant Still often needed to borrow money to embark on trips, and sometimes even to return home.[57] Banks refused him credit and dissuaded others from making him loans.[58] Catholic priest Father Chappell sometimes lent him up to $50,[59] though his family accused him of throwing money away, but friends knew that when Still had money he always settled his debts.

On one trip Charley, mystified by his father's apparently genuine lack of interest in money, assumed the role of cashier. Without success. Still said he did not like to charge as he felt he was still experimenting, and would rather treat fifty patients without making a cent and discover he could accomplish something than charge a fee and discover he did not know what to do.[60] Charley let the matter drop, but Harry, showing signs of his later business acumen, collected thirty or forty dollars owed for treatment and presented it to his father. "What shall we do with all this money?" Still responded blankly. "Well," Harry replied, "I think Ma needs something to eat."[61]

These were difficult years for Mary and the children. Blanche was teased for wearing clothes made from flour sacks and the unkind things she heard about her father would color her life with lasting bitterness.[62] When the boys tried to find work employers turned them down, saying they liked to hire staff whose family connections would draw trade rather than alienate it. In 1878 Ed and Jim tried to help, petitioning the Missouri pension office for the "injury and disability" their brother sustained during the Battle of Westport. Mary tried again in April 1882, writing Commissioner of Pensions William Dudley that the hernia her husband had suffered during the battle had left him unable to perform manual work:

> Misfortune of every kind has overtaken us. We have lost several thousand dollars by fire, and long continued sickness has brought us down, so that we have nothing left. We have a large family to bring up and educate with nothing left to do it with.[63]

Neither appeal succeeded. The Government denied responsibility, arguing that the Kansas Militia was not officially sworn into the Union forces; the State of Kansas denied accountability on the grounds that the fighting had taken place in Missouri.[64]

Kirksville provision merchant John Hannah earned Still's lasting gratitude. The grocer's wife had suffered head pain and bloodshot eyes since a fall on a washtub, and when the bone doctor cured her Hannah sent him a check. Still promptly sent it back, so Hannah paid him another way, by offering Harry a job as a clerk in his store. "Do you know you are helping me more than anyone else," Still told the grocer. "While I am away I know my family is cared for."[65]

The prophet was not without honor save in his own country. On his itinerant circuit the people called him the "tramp doctor," the "wonderful faith cure doctor," the "healing wonder." Some spoke of "the Still cure."[66] In Schell City Kathryn Talmadge overheard her mother saying that a "miracle man" was coming to town and she was determined to try his treatment. Kathryn could not remember the doctor's name, but a friend told her it was "something quiet." She recalled:

> At last came the eventful day. The town turned out to see what might appear, some from mere curiosity, some in the spirit of those who went to our Savior to be healed, and these did not go away disappointed. They found a most kindly man who worked not for pecuniary reward but for love of humanity. When Mother told the Doctor about the abscess in her side, which had baffled all medical skill, he just smiled, pressed on a rib, gave her arm a twist, and assured her she would have no more trouble. It was hard to believe, but as time passed, we all began to have faith, and the pain never returned from that day.[67]

Still eventually adopted a formal title: the Lightning Bone Setter (though with the admission that it was a "rather pretentious claim"), a designation given him in a Kansas City newspaper report of his dramatic cure of a young woman's dislocated hip.[68] His business cards now proclaimed *Dr. A. T. Still, Lightning Bone Setter*. The reverse stated:

> This is well worth your careful attention. Dr. Still has discovered that many diseases pronounced incurable are caused by partial or complete

> dislocation of the bones of the neck, chest, spine or limbs. Following is a partial list: headache, weak and sore eyes, enlarged tonsils, catarrh, sore ears, dripping eyes, loss of voice, bleeding of lungs, asthma, pneumonia, heart disease, consumption, paralysis of face, spine or limbs, goiter, piles, varicose veins, sore limbs, leucorrhea and all female diseases, fits, cold feet and limbs, general prostration, dyspepsia, gout, rheumatism of all parts of the system, liver disease, and all diseases of kidneys, etc. All the diseases above named are seldom cured until the bones at fault are adjusted.[69]

And, reflecting his growing awe at nature's power to heal, he appended the phrase,

> Man is fearfully and wonderfully made.[70]

11

MIRACLES ARE STILL PERFORMED

The Hannibal practice, in rooms rented at 814 Broadway, grew beyond Still's expectations. The townspeople initially thought him a "faith curist, magnetic and massage mountebank and medical vandal," a quack who "relied on the mind of the patient to imagine a cure." They discussed him at tea tables, in railway coaches, on the street, always in disparaging tones. Yet, as local journalist Ivy Summers observed, he "plodded along in his characteristic simple yet energetic manner totally oblivious to the tirade of abuse that was daily heaped upon him," and in time the talk turned to wondrous cures that "were the comment of the town and called forth the laudation of the press."

People spoke of a five-year-old girl suffering from spells of "intense nervousness," shrieking inconsolably, who under his ministrations made a complete recovery.[1] They spoke of an elderly black man he treated in public, surrounded by a crowd of onlookers. While walking from the railroad depot to his hotel, a sack of bones over his shoulder, accompanied by Charley and Harry each carrying a valise of yet more bones, Still saw old Mose limping along the street, and learned that he had fallen from a ladder while carrying mortar. Still stood his patient up against a dry goods box, grasped the lame leg, and performed a movement that enabled his patient to walk fairly normally.[2] No doubt they also spoke of the day he dropped in on a local dentist and looked on as a young man having a tooth extracted without anesthesia "squalled and left squalling." When the next patient, a young woman, also needed an extraction, Still offered to "control the nerves to the jaw." He exerted finger pressure to the relevant nerve, numbing it, and the dentist pulled out a "large tooth."

As word of his cures spread Still began to attract patients from neighboring counties, and the practices of local physicians began to suffer.[3] In the winter of 1882-3, Dr. J. C. Hearne, Secretary of the Marion County Medical and Surgical Association, swore out a warrant accusing him of practicing without a license or diploma.

The day of the trial was cold and misty. As the protagonists arrived, prosecuting attorney George Mahan, representing Hearne, was standing outside the courthouse, and was struck by the contrast between the plaintiff, draped in a heavy fur-collared overcoat, and the defendant, "somewhat singular in general demeanor," wrapped in a shawl. And, he soon learned, equally singular in his approach to the hearing. Before the court convened Still took Mahan to one side. "I do not have the money to hire a lawyer," he declared frankly, "and as this is a fight between doctors why not let us try the case?" Mahan had heard that Dr. Still was reputedly a "thoughtful, careful and prudent" man and that the public favored leaving him alone. Considering the proposition "very fair and square," he allowed the two doctors to argue the matter themselves.

Still told the court he had graduated from a "southern school," but had lost his diploma during the Civil War and was unable to obtain a duplicate because the establishment had since burned down. "I do not have half as many patients in the cemetery as the doctor who is complaining against me," he addressed the jury, "and hence I think my life and practice here is a general benefit to the public." The jurors evidently agreed, for the trial ended in his acquittal – a satisfactory outcome even for the prosecuting attorney. Mahan later admitted to having "but little interest in the case which seemed to me to be persecution rather than an effort to do the public good."[4]

The Hannibal Council refused to let the matter drop, though, and passed a resolution giving Still twenty four hours to leave town. He refused to comply,[5] and that summer was afforded protection from further harassment by a new Medical Practice Act that came into force on 1 July 1883. Under its terms physicians who did not hold medical diplomas or certificates from recognized medical schools were required to sit an examination administered by the newly formed Missouri State Board of Health. On 28 July the Adair County Court in Kirksville issued Still a certificate confirming his entry on the Missouri Roll of Physicians and Surgeons in compliance with the new law.[6]

On visits home Still was a common sight around town, perched on a goods box or reclining in a hammock in someone's yard with a big chew of tobacco, whittling a stick or "monkeying around with bones." In any group he was usually the one doing the talking, his sincere and logical arguments difficult to refute. Small crowds gathered to listen as he held forth in Hannah's grocery, where Harry worked as a roustabout. Sometimes he became so engrossed that he failed to return home for dinner, remaining till ten in the evening or later, and all stayed as long as he stayed.[7] People argued, more or less violently, on the merits or demerits of his treatment.

Mary and the children remained unwaveringly supportive. So, too, did Still's brother Ed who, after his wife Mary died in October 1882, began to assist Drew in his work[8] – and share the opprobrium. "At first the general impression was that we were switched off, or crazy," Ed related. "The doctors called Andrew a damned old jackass, and suggested sending him a block of hay. The preachers said it was the works of the devil. Doctors said it was too damned a fraud to be noticed. We were ostracized from any kind of fraternal feeling." With his reputation as a good surgeon Ed was "rather pitied" for siding with his brother.[9]

In 1884 Still persuaded Harry, seventeen, to quit his job and assist him full time, and during a six-month stay in Hannibal the following winter they relieved patients of "a dray load of plaster Paris casts, crutches and all classes of surgical appliances."[10] One case stood out. A wealthy businessman had fallen, dislocating his patella. A doctor cast the limb in plaster and ordered bed rest, but as weeks passed the leg continued to worsen and a friend eventually suggested he consult Dr. Still. The businessman laughed at the idea, but was finally persuaded to go and within a week was walking without pain.[11] Thinking he had done a good job Still asked for five dollars:

> To my amazement he reached in his pocket and brought out a huge roll of bills. He counted out one hundred dollars and handed it to me, saying that satisfied him if it did me. When my heart started beating again, I got my hat and took the first train for home. When I got there I walked out into the kitchen where Ma was washing dishes, and handed her the money. She looked at it and sank down on the kitchen floor, and with

tears falling from her eyes, she said she believed that at last we were going to have a home of our own.

After a decade of ostracism and ridicule, to know that his treatment "could produce results that would command such substantial appreciation" gave Still courage and assurance, and strengthened his faith that he was following the right path.[12]

In spring 1885 he and Harry traveled again to western Missouri. The crowds were ever larger, sometimes hundreds strong, the gatherings reminiscent of the old-fashioned camp meetings with people going off happy and shouting.[13] By evening Still would be exhausted, too tired to talk, and often lay awake for hours trying to work out more efficient methods of treatment to conserve his strength.[14]

In Nevada, Missouri, a Dr. Marmaduke stepped forward to ask if Still could do anything for his daughter, an inmate at the State Insane Asylum, located in the town. She had been entirely well and a competent pianist until three years earlier when a fall from a buggy rendered her deranged. They brought her home for Still to examine and with difficulty, for she was "almost raving" and unable to recognize her parents, helped her onto a bed. Still corrected the joint between the uppermost vertebra and the skull and, slowly, rationality began to return. Two hours later she washed, changed, and even played some music on the piano.[15]

Still had reached a point where he felt confident he could successfully treat "the various fevers, colds, diphtheria, croup, whooping cough, pneumonia, asthma, etc., and the innumerable so-called chronic conditions." When unsure of what to do he still occasionally resorted to drugs, though without conveying much faith in the remedy.[16] "The books say so and so," he would tell the patient. "I don't know whether they will do any good or not."[17] One case in 1885 persuaded him to stop prescribing medicines altogether.

In Wadesburg a Captain E. V. Stall presented with a large bladder stone that Still estimated, by palpation and percussion, to be two-and-a-half inches long and one-and-a-half inches wide. When the drugs he prescribed had no effect he corrected a deranged joint in the "lower spine," with the unexpected result that the concretion broke up to pass in the urine as a fine sand. The patient's speedy recovery forever convinced Still that no drug on earth could match the body's own power to heal.[18]

Not every case was curable, though. That fall his farmer friend Harvey Hildreth began to have difficulty swallowing food and was diagnosed with spasmodic contraction of the lower esophagus. The attacks were periodic, the condition progressive, and attempts to open the stricture with a bougie provided little benefit. They finally called Still, who loosened rigid neck and shoulder muscles, but was able to provide only temporary relief. One wet day in May 1886, shortly before Harvey died, the Hildreths heard footsteps on the front porch. It was Still. "I felt you people might need me," he said simply, "so here I am." The rain had turned the dirt road into an impassable quagmire, so he had walked three-and-a-half miles along the railroad track and another mile through muddy fields. For Harvey's son Arthur, now twenty-three, it gave an insight into the "real kindly spirit of the man." A friend as well as a physician.

Two years earlier Arthur had married a Kirksville girl, Margaret Corbin. One Sunday morning after the wedding, as she visited her parents, he called on Still, who lived three or four blocks away. After a brief chat Still led him around to the back of the house, where he pulled away from the wall a large open-backed goods box and from it drew a gunny sack more than half full of human bones. Picking out one bone after another he pieced them together, and explained how strains and displacements affected nerves and upset physiology. He talked at length about his new theory of disease and how, in time, it would revolutionize medicine.[19]

Soon after Harvey died, Arthur took Margaret to see Still. She had suffered from granulated eyelids since age eight, but recently the condition had deteriorated markedly, becoming agonizingly painful, and doctors pronounced her incurable. "Fungoid growths" covered the surface of the eyeballs, almost obliterating one pupil, and lumps the size of half a pea pushed out from under the eyelids. Doctors tried various remedies and periodically ground off the excrescences with blue vitriol, but they always grew back and the corneas were so foggy and vascular from the prolonged irritation that she could no longer recognize Arthur at a distance of six feet. She was advised that her only hope of avoiding a life of blindness was to undergo an operation by a noted specialist in St. Louis, but Arthur could not afford the surgery.

Still examined Margaret's eyes, then her spine. "This neck is dislocated," he said. "There is too much blood going into her head and face and it is seeking new avenues to deposit its strength, hence the production of inflammation in the eyes and lids and the development of growths." Hildreth asked if he could help her. "I can cure her," Still replied confidently, "she will be able to see as clear as an angel." But how could he do that, the farmer protested, without cutting off the growths or applying a corrosive ointment? "Arthur," he replied, "the same law of nature which has been obstructed, permitting those growths to form, when reestablished will absorb them."

Still pointed out distended veins and discolored tissue indicative of disturbed circulation, explained that the first three cervical nerves control blood to and from the eye, and adjusted the upper four neck vertebrae to "let out the excess blood." He corrected the articulations of the jawbone, saying that a displaced temporomandibular joint can often cause diseases of the mouth, tongue and throat, and, in some cases, deafness. To cut off the blood supply to the growths he lubricated a finger with Vaseline and ran the nail across the little arteries passing down the eyeball, then crushed the granules in the eyelids between thumb and forefinger. Hildreth asked how soon she would get better. "Oh, I don't know," Still said, "maybe two months, maybe six months, and it might take two years, but I can cure her." When the arteries were completely severed the eyes began to suppurate and the growths paled, thinned and, after two years, eventually disappeared, leaving the sclera a pure white. "It was all so simple, all so practical," Hildreth marveled, "that it cannot help but appeal to the reason of anyone who analyzes the whole story."[20]

Month after month, year after year, Still studied and practiced, and as kidney, liver, stomach and all manner of complaints yielded to his treatment, he became convinced he had found a method applicable to virtually all medical conditions.[21] In late 1886 he purchased a house on West Jefferson Street[22] and, when not traveling, started to practice from home. Many continued to ridicule, but a curious pattern was beginning to emerge: those he ministered to became his friends and advocates and, one by one, his former critics became his champions and supporters.[23]

Friends urged him to give his system a name. During a trip to western Missouri in 1889 W. D. Guttery, a Kirksville Teachers College alumnus now

Superintendent of Holden Public Schools, invited him to dinner. After mulling over a number of suggestions Guttery said finally, "Os means bone, doesn't it, and pathos means sorrow, disease or pain. Then put the two together and you have it." Osteopathy it became.[24]

Not everyone thought it a good name. Even Still conceded it was perhaps "not expressive enough."[25] No matter. "I did not care what others might think proper," he joked, "or what Greek scholars might say about osteo, osteon, osmosis, exosmosis or endosmosis." Since the Osage and Pottawatomie Indians had been lumped together under the designation Osawatomie, he was perfectly entitled to press osteon and pathos together to form the word "Osteopathy."[26]

One case that year, 1889, proved to be the turning point. The daughter of Kirksville's Cumberland Presbyterian pastor, Reverend J. B. Mitchell, fell and hurt her leg. Six months later, despite consulting prominent doctors in Kansas City and St. Louis, Mary Mitchell was still using crutches, unable to bear weight

floor. E. W. BOSWELL, Secretary.

Dr. A. T. Still leaves for his home in Kirksville, Mo., next Wednesday, and will return to Hannibal for the practice of his profession in September. During the four months' sojourn in this city the Doctor has performed a thousand or more cures of neuralgia, headache, rheumatism, paralysis, facial paralysis, lumbago, palpitation of the heart, etc., besides several hundred cases of dislocations of bones in the human body, many of which were accomplished in a minute's time, without the aid of instruments. Indeed, his mode of treatment and the success attending it are marvelous.

Hannibal Morning Journal, 12 May 1887.

on the ankle, and the limb remained inexplicably cold.[27] She wanted to consult Dr. Still but feared asking her father, thinking he would object. Eventually, when Reverend Mitchell was away for a few days, Mary persuaded her mother to have Still visit. He called discreetly after dark.

Still sat the girl in a straight-backed chair and made an examination. He knelt on the floor, treated not the ankle but the hip, and asked her to walk towards him unsupported. Mary stood up and advanced tentatively across the floor. The ankle no longer hurt, but the instep remained painful so he got down again, corrected a tarsal bone, then instructed her to walk up the stairs without holding the rail. She ascended easily, without pain, and soon afterwards the leg regained its normal temperature.

On Mitchell's return his wife admitted anxiously to having called the bone doctor. To her surprise the pastor did not disapprove. Overjoyed to see his daughter freed of pain, he clasped the girl in an embrace and in church the following Sunday took as the theme of his sermon *Miracles are Still Performed*. "I want to offer a prayer in which I ask every heart to join me fervently," he spoke from the pulpit. "It is no ordinary prayer. I want to invoke the blessing of Almighty God upon Dr. Still, who has restored my daughter from lameness, and a blessing upon his work which is relieving suffering and lessening the afflictions of mankind. Let us pray."[28]

The stigma of consulting Still was removed. No longer was it necessary to cross the street to avoid him. Patients could now call him without fear of discovery, and those who had praised him quietly could now do so openly.[29] He even began to attract patients who could afford to pay. In his waiting room the wealthy mingled with the poor and all found the Lightning Bone Setter eager to help.[30] Small crowds gathered on his lawn, now the stage of his public lectures,[31] and passers-by grew accustomed to seeing patients treated on benches, on porch chairs or, for shoulder or hip problems, braced firmly against one of the trees.[32]

As he waited his turn, teenager Ethel Conner recalled the first time he had encountered Dr. Still, four years earlier when he made a house call to visit his mother, suffering from neuralgia. A tall, slender, casually dressed man entered the house and sat talking with his parents, while the youth listened and wondered when the doctor would arrive. Physicians usually drove up in their buggies, got out with a rush, and entered with a pompous air of dignity and superiority. They removed kid gloves and silk hat, walked over to the patient, felt the pulse, dished out a few pills or powder, gave instructions on dosage, and advised to call again if there was no improvement. It took Ethel some time to realize that the visitor *was* the doctor. Dr. Still was courteous, reserved, and seemed sure of his treatment. On each visit he indicated whether or not it would be necessary for him to return and he was almost always right.

Ethel watched as the doctor moved from patient to patient on the lawn, apparently relieving everyone he treated, all the while explaining his treatment and repeating what sounded like passages from scripture. He threw one man's crutches twenty feet, telling him he would no longer need them. The grateful patient pressed a $20 bill into the doctor's hand, saying it was all he had and he would pay the balance later. Still promptly handed it back and told the man to spend it on groceries.[33]

A "Mrs. H." was waiting for treatment when an open wagon pulled up and the doctor bade its occupants inside. All got down except a woman in the back, in pain and unable to walk, who refused to move. Still removed the front seat, climbed into the wagon, treated a hip, and after helping the woman out asked her to walk around the lawn. She stepped forward gingerly, under protest, then, realizing the pain had gone, began shouting, kicking trees, praising the Lord, hugging Still and calling him the Christ.[34]

To accommodate his growing practice Still purchased two nearby properties, one opposite his home, the other just down the street, to convert into treatment and waiting rooms.[35] As a trickle of patients began to arrive on the daily northbound train he waited outside the depot to escort them the one hundred yards along Jefferson Street.

One day a stylish woman accompanied by a twelve-year-old boy emerged from the station and stopped to ask two men sitting on the curb for directions to Dr. Still's office, saying she had brought her son for treatment. Charley remained silent as his father stood up and said in his old-fashioned way, "I am Dr. Still." The woman turned up her nose. "I want to see the man who has become so renowned in treating disease," she replied haughtily. "He is the Dr. Still I am looking for." Still tried to reassure her that he was indeed the doctor she was seeking and instructed her to have the boy lie down on the sidewalk.

"I am Mrs. Lord of St. Louis," she asserted indignantly. Still's patience was wearing thin. "I don't care if you are the wife of the President of the United States," he said firmly, "if you want that boy examined and treated by me, have him lie down on the walk." She eventually acquiesced and disclosed that her son was suffering from petit mal epilepsy. Still corrected severe derangements of the upper neck, and after a month they returned home with no further recurrence of the problem.[36]

Still's informality surprised many a well-to-do visitor. One day he was showing a black laborer how to lay a brick walkway along the side of the house when a fine carriage bearing two elegant women drew up outside, and one called to a man on his knees, a brick in one hand and a trowel in the other, if Dr. Still was at home. "Yes," the workman replied laconically, "I am the doctor." The women protested that they were looking for the *famous* Dr. Still that everyone talked about. "If it's clothes you're looking for," he snapped back, "Mother has them hanging in the closet."[37]

In April 1891 he, Harry and Charley made one final trip to Hannibal.[38] There a man named William Stevens, whose birth Still had attended in Kansas, introduced himself. Stevens now resided in the spa town of El Dorado Springs in southwest Missouri, a mecca for the lame, halt and blind, and persuaded Still and his sons to accompany him there. They rented sixteen rooms at the St. James Hotel. The town had been a regular stop on Still's itinerary and by now his renown was such that hundreds gathered on the sidewalk. They continued on to other towns, and everywhere the crowds were so large it was impossible to treat even half the people. Still worked until exhausted, then searched for somewhere to hide and rest until morning.

In Nevada another unmanageable throng packed the square, and as the side streets filled with wagons and tents the crush became so acute that they were forced to withdraw to another location. Here a twenty-nine year old country school teacher, insurance salesman and lightning rod installer named Marcus Ward was brought to Still on a stretcher. Ward had suffered from debilitating asthma for twelve years and was so elated when Still cured him that he declared he wanted to learn the "Great Science" himself.

Their entourage was soon joined by two more enthusiastic young men: an MD named Joseph Hatten, and a cabinet maker and traveling vendor of pile ointment, William Wilderson, "wild to learn something of this method of curing disease." Wilderson thought Still's skill was a "gift" and believed he possessed the same power to heal. Still told him in no uncertain terms that his "gift" was a lifetime's study of human anatomy, and that if he wanted to be of any help he "must get *Gray's Anatomy*, begin with the bones, and get some knowledge of that science."[39] One Sunday afternoon Ward, Hatten, and Wilderson called on Still to ask if he would teach them his system. He made them an offer: $500 for one year's instruction, beginning when they returned to Kirksville.[40]

The "School of Bones" ran from mid-September to Christmas 1891.[41] The class included Charley, Harry, Herman, their younger siblings Fred and Blanche, aged seventeen and fifteen, and the three men from western Missouri. "You are now in the pursuit of a study that is as true as mathematics," Still addressed the informal gathering. "You can give a decided answer to all questions pertaining to the body as surely as the astronomer can estimate the velocity and compute the magnitude of the heavenly bodies; you have a truth from which to argue, and a fact as its voucher." He told them they could take pride in the fact that they would never create drunkards and addicts by prescribing alcohol and opium. "Despise not the day of small things," he asserted. "Your course in entering this school may provoke ridicule, but the last laugh will be the sweetest, which will be yours."[42]

Others soon asked to join the class. With patient numbers steadily increasing Still knew he would soon be unable to cope.[43] He was sixty-three, an age when most would be contemplating retirement, but tugging at him was a thought: *Osteopathy for future generations*.[44]

12

AMERICAN SCHOOL OF OSTEOPATHY

Dr. A. T. Still has in contemplation the erection of a college for the accommodation of students in Osteopathy," the *Kirksville Democrat* reported on 15 January 1892. "This is an institution that Kirksville business men should become interested in." The potential of such a venture was already apparent. "Dr. Still now has forty-three patients who are boarding at the rate of $4 per week," the paper detailed the following week. "This is a big item to Kirksville as well as to Dr. Still."[1]

To establish a medical school required a legal charter, so Still sent Charley to circuit judge Andrew Ellison to obtain one.

"Where would you teach, Charley?" Ellison asked the twenty-seven year old skeptically.

"I don't know, Judge."

"Who would do the teaching?

"I don't know."

"What would you teach?"

"Well, I don't know, Judge."

Prejudice had all but disappeared, but Ellison shared the general view that Still was a law unto himself,[2] his cures due to mysterious spiritualistic or clairvoyant powers impossible to impart to others.[3] "Charley," he said, "your father is a gifted man and when he dies this system will die with him."[4] Ellison refused to grant the document on the grounds that it would be money thrown away.

Friends advised Still that even with a charter the venture might founder under the existing state law, so he had attorney F. P. Greenwood scrutinize the wording of Chapter 110, Medicine and Surgery, of the 1889 revised Missouri statutes. "[It] is a species of legislation which upon its face looks innocent enough," the lawyer reported back, "and most surely reveals the hand of an artist of no mean ability." Greenwood told Still that the law was designed, in the words of a Missouri Supreme Court judge, "to provide for the sanitary welfare of the people of this state and to rid this commonwealth of that class of medical pretenders known by the various descriptions of empirics, mountebanks, charlatans and quacks."[5] It required every person not in possession of a "diploma or license from legally chartered medical institutions in good standing and if not a graduate to present himself before the State Board of Health and submit himself to such examination as said board shall require." The *medical institutions in good standing* were Allopathic, Eclectic and Homeopathic, the State Board of Health was composed exclusively of their members, and practice certificates were granted only to graduates of these three schools.

Faced with this seemingly insurmountable barrier, Still considered locating the college in Bloomfield, Iowa, forty miles north of Kirksville. Encouraged by an article in the February 13 issue of the *Bloomfield Farmer* citing a "rising tide of testimony" for osteopathy in the town,[6] he contacted its author, a Judge Amos Steckel, and had him organize a meeting to secure a suitable plat of land. In April a large crowd "anxious to help the movement along" gathered in the Bloomfield Opera House, and a tentative option on a ten-acre tract was offered. "Everything passed off nicely and there seemed to be no doubt as to a successful outcome," later Iowa governor B. F. Carroll wrote, "until one of our citizens, who at that time chanced to be a member of the Pharmacy Commission of the state, announced that he did not think the practice of osteopathy was permissible under the laws of the state and that he would do all that he could to prevent the establishment of an osteopathic institution in our city."[7]

Still was incensed. On May 1, after spending a fortnight with his son Fred and Marcus Ward treating patients in Columbia, Missouri,[8] he penned Steckel a furious letter. The missive began in neat orderly lines, but soon degenerated into a messy vituperative rant. Equating the lawmakers and the medical establishment to slaveholders and the Iowa populace to bondsmen, he expressed dismay over the curbing of free speech in "your great and loyal state that sent 128,000 men to destroy slavery" in the Civil War. "Those men did not fight for any class legislation, which your Dr. and Drug law are, and are not constitutional," he fumed, "they are your masters and you are their muttons." He himself would make a stand for liberty. "I am used to old slave drivers and will not let these 'Masters' kick me." He gave Steckel permission to publish his letter if he so wished, adding sarcastically, "if it be according to LAW (the word scrawled disdainfully in large letters across half the width of the sheet) and approved by the Druggist ('Whisky Smuggler')." The missive was signed, "Truly – your friend. A. T. Still, O.P. or M.D."[9]

The self-styled O.P. had reached a decision: if he had to fight he would do so in his home state. He sent Charley back to see Judge Ellison. Anticipating another grilling, Charley asked his father what the college would teach and was told "osteopathy." His son protested that the word was not in the dictionary. "Never mind," Still said, "it will be in the dictionary some day."[10] This time Ellison was persuaded to comply.

On 10 May 1892 the State of Missouri issued Still a legal charter to establish a school of osteopathy. *The purpose and object of this Association,* it read, *shall be to improve our systems of surgery, midwifery and treatment of diseases in which the adjustment of the bones is the leading feature of this school of pathology. Also to instruct and qualify students that they may lawfully practice the Science of Osteopathy as taught and practiced by A. T. Still, the discoverer of this philosophy.*[11] The following day the Articles of Association were filed in the recorder's office at the Adair County courthouse and, on the fourteenth, with the Secretary of State in Jefferson City. The stock, five thousand dollars, was divided among seven shareholders. Still and Mary held twenty-five of the fifty shares, Charley, Harry and Still's brother Edward five each, Marcus Ward eight, and Eli S. Falor (a wealthy grain farmer from Rich Hill, western Missouri) two. Still was appointed president, Marcus Ward vice-president, Charley secretary, in charge of the school's administration, and Harry treasurer.

Still had already begun canvassing for students. In April he boarded a train to visit Ed in Macon and sat beside Arthur Hildreth, bound for La Plata. "Arthur," he said, "I am looking for fifty or a hundred young men to study osteopathy. I want men who do not swear, who do not use tobacco, who drink no whiskey and who are moral, good, clean men." He wanted people of "principle and backbone" to help him revolutionize medicine and he wanted Hildreth to be one of them. He laid open his dream of an osteopathic institution – one far more modest than would actually come about. Hildreth listened attentively. He had not only seen osteopathy save his wife Margaret from blindness but also cure his niece, who had fallen from a cherry tree onto her buttocks, of dizziness, constipation and an "inability to stand." Still had adjusted the girl's fifth lumbar and inserted an index finger into the rectum to reposition a deviated coccyx, and two days later all her symptoms were gone.[12] Despite this, as the train approached La Plata, Hildreth said he must reluctantly decline the offer. "Yet there is only one reason why I am not ready to say to you today that I will study Osteopathy with you," the twenty-eight-year-old farmer explained. "I am afraid I could never learn to diagnose diseases as you do." Still looked him directly in the eye for a few moments and said simply, "I can teach you all I know."[13]

After long deliberation Hildreth decided to risk osteopathy for two years while retaining the farm as a safeguard. On the day the charter was issued, the mud too deep to drive a wagon, he walked from Troy Mills to Kirksville, a bucket of eggs in his hand and one hundred and ten dollars in his pocket. After trading the eggs he called on Still and handed over the money as part payment for tuition and a copy of *Gray's Anatomy*.[14]

Over the next weeks Still tried repeatedly to persuade Kirksville Normal School president William Dobson, whose family he had treated, to resign his post and help organize the institution. Dobson could not be swayed even by an offer of half the profits. Recruiting experienced teachers proved no easier. No one was willing to jeopardize their career on such a risky venture.[15]

Nothing could have been more providential than the appearance, that June, of William Smith, MD, a traveling salesman of medical supplies for surgical and scientific instrument makers A. S. Aloe & Co. of St. Louis. Smith had heard of neither Still nor osteopathy before arriving in Kirksville and was surprised to hear almost unanimous praise of a peculiar "bone doctor" plying his trade in the town. The only dissenters seemed to be the medical men. In his office and drugstore on the square Dr. Milburn McCarty complained bitterly that business had declined since an old quack opened a practice west of the railroad. Smith tried to reassure the physician that nothing would please him more than the presence of a quack, for it would *create* business. "But, damn it," McCarty responded, "he cures them." He knew this from personal experience, for eight months earlier Still had cured him of longstanding asthma.[16]

Smith proceeded directly to the quack doctor's cottage. He entered an unimpressive waiting room, once a parlor, with a bare floor, broken window panes and wasps making nests in secluded corners, and announced to a dozen people congregated there that he had come to see Dr. Still. A chorus of cries told him to wait his turn, and as he sat patiently he listened to dubious tales of wondrous cures. At last he was called in. Smith asked the fake about his work and, in passing, mentioned a right elbow that had troubled him for about six months. Without a word Still took hold of the arm, gave it a quick twist and said "how is that?" To Smith's surprise it felt normal again. They agreed to meet at eight that evening in the Pool Hotel.[17]

Thirty-year-old Bill Smith was "very tall, very voluble, very Scotch."[18] Born in Jamaica to a civil engineer father working on the island's first railroad, he was raised in Edinburgh and entered the Scottish capital's university medical school in 1880. After further medical studies in Manchester, London, Paris and Vienna, he returned to Edinburgh, and on 2 January 1889 received the Triple Qualification Diploma, registering him as a Licentiate of the Royal College of Physicians and Surgeons, Edinburgh, and Licentiate of the Faculty of Physicians and Surgeons, Glasgow.[19] Later that year he sailed to America to briefly practice medicine in Flatbush, New York, before engaging in his current employment.[20]

He met Still at the appointed hour. With thick dark hair, five o'clock shadow and a shapely mustache, Smith was eloquent and self-confident, and delighted in name-dropping the famous physicians who had taught him in Edinburgh: the anatomist Sir William Turner, the physiologist William Rutherford, the bile authority Daniel Cunningham, the eminent surgeon Sir Joseph Bell.[21] As the visitor reeled off this impressive pedigree Still sensed he was being made fun of, a suspicion confirmed when the Scot began questioning him on how osteopathy worked, trying to trick him into betraying his ignorance of medical science.

Smelling alcohol on Smith's breath, Still adopted the role of dumb Missourian. They walked outside onto West Jefferson Street. Electricity had come to Kirksville in 1888 and one of the new poles stood by Still's house. Feigning ignorance of how the power was generated, he lured Smith into delivering a scholarly account of the process. Smith explained how two wires led to separate vats, each containing a different chemical to produce a positive and a negative charge, and when the engine was fired up a current ran along the wires to complete the circuit. "Thus you have electric lights," he concluded triumphantly.

Still steered the conversation towards the human body. "How many kinds of nerves are there in man?" he asked.

Smith replied two, the motor and sensory, or positive and negative.

"Where is man's power of action and where is the power generated?"

"The brain has two lobes, and is the dynamo."

"Well, where is the engine?"

Smith said the heart.

"What runs the heart, doctor?"

Smith supposed the spirit of life did.

"Is it voluntary in its action, doctor?"

"It is involuntary and runs by life's forces."

"Perhaps some electricity helps to run the heart?"

Smith could only acknowledge that the body's animating power remained an unfathomable mystery.

Returning to the electric lights, Still asked what would happen if a cake of soap was dropped into one of the vats. It would play hell with it, Smith replied. "Well, doctor," Still continued (in a coded lesson on how medical drugs confound normal physiology), "I have another question I would like to ask you. What effect would two quarts of beer have on the sensory and motor nerves of a man if you poured them into his stomach?" Smith hesitated for a moment before replying that it would make a damned fool of him. Then, suddenly realizing he was the butt of the joke, snapped back, "Darn your ignorance of electricity."[22]

Having gained the upper hand Still launched into a discourse on body unity. He explained how every part depends upon every other, chemical and electrical processes entwined, and how "so called disease" results from disturbances of the body's fluids and forces. This, he said, sets up a sequence of knock-on effects in muscles, glands, digestive organs and every other part, "just like the ripples in a pond into which a stone has been thrown."

He described how nerves issue from the spinal cord to supply force to "blood vessels, muscles, and other parts of the body" and, reminding Smith that ligation of a motor or sensory nerve would result in loss of movement or numbness, asked what would happen if the vasomotor nerves were similarly cut or impeded: "Could the blood vessels act, force blood through the body and keep life in motion?" He placed his fingers on the Scot's paraspinal tissues to demonstrate where to reflexly stimulate the blood supply to, for example, the bowels and to the brain, and advised him plainly to, "get out of the old rut of ignorance" of medical thinking that had "nothing but pills and stupidity behind it."[23]

It was a warm evening and, joined by Charley, they sat on the steps of the house until midnight discussing osteopathy. Smith sat entranced. The small-town doctor's theory was "so nonsensical and chimerical," so contrary to everything he had learned at medical school, that he tried to argue the impossibility of it. "But it *is* so!" Still insisted. "There are no ifs and ands about it. I do what I tell you, and the people get well."[24] To satisfy Smith's demands for proof they spent until two in the morning calling at one boarding house after another, speaking to patient after patient. It convinced the Scot that cures were indeed being made, many of them on conditions he knew to be refractory to drugs.[25]

Smith boasted an unusual claim to fame. While at medical school in Edinburgh his departmental head Sir Joseph Bell was renowned for his uncanny powers of deduction, and the surgical amphitheater was the scene of many remarkable performances. A patient would be brought in. Bell took no case history, asked no questions and allowed no one to present an explanation, yet would state matter-of-factly that the person before him was a printer, barrister, banker, clergyman, or whatever. He described the patient's habits, where he lived, who his relatives were, and so on. This data he jotted on the registration card and he was almost always correct.

One day a man was ushered in. "You are a soldier," Bell said instantly. "You are in the Indian service; your leave will expire in about three weeks." He even named the regiment, and the astonished patient affirmed every statement. The class ganged up on Sir Joseph, demanding to know how he knew these things. "Well, army shoes usually mean army," he explained. "The pigment of the skin was that peculiar type found only in India, and certain changes in that coloring prove that he has come home for all but three weeks of the leave in that service." Someone asked how he knew the regiment, but Bell evaded this question. He made it a rule never to divulge how he reached all his conclusions, but everyone knew it was not by guesswork.

Day by day, case by case, he issued forth a stream of amazing deductions. One day the House Surgeon, Dr. Doyle,[26] told Smith he was thinking of writing stories based upon Sir Joseph's extraordinary faculties. Bell became the model for Arthur Conan Doyle's famous detective Sherlock Holmes and, according to Smith's son Cuthbert, the character of Dr. Watson was modeled upon Doyle's friend William Smith.

When Cuthbert was a teenager he accompanied his father to a lunch appointment with Doyle and Sir Joseph. By now Sherlock Holmes had become a household name, but to the youth's disappointment Bell turned out to be nothing like the great crime-solving hero he had anticipated. Tall, sparse and correctly groomed, he smoked no pipe, carried no magnifying glass, and his conversation was rather dull. Cuthbert had been instructed to be quiet and well behaved in the presence of the great man, but he burned to ask a question. "Sir Joseph," he eventually broke in, "I have read every one of Sir Arthur's stories based upon yourself. I wish you would tell me something which I may always remember as coming from you to me."

With great deliberation the distinguished surgeon took a plate and placed it on the table. He drew from his pocket a shilling and, fixing his eyes on Cuthbert, dropped it on the plate several times. "This coin is good," he said at last:

> Often persons will tell you things and you will say to yourself, 'I believe that because it sounds good.' Whenever there is told an untruth there is the knowledge on the part of the speaker of the deception, and allied with that there is always fear, and the emotion of fear invariably excites the lingual nerve, and that does not make the clear cut sound of speech any more than a false shilling would ring true striking this little plate. The secret of my deductions is most simple. It is based upon just two little sentences: God gave you ears – use them. God gave you eyes – use them.[27]

Under a full moon Still and Smith talked on the stoop of the house into the early hours, and at four in the morning the Scot returned to the Pool Hotel having agreed to teach anatomy to a small class and to study osteopathy himself.[28]

Over the summer Still hired a carpenter and erected a small clapboard structure, sixteen by twenty-two feet, across the street from his home.[29] This Lilliputian edifice he grandly named the American School of Osteopathy.

A handful of prospective students came forward. One was twenty-six-year-old Jenette "Nettie" Bolles who, in September, brought her mother from Kansas for treatment. Mrs. Bolles was suffering a progressive form of paralysis that ensued after a fall and, after consulting numerous doctors without benefit (including a visit to the Kellogg sanitarium in Battle Creek, Michigan), she heard of "a queer old doctor in Kirksville, Mo., who was making some very remarkable cures." On corresponding she was amazed to learn that the doctor was none other than their old friend Andrew Still, their family physician during the Border War. When Nettie was a baby a band of Missourians ransacked the house, stole the horses and shot her father in cold blood, leaving him for dead. The bullet passed through the upper part of a lung, missing vital organs, and under Still's care he made a good recovery.

Every day Nettie escorted her mother to Still's little cottage. With its bare boards, wooden chairs and disconsolate people the waiting room presented a dreary scene, but as the days passed Nettie listened with growing interest to "marvelous tales of the magic Dr. Still wrought with his hands in relieving pain and curing the incurable." She spoke to a dejected woman nearly maddened by an agonizing week-long headache and a few minutes later saw her emerge from the treatment room looking like a soul released from purgatory. "The pain is gone," the woman announced. "But what did he do?" Nettie asked in amazement. "Oh," she answered, "he just took hold of my neck and yanked it."

Mrs. Bolles decided to remain in Kirksville over the winter to continue treatment and Nettie, wondering how she would occupy herself, heard that Dr. Still was planning to organize a class. She called at his house that afternoon and found him sitting on a log in the back yard. Nettie asked nervously if a woman would be able to learn osteopathy. Still replied without hesitation that a woman could learn to do anything a man could. It was a deep conviction. He felt that Lincoln's equality proclamation was incomplete and that the U.S. Constitution should be amended to read, "There shall be no disabilities on account of race, color, *sex*, or previous condition of servitude."[30] Women had access to very few medical colleges at the time, but his would be open to all without prejudice.[31]

The American School of Osteopathy opened at ten o'clock on 3 October 1892. Equipped with only a U.S. flag, "a skeleton, a chart, and a *Gray's Anatomy*,"[32] the diminutive institution had nearly twenty students ranging in age from sixteen to sixty-eight, including Blanche, Fred, Herman, Harry, Charley, and Still's brother Ed. Arthur Hildreth was there, having sold his cattle, hogs, horses and farm machinery and moved into town. There were five women, including Nettie Bolles and one of the affluent ladies who had mistaken Still for a workman when he was building the brick walkway; two homeopathic doctors, father and son A. P. and F. S. Davis; and two medical doctors, Joseph Hatten and William Smith. "I can shut my eyes now and see that gathering in a small back room of the tumble-down cottage," Smith reminisced later. "Eighteen students were there, and each and every one was there not for the money there was in it, but had either been a sufferer and was cured by osteopathy or a close friend had been."[33] On that opening day he spoke of his first encounter with Still and how he had tried to ridicule the old quack, but came away chastened.[34] Smith prophesied that in ten years the school would be housed in a handsome brick building and five hundred osteopaths would be in practice. They all laughed, but it would come to pass in less than five.[35]

The course was two terms of four months each, one year apart. Every morning at eight Smith lectured on anatomy and physiology, and the students

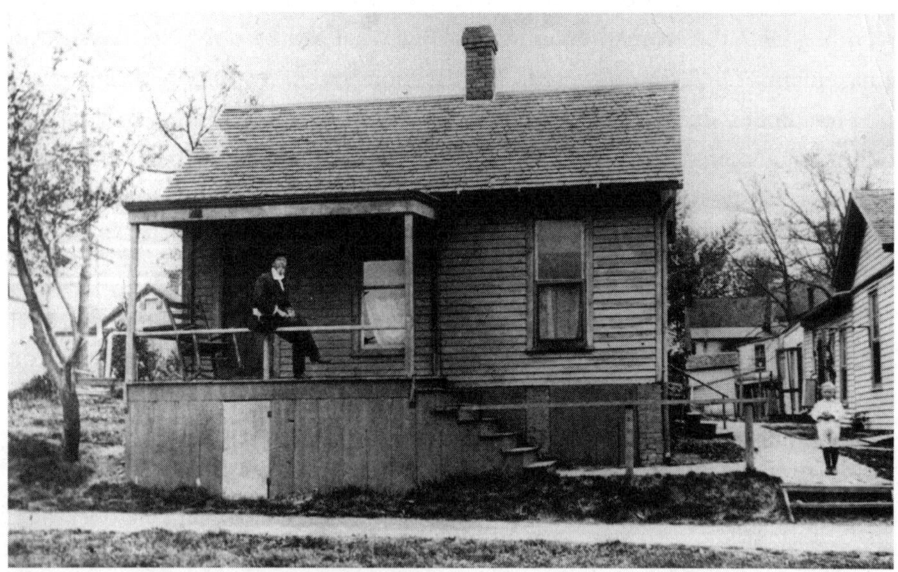

The American School of Osteopathy.

listened attentively as the musical medical terminology rolled off his Scottish tongue – ileo-colic orifice, anastomotica magna, torcular Herophili – impressing them with the names long before they knew what they stood for.[36]

At nine they entered the treatment rooms. Serving what was essentially an apprenticeship, they helped hold patients in position as Still, assisted by Charley, Harry, Ward, Wilderson and Hatten,[37] made the corrections. With the aid of the school's skeleton, known to all as "Mike," Still explained to both patients and students what was wrong and how the treatment would free nature's power to restore health. "It was good to be there then," Arthur Hildreth wrote. "It was inexpressively fine to be thrown in close contact with a man who was doing so much for humanity, who was always ready to serve the unfortunate not only with his hands but also his purse if necessary."[38]

The Missouri State Board of Health showed no such enthusiasm. It drafted a bill, to introduce before the biennial session of the state legislature in the New Year, to allow only allopathic, homeopathic and eclectic schools to grant medical diplomas, aiming to prevent ASO graduates from entering practice and force the closure of the school. Still's supporters responded by gathering five thousand signatures in a petition and, on 13 January 1893, William Smith and the two Davises (all licensed physicians) signed a sealed document before notary public William T. Porter swearing "solemnly and sincerely" that osteopathy was "in advance of anything known to the general medical profession in the treatment of disease."[39] Smith, accompanied by Judge Andrew Ellison, traveled to the State Capitol, Jefferson City, to work against the measure.

House bill No. 166 was called up on 14 February. After a lively hour-long debate, with seven representatives speaking for the ASO and three MDs against, the members voted 88 to 34 in the school's favor. "I wish I could come to your city to rejoice with you," Adair County representative Perry D. Grubb wrote Still that evening. "I think you have won a magnificent victory for right today. The American School of Osteopathy is known all over the state tonight better than ever. You came out of this fight victorious and the M.D.'s are badly beaten."[40]

The school term ended the following day. To help dispel a myth that the students could only be effective under Still's supervision he encouraged them to scatter and practice what they had learned. At the beginning of March, Harry and William Smith traveled to Kansas City, the latter carrying the American

School of Osteopathy's first diploma, a makeshift affair handwritten on a piece of card.[41] In April, Hildreth and Herman, supervised by Still's brother "Dr. Ed," headed to Elsberry and Louisiana, Missouri, to practice for one month in each town.[42]

The legislative triumph prompted St. Louis daily *The Republic* to dispatch reporter J. B. Dodge to Kirksville for a month. On April 29 the paper ran a two page article, "The American School of Osteopathy, Born Upon Missouri Soil, Will Live and Flourish, Despite the Efforts of its Enemies to Drive it From its Native Home." Dodge lambasted the State Board of Health, accusing it of drawing up "one of the most obnoxious and exacting bills ever introduced in any Legislature." By contrast he portrayed Still in a more or less favorable light: "His theory is quite simple, and when fully explained and understood ceases to be a theory and becomes a cold fact – something that must be admitted and cannot be denied."[43]

Still, however, spent the summer sunk in despondency, dissatisfied with his first attempt at running a school. Anatomy had progressed only as far as the bones and muscles of the arm and leg, insufficient to make a proper diagnosis, yet the students had emerged brimming with confidence and worryingly unaware of their shortcomings. He complained it had been a "time lost," with nothing produced but "bunglers" and "imitators." He conceded that a good imitator might be able to do *some* good, bur imitators were not what he wanted and he considered giving up the whole venture as a mistake.

His woes were compounded by an acrimonious falling-out with Marcus Ward. Despite repeated warnings by friends not to trust the ex-lightning rod peddler, Still had supported Ward, his wife and her parents for almost a year, allowed his tuition fees on credit (never to be repaid),[44] and allotted him eight of the ASO's fifty shares. At the end of the school term Ward repaid this kindness by travelling to Kansas City[45] to briefly practice "Boney-Opathy,"[46] (dropping the word *osteopathy*, he said, because the science was too "limited" and he would not confine himself to riding "in a cart with one wheel"). He then traveled to Cincinnati, Ohio, and in June returned to Kirksville to open a practice offering a combination of osteopathy and medicated baths, claiming that these ablutions could remove freckles and "sallow splotches," expel "lime deposits," and even dissolve tumors and abscesses. And, the ultimate heresy, he also prescribed drugs, accusing Still of becoming "fossilized" by confining himself to manual treatment.[47]

A grudge lay behind Ward's extraordinary behavior. In a letter published by the *Kirksville Weekly Graphic* on June 30 he alleged that Still had subjected him to "vile abuse," called him a "fourth class operator" (through jealousy, Ward maintained, "because most of the patients preferred me to him"), and "mistreated" him by trying to cut him out of the organization. He further maintained that Still had demanded a 20% royalty on earnings made by students practicing in Missouri, Kansas and Iowa.

J. B. Dodge sprang to Still's defense. The reporter slammed the "jack leg one-horse real estate agent" for base ingratitude, dismissed as "bosh" the claim that

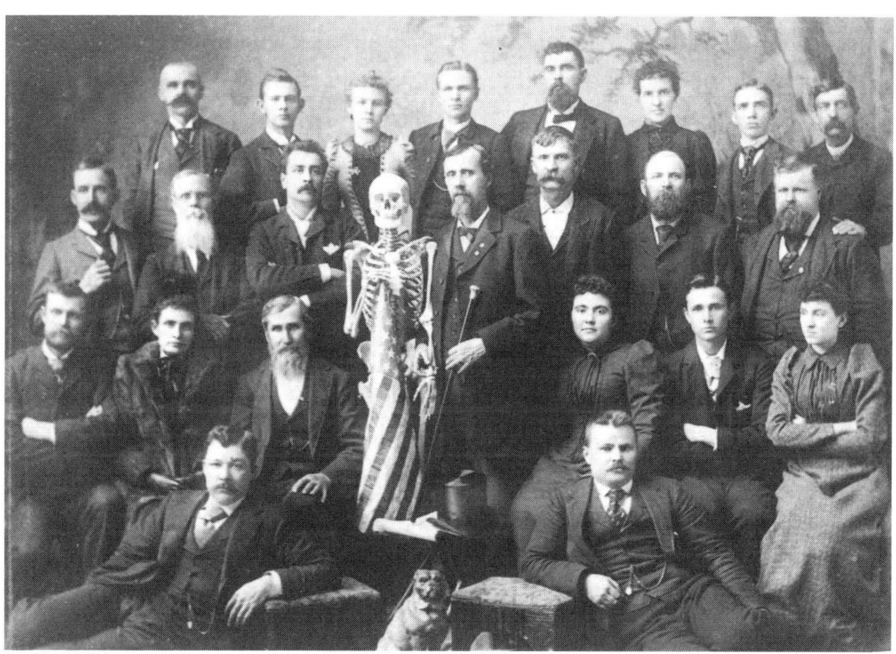

First class of the American School of Osteopathy.
Top row (left to right): Obie Strothers, Arthur Bird, Blanche Still, Herman Still, Frank Polmeteer, Mrs. Gentry, Mason Peters, Dr. Hall. Second row: Arthur Hildreth, A. P. Davis, William Smith, A. T. Still, Marcus Ward, Millar Machin, Joseph Hatten. Third row: F. S. Davis, Mrs. M. S. Peters, Edward Still, Nettie Bolles, Fred Still, Mamie Harter. Bottom row: James Hill, Harry Still.

Still had demanded royalties, and challenged Ward to deny that "the real reason Dr. Still would have nothing more to do with you was because he caught you in two point blank falsehoods."[48] Dodge elaborated no further, but an undated note in Still's hand perhaps hints at the nature of the wrongdoings. "Ward will pull out for K. C.," it states, "and work and steal from Smith."[49] Whatever the truth, the episode ended in Ward's dismissal.

During the summer Charley, who had remained in Kirksville to help with the clinic practice, was invited to Minnesota by a wealthy patient he had cured of sciatica the previous winter. O. H. L. Wernicke, president of the Altman-Miller Harvesting Company, arranged a temporary practice in the Windsor Hotel, Minneapolis. Charley and his wife Anna, married just over a year, arrived there on July 16.[50]

A few days later Charley received a letter from Dr. Thomas McDavitt,[51] Secretary of the Minnesota State Board of Health, serving notice for practicing medicine without a license and threatening legal action. Wernicke put Charley in touch with his lawyer, the Hon. F. F. Davis, who advised Still's son to continue working and to notify McDavitt in writing that all further correspondence should be transacted through his attorney. Charley, expecting to pay perhaps $5 for Davis's services, was shocked to receive a bill for a whopping $150. But he heard no more from the State Board.

In September he accepted a further invitation to practice in Diamond Bluff, Wisconsin, on the east bank of the Mississippi River, and there received a visit from his parents, en route to Chicago for the 1893 World's Columbian Exposition. Still delivered an address to a "large and enthusiastic audience," treated a few patients, fished with Charley, and they all traveled together to the "Fair."[52]

Organized to commemorate the four-hundredth anniversary of Columbus's discovery of the New World, the Exposition was the most spectacular cultural and entertainment event the world had ever seen, and attracted 27 million visitors between May and October. America was in the throes of social and cultural upheaval. The notion of progress, previously epitomized by moral and political innovations, was being increasingly linked to science and technology, especially electricity, and with it were emerging giant corporations, a powerful business elite, and the beginnings of the consumer society. A vast site resplendent with grand buildings in Beaux-Arts style boasted an elevated railway and a complex of canals and lagoons fed by Lake Michigan plied by electric launches. Visitors could view tens of thousands of exhibits, attend lectures on a multiplicity of subjects, and indulge in every kind of amusement imaginable.

On his return from Chicago, Charley was invited by Minnesota senator Peter Nelson to practice in the town of Red Wing on the west bank of the Mississippi.[53] He had treated Nelson in Minneapolis for limb and speech problems following a stroke, and the senator's improvement gained him a powerful ally whose help he would soon need.

That November, Charley was called to treat the president of a business college, a Professor Curtis, hurt in a fall. Worried that failure in such an important case would ruin his reputation, he wired his father to come and attend the case himself. Still arrived by train and was escorted to the patient by Senator Nelson and Representative August Peterson, who looked on as he adjusted a hip, a sacroiliac joint and some vertebrae, and freed Curtis of pain. Before Still returned home Nelson and Peterson took him for a ride around town in a surrey.

Pinned to many front doors were small cardboard signs that Still learned were quarantine notices: *Keep Out! By Order of the State Board of Health. Contagious Diphtheria.*[54] The epidemic, with a mortality rate of up to fifty percent, was claiming an average of one fatality a day in Red Wing. Still asked the two politicians why they had not asked Charley to treat the cases. Peterson replied that he did not know that diphtheria was treatable by osteopathy. Neither did Charley, and before his father left he asked for a hasty briefing.

The disease, marked by inflammation and the formation of a leathery membrane on the tonsils and palate, blocked the airways and caused suffocation. Toxins produced by the recently discovered agent of the infection, *corynebacterium diphtheriae*, entered the circulation and damaged the heart, nervous system, kidneys and other organs. In addition to these symptoms and signs, experience had taught Still that the disease gave rise to a characteristic pattern of contracted muscles from the neck to the diaphragm, producing fluid stagnation and a fertile breeding ground for bacteria. "By playing along the lines of sensation, motion and nutrition – if you do not play ignorantly," he told Charley, "you will win the reward due your intelligence, and lose not a single case."[55] This meant loosening joints and muscles, with the aim of freeing nerves and vessels to enable the body to "excrete poisonous products as fast as they accumulate" and allow nature's perfect remedies to destroy the germs before complications created by their toxins could arise.[56]

That evening Charley was thrown in at the deep end. Peterson asked him to call on a farmer, Charles Moline, whose sister's five children and a servant girl had the disease, while a sixth child had already died in a Minneapolis hospital. "I worked with those children all night," Charley related. "I was afraid to quit treating." By morning all his patients were heading towards recovery. As word of his success spread he soon became overwhelmed and wired Kirksville for assistance. Still dispatched Harry and student Charles Hartupee to Red Wing to keep the office open while Charley concentrated on the diphtheria cases.

While making a house call across the river in Wisconsin, Charley got caught in a blizzard and was unable to return to treat a boy with the disease, who subsequently died. Since Charley was not a qualified physician, the health officer refused to let him sign the death certificate and called a doctor from Red Wing to issue the burial permit. Two days later the State Board of Health had Charley arrested, indicted on charges of practicing without a license and of failing to report a case of contagious disease within twenty-four hours. The Justice of the Peace, in a "very ugly mood," refused to accept a cash bond and had Charley imprisoned in the county jail. Nelson and Peterson intervened, however, and secured his release.

The community united against the medics. At the trial so many crowded into the Justice's office that they were forced to transfer the proceedings to the courthouse, and when Charley and his defense lawyer walked down the aisle accompanied by Nelson and Peterson they received such a rousing ovation that the prosecution witness, a Dr. Anderson, feared to enter, giving his attorney no choice but to dismiss the case. Dr. Charles Hewitt, director of the State Board of Health, attempted to press Governor Knute Nelson to reopen the prosecution but, unbeknownst to Hewitt, the governor, Secretary of State Brown and State Auditor Bierman had all been treated by Charley.[57] The matter was closed.

Still proclaimed a victory for constitutional rights. Branding the Minnesota State Board of Health the "State Board of Ignorance," he condemned the doctors for their narrow self-interest and praised the largely Scandinavian community for their courage. "They declared that the people were the law, and the statute the tool," he asserted. "The statute is a money-making provision and when the people arise they are the law of the country. Americans will not have their liberty abridged."[58] When the story hit the newspapers Charley was inundated with work, one Red Wing daily reporting that fifty-six patients from out of town were waiting for treatment.[59]

The new diphtheria antitoxin, already available in Europe, reduced the death rate in children to five percent. Despite his inexperience, Charley fared even better. Of over sixty cases he treated that winter he lost only one, the boy who died during the snowstorm.[60]

13

FIND IT, FIX IT, AND LEAVE IT ALONE

His first attempt at running a school taught Still a fundamental lesson: to turn out successful practitioners he must teach his students how to think *osteopathically*, not medically.

They must understand that osteopathy is, first and foremost, a philosophy. And all their reasoning on health and disease must be guided by this philosophy. Medicine is grounded upon scientific materialism; osteopathy, while embracing all verifiable scientific facts, challenges the ultimate authority of science, declaring its materialist suppositions unsatisfactory when applied to the living being. The whole edifice of osteopathy rests upon an observable, *spiritual*, truth unexplained by any known scientific law: organic nature strives inexorably to express health.

Osteopathy's spiritual foundation makes it virtually impossible to define. Still usually resorted to explanations or descriptions, rarely the same twice, ranging from the practical to the transcendental. Anything from, "It means to know the normal in health, the abnormal in disease, and the process of adjusting the abnormal back to the normal,"[1] to, "Osteopathy is God's law, the law that keeps life in motion."[2] Perhaps most comprehensively:

> All mysteries are hidden in Nature, all facts are found in Nature, all discoveries are made in Nature. Then does it not follow that Nature's unchangeable laws must be followed in order to find what you seek? Osteopathy is founded on Nature. Osteopathy is natural. Osteopathy is *nature*.[3]

Nature understood as a union of the Knowable and Unknowable; body, mind and the spirit of life united by a law beyond human comprehension, "the law of matter, mind and motion, blended by the wisdom of Deity."[4] A deity less Christian than American Indian, Creator and creation inseparable, the divergent attitudes of the white and indigenous races towards nature mirrored by the divergent attitudes of medicine and osteopathy towards the ailing human body: try to control it with limited knowledge; or humbly listen to, learn from, and harmonize with its superior wisdom.

In summer 1893 Still moved the small classroom from the opposite side of Jefferson Street to stand next to his home.[5] To replace William Smith, who had decided to remain in Kansas City, he appointed sophomore Nettie Bolles, a holder of two bachelor's degrees, to the post of anatomy lecturer.[6] Many locals, seeing what the first group had achieved, wanted to enroll as students.

One was Charley's boyhood friend Edwin Pickler, now Kirksville's postmaster. At the Post Office people from all over the country spoke openly about their maladies, hardly a day passing without some surprising cure being discussed, and Ed was struck by how they endorsed their treatment in such a "peculiarly unanimous" way.[7] When his friend George Tull quit his photographic business to study osteopathy, Ed decided to do the same. He called on Still the next morning.

The interview was a lesson in itself. "You want to make some money, don't you," the founder surmised, and Ed said, why, yes he did. To his surprise Still advised him to stay out, for a desire for wealth or status was no reason to become a doctor. It was a sacrifice and a responsibility; your heart must be in it, with a genuine calling to alleviate suffering and be of service to your fellow man. Pickler left thirty minutes later with a radically different impression of the profession he was about to enter and a conception of his duties as a physician he would never forget.[8]

Another matriculant was Effie Koontz. Three years earlier, while at college in Carthage, Illinois, she had slipped while carrying a tub of water down an icy flight of steps and was found unconscious, clothes frozen to the ground. The fall left debilitating strains of the lower lumbar and sacroiliac joints, a barely usable right arm, and a soft lump the size of a saucer in the mid to low back. A catalogue of ailments followed: constant headache, constipation,

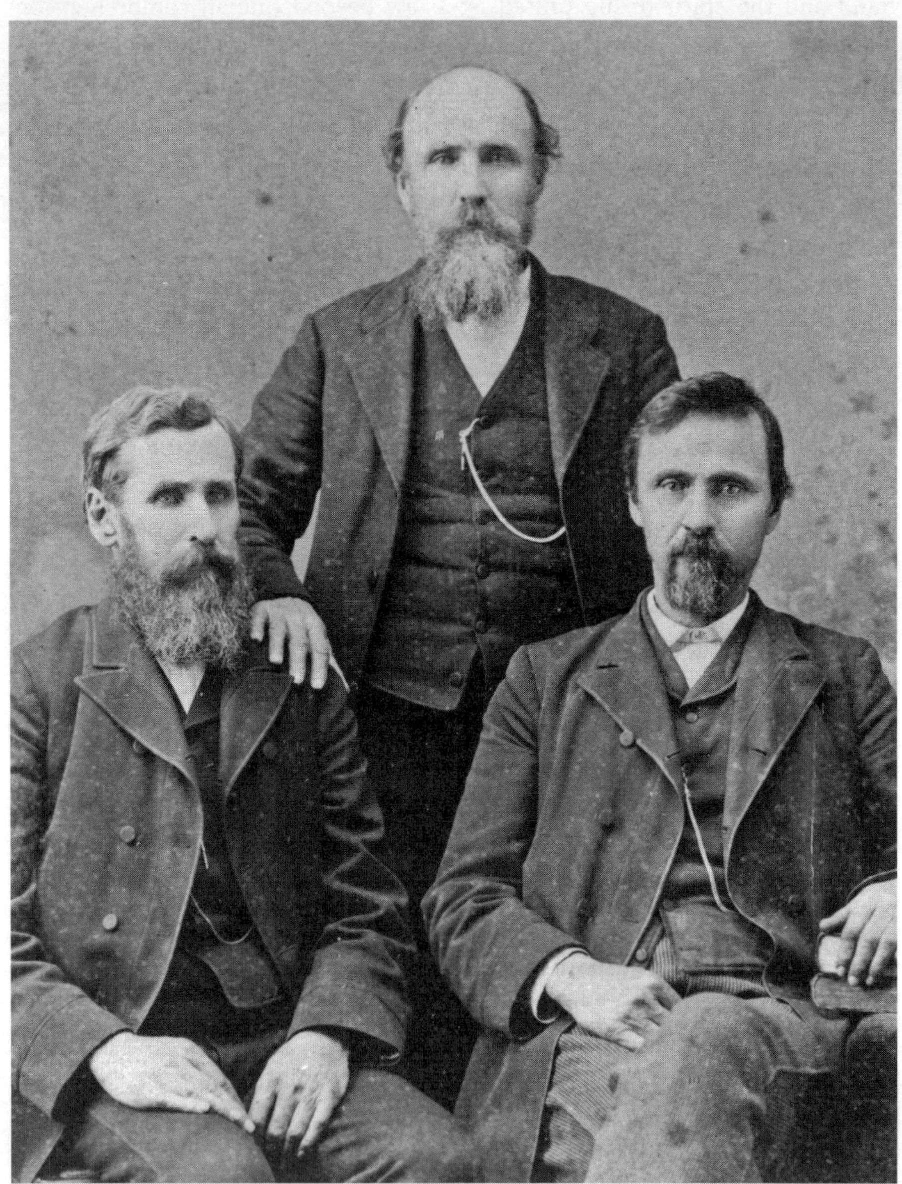

(left to right) Edward, James and Andrew Still.

menstrual pain, nephritis. Her weight fell to eighty-five pounds and doctors pronounced her case hopeless. Forced to drop out of college, she returned home to Missouri.

In September 1892 Effie persuaded her parents to take her to see Still. The twenty-one mile journey to Kirksville was exhausting, every jolt of the buggy excruciatingly painful. She was helped into the bone doctor's office, lifted onto the table, and after a few preliminary questions Still ran his fingers along her vertebrae. "If you were setting out onions," he said by way of diagnosis, "you would say this one is out of the row." After a very gentle treatment he instructed them to return in a month.

Next morning Effie had no headache for the first time in two years. At the second visit Still invited her to stay in his home over the winter to continue treatment and, too sick to climb the stairs, they set up a bed for her in the corner of the living room. When Still's brother Ed came to test her urine Effie overheard him say, "Drew, you might as well give it up." But Still was not one to give it up. He treated her frequently, placing his hands under her back and rolling her from the bed across his knees. As he worked he usually kept his eyes closed, but when treating the spine monitored her facial expression intently, for her injuries were so severe that she occasionally fainted. When Effie returned home in the spring she was able to walk with only occasional pain, and in time made a slow but complete recovery. That summer Still made her an offer: if she would like to study osteopathy he would waive the tuition fee.[9]

Of thirty new students perhaps the most unlikely was Still's brother James. Now living in Trenton, Missouri, Jim had shunned his brother for nineteen years until persuaded to visit Kirksville on his way to the Chicago Exposition. The once staunch advocate of medicine had been entertaining his own doubts about drugs,[10] and after a reconciliatory meeting both he and son Summerfield decided to join the class.[11]

With its tiny clapboard schoolroom, informal teaching and disorganized classes the institution was decidedly embryonic, but these early students would later realize their enviable privilege at having received Still's teaching at first hand, pure and unadulterated. "Those days," one reminisced, "were wonder days in Kirksville."[12] All pervasive was an infectious enthusiasm, a pioneering spirit and a determination to master the practice.

This year, from the outset, Still drummed into them how to think *osteopathically*. One freshman recorded his introductory lecture:

> The first step in Osteopathy is a belief in our own bodies. The next step is to advance that belief to an intelligent understanding. You will learn that the body is self-creative, self-developing, self-sustaining, self-repairing, self-recuperating, self-propelling, self-adjusting, and does all these things on its own power. It will use only those things which belong in the realm of foods. I want to impress on you in the beginning of your study of Osteopathy with the things you must know to make a success of it. First, Osteopathy is not a system of movements [techniques]; second, neither Osteopathy nor its application to the patient is something that can be passed around on a platter. One must delve and dig for it themselves; third, its application to the patient must be given by reason and not by rule. Osteopathic physicians must be able to give a reason for the treatment they give, not so much to the patient, but to themselves.[13]
> Neither am I operating a school to teach a lot of parrots, or turn out just another doctor. The field is already overcrowded with those who for these hundreds of years have treated the patients by rule rather than reason.[14]

Radically different philosophies gave medicine and osteopathy fundamentally different concepts of etiology, diagnosis, prognosis and treatment. With characteristic sarcasm Still contrasted the two:

> The patient tells a doctor where he hurts, how much he hurts, how long he has hurt, how hot or cold he is. The medical practitioner then puts this symptom and that symptom in a column, adds them up according to the latest books on symptomatology, and finally he is able to guess a name by which to call the disease. Then he proceeds and treats as his pap's father heard his granny say their old family doctor treated 'them sort of diseases in North Carolina.' An osteopath, in his search for the cause of diseases, starts out to find the mechanical cause. He feels that the people expect more than guessing of an osteopath. He feels that he

> must put his hand on the cause and prove what he says by what he does; that he will not get off by the feeble-minded trash of stale habits that go with doctors of medicine. By his knowledge he must show his ability to go beyond the musty bread of symptomatology.[15]

Unraveling the mystery of disease and reversing its course demanded an understanding of the complex mechanical relationships between anatomical derangements and physiological sequelae. Osteopathic etiology was not physiological but anatomical, the symptoms and signs of disease, all-important to the medical doctor, simply the result of a failure of the nerves to regulate the circulation of blood. Osteopathy provided an exact method of treatment that, if properly applied, enabled the blood and tissues to administer nature's perfect remedies, in the optimum dose, without side-effects.[16] The practice was not guided by rules of prescription but by two complementary *principles*; one explicit, the other implicit: *cause and effect* and *nature's inexorable drive to express health*.

To reason from effect to cause called for an intricate knowledge of anatomy. Still insisted his students possess a skeleton or at least a spinal column,[17] advised them to keep *Gray's Anatomy* under their pillows at night,[18] and repeatedly emphasized that the osteopath's "first lesson is anatomy, his last lesson is anatomy, and all his lessons are anatomy."[19]

This did not mean, as a later myth held, that he thought physiology unimportant. This misunderstanding derived from a widely repeated story of the day he strode angrily into the little classroom and chalked on the blackboard the words *No Physiology*. Over time the rest of the story became forgotten. "Let the piffle and poppycock go," he continued, before launching into a diatribe on the shortcomings of the physiology *books* of the day: "compilations of many theories, few facts, and quotations from other authors; a mass of contradictions, uncertainties, confusing references to differences of opinion, and laden with disclaimers like maybe, possibly, and however."[20] Physiology itself, he stressed, was "as much a part of anatomy as a wing is part of a chicken," and no osteopath could hope to be a success without it.[21] In Still's usage the word *anatomy* always included its "branches": physiology, histology and biochemistry.

Cases with similar symptoms and signs might have entirely different anatomical causes, therefore the students must not think in terms of medical conditions – named diseases – but of *conditions of the body*. Still insisted that an abnormal condition of the body is found in "all diseased persons."[22]

These abnormal conditions became known as *osteopathic lesions* (not to be confused with the medical definition a lesion as a pathological change in the tissues).[23] "An osteopathic lesion is a perverted state of a joint," a student explained,

> in which the bones are held in false position by angulation and ligamentous tension. A false position is produced when, at the limit of its normal movement, a bone is subjected to further stress. The secondary movement that then occurs goes as far as the shapes of the bones allows, until they become jammed against each other. At the same time the ligaments are under heavy tension. The angle of the ligaments is changed, so that they do not draw in the direct path of return, but at an angle, and so may act to prevent that return, and may actually increase the deviation.[24]

Osteopathic lesions often caused discomfort, but their real significance lay in the physiological effects they produced. Still taught that nerve irritation at the intervertebral foramen can generate different symptoms and signs depending upon which tracts within the nerve are primarily affected: sensory tracts producing pain, tingling or numbness; sympathetic tracts, by causing constriction or dilation of blood vessels, disturbing the supply of oxygen and nutrients or polluting the tissues with metabolic wastes; motor tracts causing muscular cramps, asthmatic spasms, constipation, hiccough or, through excessive relaxation, pendulous abdomen, sagging colon, prolapsed uterus, hemorrhoids, and many other problems.[25] The initial physiological imbalance may be minor, with symptoms and signs appearing much later, but every lesion places a burden on vitality, immunity and powers of recovery.[26] Osteopathy was therefore not only curative but also powerfully preventative, and Still believed that early correction of lesions might significantly increase life expectancy.[27]

He made clear, though, that his science would be far from complete "were it only concerned in irregularities in the framework."[28] Osteopathic lesions could be *primary* or *secondary*. Primary lesions were structural abnormalities; secondary lesions were other factors that caused or maintained abnormal function, originating elsewhere and registering reflexly in the spine through sensory nerve irritation.[29] The list included mental shocks, bereavement, loss of property or friends, poor diet, overeating, extremes of weather, poisons – including microorganisms and their toxins – and medical drugs. Dr. Still "never taught that *all* diseases were due to displacements of bony structure," student S. H. Kjerner wrote:

> but distinctly stated that changes in relationship of bony structure may be due to conditions at the peripheral end of nerves acting as irritants, [the] results of which may be contracture of muscle, which in turn bring about the osseous conditions. Among these conditions we have abuse of function of various kinds, such as occupational conditions, lowering of resistance through loss of sleep, fatigue, abuse of digestive organs etc. We were told that these vertebral conditions brought about a situation which resulted in lowering resistance of a part that in turn permitted bacteria to become effective, and how we practitioners could bring about a normal state by removing the conditions which interfered with the normal functions of the part.[30]

To identify and correct lesions demanded mastering the art of *palpation*. "There was no sidestepping the tactual requirement," one student wrote. "It was a behest without a single reservation."[31] The feel of the tissues provided a window on the underlying condition and revealed a wealth of diagnostic information otherwise unsuspected. Abnormal joint position, muscle tone, range and quality of movement; altered tissue resistance, resilience, elasticity; variations in ligamentous tension, tendinous freedom, surface temperature, skin reaction, and other qualities – these changes, often subtle, were invariably accompanied by soreness or sensitivity. Palpation dictated where and how to apply treatment, and indicated when it had been successfully completed.[32]

It took time to develop sensitive fingers, and for two or three months the novice went through an inevitable period of fretting that he would never be able to feel very much.[33] Still was patient, but insistent and firm. Palpation was an art to hone over a lifetime. Even now he strove to improve his own skills, his fingertips continually searching out the details of anything within easy grasp.[34] The students copied his habit of studying a joint, muscle, nerve or artery of one hand with the other, and to refine their sense of touch devised a challenging exercise, placing letters or numbers made of thread under a piece of cloth and trying to read them by touch, using progressively thicker cloth as their proficiency increased.[35] As their hands evolved into instruments of unanticipated sensitivity, early frustrations and worries slowly matured into confidence.

Once the philosophical, anatomical and palpatory foundations were laid Still took the students under his personal supervision. He was never authoritarian. To him all were equal, but like the Shawnee he expected age and ability to command respect. His attitude towards the students was paternal; he called them boys and girls, they called him Pap, and they mixed on intimate and friendly terms. Six days a week they congregated at six-thirty in the morning, worked until six in the evening, returned after supper for an evening lecture, and before retiring mastered the next day's lessons.[36]

His early morning class was eagerly awaited, the topic of his "homely sensible talks"[37] always something of immediate interest, often inspired by something that had just happened in the treatment rooms. "Our school-house was a little one room house in Dr. Still's side yard," Alice Patterson reminisced,

> and the dear old Dr. gave us a lecture every morning of our lives for the two years. I would not exchange the training for worlds. I shall never cease to be thankful for the great privilege we had. These lectures from Dr. Still were brimful of the beautiful truths we were all so greedily seeking, and they were given in his unique way, and with that earnestness and enthusiasm so characteristic of him, and we all caught that all abiding inspiration and determination to work without ceasing, and with love and joy in our hearts, and confidence in the Eternal truth and efficacy of this Science.[38]

Handling a few vertebrae, moving them first one way and then another, he described the physiological effects that might result from various abnormal positions,[39] continually illustrating his point with a diagram or part of a skeleton, or on a member of the class he called forward.[40] Sometimes enthusiasm carried him away, an explosive utterance sending his false teeth clattering to the floor, to be promptly retrieved by a student and clapped back into his mouth entirely without embarrassment.[41]

He never used a textbook[42] and wanted no note-taking by rote – he said he was talking to their heads not their notebooks.[43] He advised them to read widely, but with a proviso: it was not how much they read that mattered, but how much they were *thinking* while they were reading. "Study all the books you like," he advised, "but remember that many of them are merely products of man's misinformed mind. Better study from the book of nature – study it as I have studied it."[44] He asked that when they studied bones, muscles and tendons they learn not just bare facts but try to comprehend the sublime design of every part. Consider the biceps, he said, no engineer could duplicate its mechanical perfection, with no lost motion and every action performed without strain. He never failed to impress upon them that man was a machine.[45]

At first some struggled with his "oddities of word and action"[46] – unexpected phraseology, imagery, ellipsis, and messages cloaked in metaphor and allegory, often to the point of obfuscation. During Nettie Bolles' very first lecture he entered the room to deliver a brief, perplexing message: "Good morning children. Today you will learn there is a yellow dog; tomorrow you will learn he has a blind eye; the next day you will learn he has a bobbed tail." Then, without further elaboration, he quietly left.[47] However obscure the words, though, they soon learned that Dr. Still never indulged in idle chatter. His object was to spur the imagination so that the lesson would not be forgotten; if what he said sounded like hocus-pocus it "generally proved to be due to a lack of interpreting power."[48] Sometimes he would say, "Boys, think that over at your leisure. If you find anything in it, tell me what it is the first time we meet"[49] – and if they found nothing they always found him anxious to explain. The yellow dog riddle turned out to be a lesson on *brevity*: he told them he was striving to teach "a practical knowledge of how man is made and how to right him when he gets wrong, and not humdrum your brains out with old theories that are of no practical use to man or beast."[50]

To fully grasp the osteopathic concept entailed a lengthy period of adjustment, a purging of culturally ingrained beliefs and habits of thought, and a rejection of the deeply conditioned notion that experts and authorities know best. Still told his students it mattered little what kings, queens or professors said; what mattered was what they personally knew.[51] "Truth belongs to no one section of the world," he said. "It is the inner spiritual flame that burns at the center of every life."[52] They must learn to trust their own judgment and take nothing as truth – not even from him – unless it filtered through their "God-given reason."[53] He persistently oriented them away from the cleverness of man and towards the wisdom of nature:

> I want men and women to study Osteopathy who reason and think for themselves. It is never a question as to what the remedy or the treatment will do to the body, but what the body will do with the remedy or treatment. You will find that the same natural law when obstructed that produces a condition or allows one to exist, when reestablished will take it away. You will find that it is only when by knowledge, by sight, by sense of touch, you have become so familiar with that which is normal, you will be able to recognize and normalize that which is abnormal.[54]

Little by little, as they applied his principles and attuned to his philosophy, they passed through the same sequence as he had: curiosity, conviction and eventually certainty. "I am talking to you as though you were osteopaths of many years' experience," he told one group, "many days of experimenting, and have placed your hand on the side of Christ and found the scar, and have no further doubts."[55] But skepticism invariably formed part of the process.

Arthur Hildreth listened doubtfully as Still lectured that eczema can be caused by lesions of the upper cervical or upper thoracic joints, the consequent nerve irritation affecting the vasomotor center in the brainstem to alter the circulation throughout the entire body. "Wait a minute," Still suddenly stopped, groping for words to explain his meaning, "I'll be back."

He reappeared a few minutes later bearing a bronze, tan and white duck. "Here, look at this fowl," he said, placing the stuffed bird on the desk,

> and get this fact into your heads if you can that this perfection, the beauty of this fowl, is maintained by the natural law of supply and demand

> within its body. So long as the nerves and the circulation within that fowl perform their natural function, and needed materials can reach their intended destination in a normal way, the beauty will continue. In other words, every grain of wheat, every kernel of corn or any other variety of food carries with it the building materials to keep up and carry on the beautiful perfection you see before you, provided there is no physical interference. It is the same magnificent law working within the human body with which you are to deal. There cannot be eczema if the body is normal.[56]

Hildreth found the last statement hard to accept – until a year later when he was presented with a sixty-year-old woman with appalling eczema from head to toe, so bad he dreaded touching her. He corrected lesions of the first to third cervical and fourth to sixth thoracic vertebrae and, to his astonishment, over a period of weeks the scales and eruptions peeled and cleared, leaving pure unblemished skin.[57]

Other students found it hard to believe that correcting joints and loosening muscles could affect organs deep within the body, so Still devised a simple exercise to demonstrate the principle. To stimulate the spinal center related to the eye, one student applied firm thumb or knuckle pressure to another's upper back, one inch each side of the spine, and moved the contact up or down for a few seconds, while the other person looked in a mirror and observed his pupils dilate.[58] The same principle, employing what later became known as somatovisceral reflexes, informed much of Still's treatment. For an acute case of appendicitis he applied *inhibition* – gentle, sustained pressure – to the muscles adjacent to the eleventh and twelfth thoracic vertebrae. This, he taught, would affect the spinal center related to the appendix, normalize the circulation, and calm the inflamed organ.

One student whispered to his neighbor that he would need to see this to believe it. Six months after graduating he was called to the home of a forty-year-old man with acute appendicitis. Two medical doctors had advised immediate appendectomy, but the patient's wife wanted him to try osteopathy before submitting to the knife. The graduate applied Still's teaching and inhibited the tissues at the eleventh and twelfth thoracic. To his amazement the pain eased, the vomiting ceased, the rigid muscles over the appendix relaxed, and within thirty minutes the man, who had not slept all night, fell asleep. One further treatment that afternoon permanently resolved the problem.[59]

After the morning class the students spent from nine until noon in the "operating" rooms, acting as assistants until proficient enough to handle their own patients. Daily exposed to a wide range of chronic disorders, they acquired a wealth of knowledge in a short time. Still personally supervised every case, never too tired or too busy to bring out its salient points.[60]

The consultation began by listening closely to the person's story to ascertain what had precipitated the decline in health – perhaps a fall, a jar, a strain, a postural or occupational stress, an illness or an operation.[61] Still insisted his operators treat every patient with consideration and respect, not as a collection of symptoms and signs but as a fellow human being suffering. "Do not put your hands on a patient," he admonished, "until you first know the anatomy under your fingers, the physiological changes that are taking place, something of the pathology that may be there and, more than all, that a living soul is within."[62] In all adjustments of the body from the abnormal to the normal they were dealing with *life*, and should apply their energies "to keep that living force at peace, by keeping the house of life in good form from foundation to dome."[63]

The dictum for treatment was *Find it, fix it, and leave it alone. Nature will do the rest* – a restatement of osteopathy's two complementary principles.[64] "The osteopathic doctor's only hope is that nature will do the work, otherwise it will not be done," Still stressed. "All he can do is line up the body, and his success as a doctor will be in proportion to the degree of his ability to detect and adjust all physical variations to the normal, and leave his work in the hands of the chemist of the laboratory of animal life."[65] Nature healed, not man, and to acknowledge that fact inculcated humility, a sacred regard for the patient, a reverence for the mystery underlying Creation, and a love of all mankind.[66] In theory, anyway.

Ed Pickler's first patient was "one of the sorriest and dirtiest specimens of humanity" with an ankle problem. When the man removed his shoe Still caught the student's involuntary expression of disgust at the odor and immediately called him outside. "You must not expect all your patients to be clean and well dressed," he said firmly. "This man needs care and cannot pay for it. Don't you think he should be taken care of?" Pickler replied that the man should give his feet as much care as he expected them to give. Still laughed, "You will find many occasions when a clothes-pin would be welcome for your nose. Remember that the best doctor is the one who will give especial attention to the disagreeable work, and not shirk it because it happens to be distasteful to him. Now, let's go in and tell this man to renovate his feet." Still explained his diagnosis and treatment plan, and instructed the man to bathe his feet in hot salt water for fifteen minutes night and morning, and to return the following day. Over the next few days he asked Pickler gravely how his patient was doing, and if the foot was getting "stronger."[67]

The aim of treatment was not simply to normalize deranged structure but, more importantly, to free nerve and blood supply. "The rule of the artery and vein is universal in all living beings," Still taught, "and the osteopath must know that, and abide by its rulings, or he will not succeed as a healer."[68] The treatment must liberate the forces and fluids of the affected part, and thus enable the endogenous *body ferments* to "dissolve and carry away all detained matter and hindered substances, that nature can build anew the depleted surroundings."[69]

Hugh H. Gravett failed to heed this admonition. Presented with a bedridden man with inflamed knees, the student tried to treat the symptomatic area, but the patient found it too painful. Gravett went to Still to complain that the man had "inflammatory rheumatism" and could not bear to have his knees touched. "Of course he can't," Still responded in exasperation. "Neither could I let you poke your fingers in my eyes. How often must I tell you osteopathy is for invalids as well as athletes? I see though you have learned enough from Bill Smith to give it a name." Still turned to the blackboard, drew a pair of legs, and beneath them chalked the words *Mud Puddle*. "Suppose," he said, "I know where to go in the spine and open up a faucet that will send to the knees a supply of fresh clean water and with it the 'House Cleaner's Lymphatic?' Suppose I know where to go and open another faucet that will let the fresh supply through and carry the impurities back to the eliminating organs? What will happen to the mud puddle?" Gravett answered sheepishly that it would clear up. "So will the patients knees." The student made the further error of asking how he should proceed. "You damn fool," Still responded, "what have you been doing with your time while you have been in school? You handle that case or I will turn it over to someone more competent." Though Missouri was known as the Show-Me State, Gravett remarked, "there was no show-me-how-to-do-it with Dr. Still."[70]

No two cases were the same so nothing should be done by formula, and day by day Still pounded this message home.[71] He did not teach specific techniques and actively discouraged anyone from copying his methods; he expected his operators to work out for themselves the modes of treatment they found easiest and most effective.[72] "Each case is a law unto itself," one student elaborated, "having some peculiarity of its own which forces the practitioner from a routine line of treatment. To a large extent this causes technique to be largely individual."[73] Still told them that if they knew the construction of the engine and how to control the fluids and forces that govern its action, it would not be necessary to have someone demonstrate "how to use the monkey wrench and screwdriver to repair it."[74] They must possess the skill to perform the correction, but learning to adjust joints by routine stultified the reasoning faculties and blunted the palpatory art.[75]

Still might occasionally place a novice's hands over the joint and carry them through the adjustment, saying "do it this way,"[76] but beyond that he merely issued a universal guideline: "Be sure of your anatomy and be specific in what you wish to do, then simply apply the principle of lever and fulcrum."[77] This meant a fixed point to stabilize the body or limb (perhaps a table, chair, stool, wall or tree); a bone to use as a lever; and a fulcrum over the structure to be adjusted.[78] The key was to apply the fulcrum with maximum precision and minimum force.[79] Specificity was imperative; recovery could not be expected without removal of the exact cause.[80] Sensitivity, too; they must never hurt the patient nor bruise any delicate structure. "An intelligent head," Still said, "will soon learn that a soft hand and a gentle move are the head and hand that get the desired result."[81]

The students observed his method of treatment. "I have seen him many times take hold of a patient, and tell you as he did so what was wrong with the body," Ethel Conner wrote. "He usually did little exploring with his fingers; he knew what he wanted to do and where to find it and his movement in correction was lightning-like in swiftness. There has never been a technic like his because there has never been a mind like his to know intuitively what to do."[82]

In making the adjustment Still generally employed "a rocking action and leverage," turning the joint in the direction of greatest ease, an "indirect" technique they called "exaggerating the lesion."[83] Sometimes he resorted to "direct" techniques, turning the joint sharply towards the restriction to make a sound like a "pop" – but he cautioned that "snapping and popping of the bones" was no evidence of an effective treatment, and told his operators not to inculcate that idea in their patients.[84] The abnormal condition might remain due to lesions elsewhere drawing the spinal column out of line, causing tightness of muscles, ligaments or connective tissues as they compensated for the alteration in posture.[85] These additional problems must be corrected before the joint could be expected to remain in place.[86]

The number of visits and the interval between each depended on the case. Some needed only one or two treatments, others courses lasting months or more. For chronic conditions it was often necessary to relax muscles, stretch shortened ligaments and calm irritated nerves before attempting to free the offending joint,[87] otherwise the adjustment might not hold. Still occasionally took weeks or even months to do this, especially for joints with a large range of motion.[88]

Healing was a process. With each visit, he instructed, "you are warranted to go further with your treatment, because the surrounding tissues and delicate fibers have had a chance to be relieved from dead and inactive fluids, and have taken on some nourishment."[89] He warned his students not to presume that every case was curable, for many sought help only after disease had already wreaked irreversible damage. Recovery depended on the general state of health and the regenerative potential of the part – and, not least, on the competence of the practitioner. "If success does not attend your efforts," Still cautioned, "it is not the fault of the science, whose working is exact, but of yourself."[90] But he insisted that osteopathy always worked if the case was taken in time and the patient was not poisoned by drugs, enfeebled by age, or weakened by wasted vitality.

Still also warned patients not to expect his operators to do everything. They must share the responsibility for their health. Nature healed, not the doctor, and nature had no substitute for sleep, rest and right living.[91]

One afternoon he invited Ed Pickler to accompany him on a house call. The student tagged along enthusiastically, anticipating learning something useful for practice, but when they arrived at the house Still told him to wait outside, and on the way back said nothing about the patient. The following day he asked Ed to accompany him again. This time, before visiting the patient, they walked out into the pasture north of the school and sat under a tree. Still now discussed what he had found the previous day and gave his diagnosis, but no more, so Ed asked how he would treat such a case. "I would treat it as my reasoning faculties told me it should be treated," Still replied. "Your brain was given to you to use and you must use it if you are going to be successful." It was not enough to copy what he, Harry, Arthur Hildreth or anyone else did. "When you get into practice and run up against something that stumps you," he said, "you won't have the chance to run to 'Pap' and ask him what to do. Now, we'll go see this patient and I want you to show me how she should be treated." Afterwards they spent most of the afternoon talking about osteopathy. "Now, you perhaps think I have not said much," Still said finally,

> but I have told you enough to keep you busy the rest of your life. Don't forget how much is before you. Don't hesitate to trust your own judgment and reason, and remember you are just as apt to make valuable discoveries as anyone else. I could not wish you any better luck than when you start practicing you may come up against hard problems that you have to solve. Go to a small town, live on corn bread and sow-belly if you have to, but sleep with your anatomy under your pillow, and don't forget you are supposed to have a brain inside your skull.[92]

14

A SECRET PROCESS OF TREATING HUMAN ILLS

On Friday, 2 March 1894, a capacity audience crowded into Smith's Opera House in Kirksville for the American School of Osteopathy's first graduation ceremony. The event was significant not only for the seventeen to receive diplomas but also as the first unified show of support for Still, whose address was greeted with round after round of enthusiastic applause.

Local dignitaries praised the school and urged united action to help it flourish. Attorney F. P. Greenwood condemned the injustice of the Missouri medical laws – "obnoxious and offensive to free institutions and a free government; kept alive only by ignorance, prejudice and self-interest" – and asked the people to assist in having them expunged from the statutes.[1] The *Kirksville Democrat* backed Greenwood's call and, extolling the "financial good" Still promised the community, pressed for the erection of a "handsome, commodious building."[2]

The three small cottages had become woefully inadequate to cope with a growing multitude of patients descending upon the town. "I was dumbfounded by what I saw," one visitor related. "I was carried back in spirit to Biblical times, when the lame, the halt and the blind lined the roadways seeking restoration to health." Suffering humanity thronged the porches of boarding houses and moved in a constant flow to and from Still's fledgling institution.[3]

Awareness had dawned on the community that something important was occurring in their midst, and with it the realization of a communal failure to recognize Still for who he really was. "For twenty years we had seemed to know him and had held him off," Normal School president John R. Kirk wrote. "We were slow, very slow to admit the victory our neighbor had achieved. But we did admit, and accept and approve. We shared with him the honor. We took him over. He was an asset to our town, and the world knew what our town had done, and knew our town." The crazy crank was now celebrated as "unostentatious, kindly, obliging, generous, whole-souled, sympathetic, public-spirited, humane," a fighter who had endured monumental obstacles, opposition and envy to emerge an "unstained, unscathed, heroic man, sweetened in spirit."[4]

To help promote a better understanding of his science, in May 1894 Still launched a monthly *Journal of Osteopathy*. The four page quarto, edited initially by Blanche,[5] was sold by subscription, sent in answer to letters of inquiry and scattered widely. In Trenton, Missouri, one enthusiast distributed a copy to every afflicted person he saw. A woman who wrote to the ASO on perfumed, violet tinted stationery, "ordering a dollar's worth of osteopathy, saying she had heard so much of the remedy she wished to try it," was sent a year's subscription.[6] "Occasionally an M.D. would come in contact with a copy," reporter J. B. Dodge joked, "and really his eyes would 'bug out' till you could scrape them off with a stick."[7]

As word of osteopathy spread, Kansas City, Macon, Moberly and Sedalia, Missouri, and Des Moines, Iowa, made generous offers of land and money to entice Still to relocate.[8] In response a number of Kirksville residents, alarmed at the prospect of losing their lucrative commodity, arranged a meeting in the Mayor's office on May 28 to "devise ways and means" of persuading Still to remain. Lauding him as "the greatest healer of modern times," they praised his integrity, ability and skill; promised their "most hearty support;" and resolved unanimously the "advisability" of helping him erect an infirmary. A finance committee was appointed to solicit subscriptions of money and a suitable plat of land,[9] and on June 2 a delegation called at his home to tender a "free-will offering of $2550, and his choice of several building sites with Kirksville's compliments." Judge Ellison acted as chief spokesman and, the *Kirksville Journal* reported, "he did the job very brown."[10]

Still "responded with much feeling," but the hypocrisy was not going to pass unnoticed. Until comparatively recently he was barely tolerated; now they were deferential because of the money he might generate the town. He said he would stay, but made clear his decision had nothing to do with their blandishments. (Unbeknownst to them he had already rejected all the other proposals anyway.) He declined the offers of land, ruled out the possibility of a joint venture, and announced that he would build a combined infirmary and school on his own property with his own funds. "Told them I wanted to pay every farthing in the structure," he scribbled privately. "I thought if I owned it I would be boss. If anyone else owned stock in the building I would lack that amount of having perfect control."[11] With money pouring in from patients and students he purchased a sixty-one-acre lot with a brick house next to his home, plus an adjoining five-acre lot,[12] and commissioned Ed's son Thomas, a qualified architect, to design the building.

These events were overshadowed by tragedy. The previous fall Still's son Fred was crushed by a horse against the wall of a barn, a fractured rib puncturing a lung, and in a weakened state he contracted tuberculosis. A week before Christmas, Mary accompanied him by train to California to recuperate at his physician uncle Thomas's ranch in Lapanza, San Luis Obispo County.[13] But despite the warm climate Fred continued to deteriorate. "Dear Bro. Harry & the rest," he wrote home on 23 March, "my pen shakes pretty bad as I am very nervous." He complained of a cough and other distressing symptoms. "That swelling on the side of my neck is there yet, it seems like a goitre. I have to sit with a pillow under me almost all of the time as the coccyx & one or two lumbar vertebra are turned in such a position as to render it painful to sit on a hard chair but when my stomach gets out of fix, as it has been doing for sometime past (the spells last about a week or more), when I have them I am in terrible pain and my bowels run off terrible bad. I hardly know what to think & want Pa's opinion."[14]

They returned home in the spring, but even Still was unable to help.[15] On Friday, June 8, with the family gathered around the bed, Fred died.[16] Twenty, studious, thoughtful and good looking, he had been considered osteopathy's "brightest star,"[17] his mind set on continuing the work his father had begun. "We often think of our beloved dead," Still wrote soon afterwards. "Why do we? Because of ties made from the fiber of the soul. Each strand found in the cord of love is so pure that the acids of time never corrode."[18] He showed little outwardly, but it was said that the loss of Fred changed his world. A fortnight after the funeral he went to visit Charley in Red Wing, taking Ed Pickler for company.[19] Still remained "serene," Pickler noted, "though his heart strings must have been wrung, for I believe Fred plumbed the very depth of his affections."[20]

On returning home Still immersed himself in the infirmary project and, on August 6, his sixty-sixth birthday, laid its foundation stone at 800 West Jefferson Street on the original site of the old clapboard schoolhouse. In an open letter to the *Kirksville Democrat* he thanked the townspeople for their generosity and detailed how their $2550 donation would be spent: "Not a dollar of the above money has been used for the new building. As I have unaided and alone developed the Science of Osteopathy I wish the new building to be the work of my own hands, and thus let no other individual have any claim on it whatsoever." Since the cash had been raised "for the benefit and the upbuilding" of the city he would invest it in a modern twenty-four-room hotel, the Still Boarding House, for the accommodation of patients.[21]

With the infirmary under construction Still decided not to begin a new class that fall, but was soon persuaded otherwise by a twenty-one-year-old University

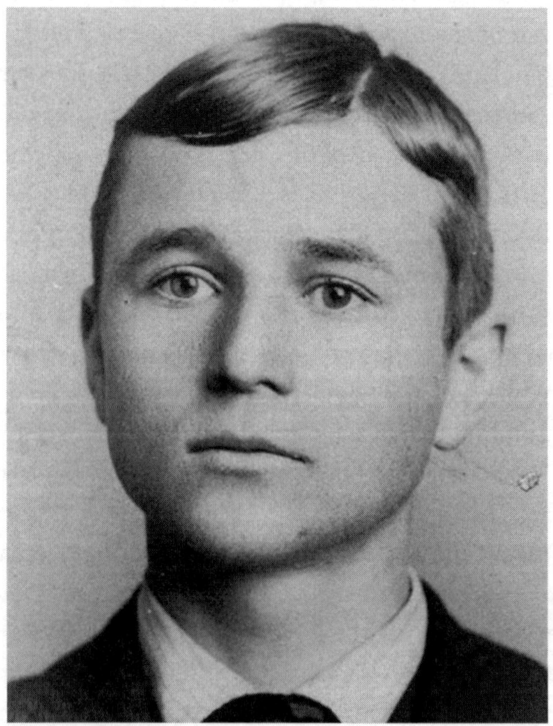

Fred Still.

of Wisconsin student. That March, Carl McConnell had fallen heavily onto his buttocks during a baseball game, and over the subsequent weeks suffered a progressive deterioration of vision that eventually forced him to drop out of college. For five months his wealthy parents took him to a number of renowned eye specialists around the country, who diagnosed "the beginnings of optic nerve atrophy" and pronounced his condition hopeless. In August, as a last resort – more as an experiment – he consulted Charley in Red Wing.[22]

The eminent physicians had limited their examination to McConnell's eyes. Charley, regarding the visual deterioration as an effect, sought its cause in disturbed nerve and blood supply, and directed treatment not to the eyes but to strained joints and contracted muscles in the neck.

Between treatments Carl accompanied Charley on his house calls and listened interestedly as families spoke of the good work Still's son was doing. The recoveries of the diphtheria patients made a "deep impression," instilling "confidence in, and enthusiasm for, osteopathy," but it was the restoration of his own eyesight after two months of treatment that persuaded McConnell to quit university and study the science himself. In October he traveled to Kirksville, called at the little school, and was directed to the office of its secretary and business manager.[23]

This was no longer Harry who, as an inveterate worrier, had found himself unsuited to the task and quit in the spring.[24] His replacement, freshman Henry Patterson, was an ideal candidate for the position. Raised on a Kirksville farm, he had previously worked as a real estate agent, sold cyclone insurance, acted for twelve years as a Notary Public, and served one term as Adair County Treasurer.[25]

Patterson told McConnell that because of the building work they did not have time to organize a new intake of students and he would have to wait until the following year. Undeterred, Carl proceeded directly to Still's home and found him drinking at the well. Still greeted him with customary informality and after an equally informal interview – a walk in the woods[26] – acquiesced to beginning a new class.

The six original students (a dozen more joined a month later) included Joseph Sullivan, a steam heating contractor from Sioux City, Iowa.[27] That April Sullivan had brought his wife to Kirksville for treatment of an unexplained malady, initiated by a fall two years earlier, diagnosed by various doctors as either locomotor ataxia or Landry's paralysis. When they gave her only three months to live, in desperation (and privately pessimistic), Joe took her to see the "Bone Doctor of Missouri." She arrived at the Wabash depot on a stretcher in the baggage car.

As the couple sat in Still's spartan waiting room they saw a "remarkable appearing man" in shirt sleeves dodging in and out of the treatment rooms and noted, as did many, a passing resemblance to Abraham Lincoln. (Parallels with the great emancipator were cemented a few days later when they heard him lecture, "I helped to free the colored man from slavery and am now engaged in freeing the white man from slavery – the slavery of drugs.") They were eventually called into a treatment room and Sullivan looked on as Still, surrounded by a group of students, tended to his wife.

The examination took less than five minutes. The doctor used no stethoscope – in fact no instruments at all. With Mrs. Sullivan's back exposed he ran a hand up and down her spine, and settled on the ninth and tenth thoracic vertebrae. "This girl must have been kicked by a mule," he addressed the students. "Fix her back, and she will walk again." As he turned to leave Sullivan called him back and proffered a sheaf of paper. "What's this?" Still asked. It was a meticulous history of his wife's medical treatment, gynecological examinations, massage and dietary measures, embellished by the ideas and deductions of her doctors Sullivan suggested it would help him better understand her condition. "If I looked at that," Still laughed, pulling on his beard, "I would not know anything about the case." What about diet, Sullivan persisted, since his wife was barely able to eat anything. "Go up town," came the professional advice, "and buy her a couple of bags of popcorn." This Sullivan did and by evening, to his surprise, she asked for two more.

Still advised a lengthy course of treatment, but Sullivan said he could not afford it; his money was already exhausted by medical bills and he would be unable to work if he remained in Kirksville. Still took them under his wing, encouraging Joe to enroll as a student and supporting them financially for the next three years. After eighteen months of treatment the young woman made a complete recovery. "Imagine my state of mind after going broke paying for ponderous medical consultations, technical examinations, dietetics," Sullivan wrote. "I grant these people had been sincere, but I was forced to conclude they had been a hindrance instead of a help, and results justified my belief." As for the prescription of popcorn, it turned out to be a coded lesson on fad diets. In class Sullivan listened as Still compared digestion to the manufacture of a shoe. What would the foreman do, Still asked, if twenty machines were involved in the process and one was malfunctioning? Would he tell the workers to do their best with the remaining nineteen or have the faulty one repaired? Unless the nerves to the digestive system are unobstructed, he said, a special diet will be as helpful as "greasing the spokes of a wagon wheel."[28] But if digestive organs are working correctly, all most people need is a balanced diet of plain nutritious food.[29]

As the infirmary took shape the town fulfilled its promise of support by hiring one hundred and fifty laborers to grade the nearby streets,[30] while Still turned his attention to the thorny issue of the state medical laws. The existing Missouri statutes stipulated that medical practice licenses could be granted only to graduates of allopathic, homeopathic or eclectic schools, and the State Board of Health had no intention of extending the same privilege to ASO graduates, as a scathing attack on Still by one of its members demonstrated:

> Concerning his institution . . . I would say that we cannot endorse or recommend it to the afflicted, but on the contrary we condemn it, and his mode of advertising, by articles in the public press of a character that tends to mislead and deceive the public, to wrongfully impose upon the fears, weaknesses or ignorance of the sick or credulous, and to defraud the people by false and impossible claims in regard to the treatment of disease or deformity. And we are further surprised that such an institution should be advocated by good citizens . . . where young men and women from all parts of the state come to be taught and imbibe such doctrine as the 'Bunco man of Jamaica' puts forth; 'a snake's head, a lizard, a chicken gizzard and a rabbit's foot cure all ills.'[31]

Still went on the offensive. On 30 October 1894 he had the Adair County Court issue a revised charter for the ASO: *The object of this corporation is to establish a College of Osteopathy, the design of which is to improve our present system of surgery, obstetrics, and treatment of diseases generally, and place the same on a more rational and scientific basis, and to impart information to the medical profession, and to grant and confer such honors and degrees as are usually granted and conferred by medical colleges.*[32] The document effectively entitled the school to award the MD degree, a course many urged him to follow as a means of obtaining practice licenses. Still's response was unequivocal: his graduates would be "ashamed to place M.D. after their names." The ASO qualification would be DO, Diplomate in Osteopathy.[33]

He had a bill drafted, to introduce before the forthcoming session of the Missouri General Assembly in the New Year, to have the state medical laws amended to grant osteopathy equal status to the three recognized systems, and formally requested those who desired osteopathy's "growth and perpetuity" to assist by writing their State Representative at Jefferson City, declaring "truthfully what you know and can say about the science." Should the legislative attempt fail, he vowed, "we shall neither feint nor fall by the wayside, but move onward in demonstrating that osteopathy is a science."[34] He recognized the magnitude of the task ahead:

> The theory taught in this school is that diseases can be successfully treated without drugs. Opposed to this theory stands one of the most influential, powerful, and learned professions; backed by an array of authors, colleges, professors and teachers; added to which may be classed the most scientific experts and theorists; as well as man-kind in general. Like other discoveries this science conflicts with the theories and ideas advanced by all other schools and authors. This conflict will cease when the votaries of Osteopathy succeed in convincing the intelligent mind that it is a science guided, directed and controlled by natural laws.[35]

An outbreak of measles in October 1894 served to corroborate this contention. "The usual fever that accompanies the disease was controlled from the start," the *Kirksville Weekly Graphic* reported on forty cases treated by Still and his operators, "and the patients recovered so rapidly as to hardly realize they had been sick." It added that not a single death had occurred in "hundreds" of patients treated for other types of fever.[36]

By Christmas the A. T. Still Infirmary stood complete. Situated on a slope and fronted by a paved macadam driveway, the sandstone and brick structure in Old Colonial style emphasized quality throughout. The main entrance, sheltered by a broad veranda, accessed an "artistically painted" second floor hallway that ran the length of the building, and from it issued Secretary Patterson's office, men's and women's waiting rooms, a library and ten treatment rooms. The basement accommodated seven more treatment rooms, a barber shop and an immense boiler room. The third floor housed Still's private office, a carpeted classroom with "skeletons and manikins of considerable number," and a 250-seat auditorium delicately painted in white and gold, lit by eighty-five incandescent lights, named Memorial Hall in honor of Fred. The top floor contained a dissection chamber, and all thirty rooms were connected by an elaborate "electric enunciator." The building was crowned by an American eagle with wings outspread, symbolizing freedom.

At a final cost of $16,000 and Still possessing only $750 at the ground-breaking many thought it a reckless venture, but with patients arriving in droves and his chaotic finances managed by the able Henry Patterson the infirmary was inaugurated on 10 January 1895 without debt. That evening over 1500 visitors "surged around the building" before crowding into Memorial Hall to attend the dedicatory exercises and a musical program.[37]

"Osteopathy has fought and fought hard for every step gained," Still declaimed in a defiant speech. "Its path has not been strewn with flowers but lined with stones of opposition. . . . I tell you that it means all that medical doctors have tried to express by the word remedy for hundreds of years. It succeeds where they fail because it is bound to the laws of Deity. . . . Osteopathy is an unerring law, but it is not a new law for all law is eternal. You rode into the world on the law of life and you will ride out of it on the law of death, and no man knoweth which of these laws is the stronger."[38] He took another swipe at the businessmen who had sought to profit from the institution. "Every brick from foundation to dome is free from the odium 'joint stock company.' It was not built to boom and sell town lots, nor was it built to obtain money, but to teach the principles of osteopathy."[39]

With the infirmary now open, Still turned his attention to the forthcoming legislative contest. To lobby support among the lawmakers he dispatched the affable Arthur Hildreth to the State Capitol, Jefferson City, accompanied by Kirksville attorneys F. M. Harrington and Henry F. Millan.[40]

The lawyers introduced Hildreth to the leaders of the House and Senate, spent a couple of days instructing him as best they could, then left the ex-farmer to his own devices. "Feeling very green and unprepared for the undertaking," Hildreth approached the situation the only way he knew: practically. Few members had even heard of osteopathy, so he broke the ice by offering free treatment. The first to accept was State Auditor James M. Seibert, suffering from "rheumatic gout" and walking with crutches. Three weeks later, walking unsupported in comparative comfort, Seibert invited a number of House and Senate members to dinner to tell them how much osteopathy had benefited him, and suggested they present a bill to legalize the practice.

Hildreth was soon in demand to treat a wide range of conditions, from sore throats to nosebleeds, colds to constipation, sciatica to "all types of ailments, acute as well as chronic." He found the members by and large reasonable and impartial, genuinely wanting to make the correct decision, but prey to the influence of medical lobbyists.

Ten representatives from southern Missouri remained determinedly opposed to osteopathy. To try and win their allegiance Hildreth wired Still to have sent to the State Capitol a farmer, an enthusiastic supporter of the science since his wife's cure, to meet one of the southern members. To their mutual surprise the pair knew each other well; the representative had once worked for the farmer and they were delighted to see each other. Through this providential circumstance all the dissenting members came to support the bill.

Hildreth made a brief visit home in February, and on the return journey was accompanied as far as Moberly by Still, who was eager to discuss a new reason why legislation was important. A handful of ASO students, bearing paperwork proving only that they had attended lectures,[41] had entered practice without completing their studies and the press were printing stories about the public being fleeced by these untrained, incompetent charlatans. A man who had previously worked as Still's hostler had recently opened an office in Moberly with no qualifications other than having looked after the founder's stable, buggy and horses.[42] "Arthur," Still confided tearfully as the train approached the town, "little did I dream that the child of my brain could ever be used to rob honest people of their hard-earned dollars."[43]

On 14 March 1895 the osteopathic bill came before the legislature and, despite strong opposition from medical doctors and the State Board of Health, was passed 88 to 29 in the House and 25 to 3 (three MDs) in the Senate. "Osteopathy Triumphant" the *Journal of Osteopathy* rejoiced. "The osteopath is now on a legal equality in Missouri." Still instructed ASO graduates to present their diplomas to the Adair County Clerk for a certificate of registration granting them entitlement to practice.[44]

The announcement was premature. To become law the bill required the signature of the Missouri governor. If he failed to sign within ten days the measure would be passed automatically, but during this period he held the power of veto.

Day nine fell on the last day of the legislative session, with adjournment set at 8 p.m. At 4.45, in what appeared to be a premeditated move, Governor William J. Stone exercised his power and vetoed the bill.[45] "Osteopathy, whether called a science, an art or by some other name, is a secret," he addressed the General Assembly:

> Only those initiated into its mysteries know what it is or would know whether any person professing to practice it was acting in good faith or otherwise. What would prevent the filling of the state with people practicing any secret art under the pretense of Osteopathy and under the protection of their diplomas? The principle of giving statutory recognition of and sanction to a secret process of treating human ills does not receive my approval. I do not believe any such thing should be designated in the law as a science, or that any mysterious contrivance or practice should be recognized by legislative endorsements.

And:

> The bill does not require any course of instruction in anatomy or physiology or knowledge of any science or knowledge of anything except osteopathy.[46]

Many of the members had already left, making further action impossible until the next legislative session, two years hence.

Hildreth was crushed. "I shall never forget the feeling that came over me," he wrote. "I felt as if a knife had been stuck through me."[47] The following afternoon he returned to Kirksville and walked from the Wabash depot down West Jefferson Street past his own home and on to Still's to offer consolation. Still had gone into town, so Hildreth went home and waited by the window to intercept him on his return. At last he spotted Still walking up the street and went out to meet him. "When he saw me coming he began to laugh," Hildreth recounted:

> and instead of my being able to console him, I found him much more able to relieve my suffering. His first remark was, 'Well, Arthur, that is all right and for the best. The next time we will pass our law, and it will be signed, and when it is, it will be a much better law than this one was.' I asked him to come into the house, and he said, 'No, you come with me,' and he led the way around back of my house where we were sheltered from the raw northwest wind just a little, and there upon that bleak, raw evening we had one of the very best talks we have ever had in our lives (and we have had many); it was there on that day that he unfolded to me why he never worried nor fretted in our darkest hours. Even when it seemed the whole world was against his discovery, he would work and act with the utmost confidence in the ultimate outcome.

"Listen, Arthur," Still concluded enigmatically, "years ago I was promised no matter how dark conditions seemed to be, and no matter how hard the storms of internal strife or outward opposition seemed to rage, that all the rubbish would be wiped from our pathway as if but chaff, and in the end Osteopathy would reign triumphant."[48]

15

FLATULENCY AND PAUCITY

All knew that William J. Stone had been pressured by medical lobbyists. "The governor was an ardent politician," Senator Alfred N. Seaber of Adair County, who introduced the bill in the Senate, declared, "the drug doctors got in their work on him, and the result was a veto."[1] The *Kirksville Journal* called the episode "a rank bit of executive interference with the will of the people, a master stroke of peanut politics."[2] The *Brookfield Gazette* was more lighthearted, suggesting that Dr. Still might like to examine the Missouri governor to see if he had any "bones out of place."[3]

Still's own response, uncharacteristically, lacked any trace of humor. "We made a hard fight for legal existence," he spoke in Memorial Hall, "and gained a glorious victory in the two law-making departments of our state – our representatives and senators being wise enough to see the best interests of the people and bold enough to advocate them. But at the last hour in the day a man of great prejudice, who had been exalted to the high office of governor under the mistaken supposition that he was capable of filling it to the honor of our grand state . . . sent in his veto accompanied by false and insufficient excuses." Still slammed the governor's action as a betrayal of the people of Missouri and predicted that in the November 1896 elections he would be thrown out of office.[4]

Over the following months Still's talks and articles bristled with anger. He saw the governor's abuse of power as a symptom of a deeper malaise: a corrupt ideology that placed business values above morality and led to the concentration of money and power in the hands of a privileged few. He condemned "the flatulency and paucity on the part of would-be leaders and statesmen," and called for politicians to place their true convictions above party policy. "Policy is the soft soap of liars and hypocrites," he declaimed, "which a man never borrows or pays unless he doubts his own merits. A just and wise man needs no such help."[5] He challenged "the million heirs, syndicates and officers of corporations" to "rise above avarice and greed," and aspire to integrity and honesty. "If we were less a nation of liars and frauds, and governed by principle instead of selfish policy, more would be accomplished in restoring contentment, happiness and prosperity than all the sermons, discussions of finance, commerce and politics can do from now until the end of time."[6] Above all, he called for adherence to "God's eternal laws":

> The path of life is along the line of true, fraternal citizenship, and when we, in all our business and social relations with each other are governed by these laws, and realize that within ourselves we have the power to strengthen, build up and support each other, thereby enabling all the living to provide for themselves through life, we shall have learned that life should not be lived for self alone.

Generosity and gratitude, mutual support, cooperation. Two decades of seeking truth had convinced him that finding health and happiness demanded adopting an essentially American Indian philosophy. But Still feared that American culture was so entrenched in materialism, so focused on competition, so fixated on money and power, that "nothing short of that immutable law of rewards and punishments will ever force this desired step forward."[7]

He deplored the misuse of the legal system by the rich and powerful to protect their own interests. The existing medical statutes were a prime example. Though promoted as measures to help protect the public from quackery, their wording, he charged, had been "so skillfully and artfully" drawn up that only the MDs themselves understood their true design. He urged the public to demand their constitutional rights:

> The last quarter of the century has taught the American people (often too late), that by hasty and dishonest legislation, under the specious plea of 'for the good of the public,' the citizens have been robbed of

> their inalienable rights, and the same transferred to monopolies. If the real scope and design of such laws had been generally known and understood, not one could have been passed by any law-making power, either state or national, without raising such a storm of indignation amongst American freemen, that the enactors of such laws would have been hurled from power.[8]

Not by accident had Still named his institution the American School of Osteopathy. Through respect for the noble values of United States Constitution, for the right of every American citizen to freedom and equality, he had fought for the abolitionist cause in Kansas and for the Union in the Civil War, but in these latter days, he complained, few paid more than lip service to liberty.[9] American society, structured in hierarchies of rulers and ruled, experts and laymen, fostered dependence on authority rather than independence of thought, especially in the more cultured parts of the country. "Their religious and social customs are very much after the law of servility, which demands and legislates to obedience," he wrote of the Eastern states. "There is still in the East some of the same intolerance to man's freedom of thought as was shown in the reign of Henry VIII."[10]

Still warned his students of the snares, trials and pitfalls they would face on entering practice: "Geese will hiss at you, and from their somber roosts, old and musty owls will hoot at you. Even the governors will be hired to bray at you. The press will look wise for a time and say, Amen, good Lord, good Devil! Let me ride on that boat if it has plenty of cash."[11] Graduates joked (with a large measure of truth) that they worked in pairs so that when one was in jail the other could keep the office open. In state after state they faced harassment, arrest, trial, fine and incarceration.[12] Still accused the MDs of professional jealousy and of bringing prosecutions "not for malpractice but for curing."[13]

This was precisely what happened to Herman. Independent, shrinking from routine, often disappearing for days without explanation,[14] Harry's twin had little to do with the infirmary, preferring to promote osteopathy by establishing practices in scattered locations to pass on to other graduates. After Fred's funeral he opened a practice in Muscotah, Kansas, before moving on to Sioux City, Iowa, and, in late 1894, to the wealthy Chicago suburb of Evanston.[15]

Here he was presented with a young girl, lame for two years after an injury and still walking with crutches despite twelve months of almost daily medical attention. When Herman restored the child to health in four visits by treating a hip, the Illinois State Board of Health had him prosecuted, fined $100, and threatened with a jail term for default. "If Christ should appear on earth again and cleanse another leper or cause the blind to see or the lame to walk," Still fumed, "for such effrontery and mendacity he would find the State Board of Health suing him for unlawfully practicing medicine without a license; though he may but have laid on hands and said, take up thy bed and walk." He condemned such "illiberal, nefarious laws" as a "foul blot on the escutcheon" of Lincoln's noble state, and called for its citizens to have them repealed.[16]

To Still's surprise the challenge was taken up and a bill introduced before the Illinois legislature. On June 13 the Senate passed an act permitting the practice of osteopathy as part of the profession of medicine, but the session ended before the measure could be debated by the House, leaving a degree of ambiguity.[17]

In Missouri, meanwhile, osteopathy continued to flourish. Kirksville's population grew to five thousand, vacant lots filled with new hotels and homes, and hundreds took in students and patients as lodgers.[18] A flood of sufferers were arriving from all parts of the Union, many as a last resort after doing the rounds of the country's medical centers and some even those of Europe.[19] "The scene about the Infirmary from early morning until noon beggars description," the *Kirksville Weekly Graphic* reported. "From over the hills, in every direction, patients can be seen wending their way, some in carriages, others in invalid chairs wheeled by attendants, while many are painfully hobbling along on crutches. There are invalids from almost every corner of the United States, and of every degree of infirmity. . . . All day long there is a constantly moving stream of humanity going to and from the building, while every train brings in a new detachment of patients." And with each practitioner administering around fourteen treatments a day, "the ten operators are kept moving pretty lively."[20] Still, too, acting as consultant, overseeing scores of cases a day.

The staff were already stretched when Harry left for Chicago to take over Herman's Evanston practice, his brother leaving to break new ground in Crawfordsville, Indiana. In July, Still persuaded Charley to return from Red Wing to take charge of the school's administration.

Under Secretary Patterson's management the infirmary was a paragon of efficiency. Telephones rang, typewriters clicked, and from 7 a.m. to 1 p.m. electric bells called patients into the "operating" rooms. Examination was free, assessment frank, and treatment charged at a uniform fifteen dollars a fortnight or twenty-five a month. Patients were required to strictly abstain from alcohol.

Most arrived knowing little or nothing about osteopathy, many assuming its founder to be a faith doctor, magnetic healer, Christian Scientist, masseur or hypnotist.[21] Still joked that some believed he carried some kind of conjuring machine up his sleeve that squirted out a healing fluid. When he tried to explain how osteopathy worked at least one person dragged him off into a corner, imploring him with a wink and a whisper to tell the truth.[22] Graduates encountered similar mistrust. In Detroit a patient asked one practitioner his

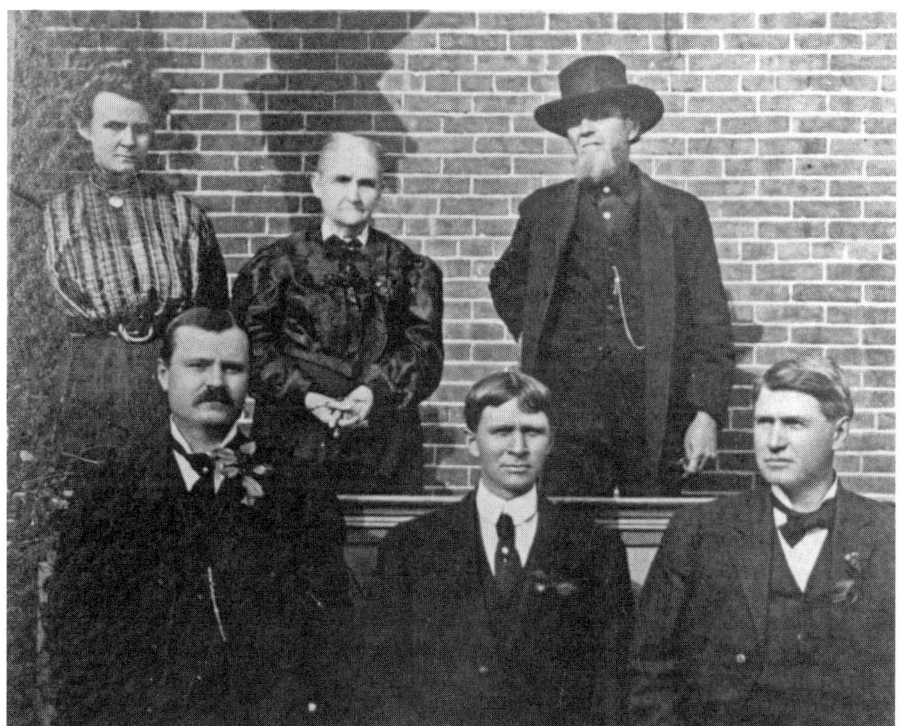

Top row (left to right): Blanche, Mary Elvira, A. T. Still.
Bottom row: Harry, Herman, Charley.

fee to pray for someone; another carefully inspected the treatment table for hidden electric wires. Quick results often generated suspicion, too, leading some patients to fear "there had been some rabbit's foot business worked upon them."[23]

But osteopathy was no "magical secret" as Governor Stone had charged. From his early schoolhouse talks to the *Journal of Osteopathy* Still had constantly striven to educate and empower. To him the regular system was the more secretive, and he detested its use of obfuscatory classical terms that gave physicians a mystique of erudition and superiority. (As someone put it, "He disliked the lingo that hid the inefficacy of a prescription from a trusting patient.")[24] Ignorance made patients dependent on doctors who explained little or nothing. "The great mass of people are like little robins," Still observed, "they open their mouths and gulp whatever the doctors advise."[25] Concerned that many were turning to him with the same blind obedience, he set aside Wednesday mornings for a lecture in Memorial Hall, inviting students, patients, townspeople and visitors to attend.

Returning the meaning of doctor to its original Latin *docere*, to teach, he explained how the human body worked and challenged all to expose osteopathy's fallacies if they could find any.[26]

"What does medicine do for you?" he detailed the shortcomings of the regular system. "By temporarily allaying the misery it often begets a worse thing and fills the system with poison. In administering drugs the physician is never sure of the results, and can only stand helplessly by, and await developments, trying another remedy when one fails." His attack was not personal, he insisted; he had "no desire to make war on the doctors themselves," only on "their fallacious theories."[27] Theories rooted in a materialist philosophy and perpetuated by tradition. "It is the system that is wrong. As the child follows the advice of its mother, so the medical student heeds the teaching of his Alma Mater. From her walls he goes out instructed to give so many drops of a certain liquid to excite the nerves, and so many drops of another liquid to quiet them, and so on all the way through, the path is laid out for him to follow."[28]

Instead of countering physiological abnormalities with drugs, medicine should ask what brought about these abnormalities in the first place. Doctors should recognize that the body constantly strives to express health, and that every cell requires an unimpeded nerve and blood supply to function normally. The role of the physician should therefore be to try and ascertain the cause of disturbed circulation in the ailing part. Switching continually between fun and seriousness ("such a seriousness as would crack rocks and congeal the limpid air with purposefulness"),[29] he encouraged his listeners to teach themselves anatomy in order to better understand the causes of their problems and become more self-sufficient in matters of health. "How many families have a boy or girl who can tell the names of the bones in the lower limbs?" he addressed one audience. "How many bones in the foot? How many more bones in the right foot than are in the left? And which side of Adam the rib was taken from which to make Eve? Whether his liver looks like a bucksaw or an owl? And which leg the liver is in?"[30]

With a liberal sprinkling of metaphor and mechanical analogy he explained how disease begins with disruption of the body's forces and fluids. "Now suppose we would call these lights in the center of the room the spinal cord," he gestured. "By turning off the lights, we represent to a reasoning man a stroke of paralysis. [In his usage the word "paralysis" generally signified reversible nerve interference.] To an osteopath it suggests a principle, a reason, a foundation on which to build." An assistant extinguished the center lights. "While these lights are off, suppose you try to make them burn by digging around the corner of the house, pouring things into the chimneys or into any other available place. Would that help matters? Would any intelligent electrician who knew the ABC of his business expect to renew the lights by any such process? There is only one principle by which that paralysis can be cured," he declared triumphantly as the lights were switched on again, "and that is to open up from the battery the electric wires on which it will travel, which are now obstructed."[31]

He compared the blood and lymphatic vessels to plumbing. "Dr. Sullivan, you have been a plumber for many years," he singled out the former steam heating contractor, "suppose you would find that at some point the water was not conducted on to the next wash-bowl. You would say there was a break or dent in the pipe, wouldn't you. How would [a customer feel if they] were to call you up and say, 'Sullivan, what is the matter with the pipe, it won't let water pass through, I can't get any water out of it,' and you were to reply,

'There is something peculiarly wrong. It is probably organic disease of the valves of the heart,' and recommend an injection of morphine. That is about the sense that you are answered with when you pay your money and ask the doctor for advice."[32]

The theme of treating effects had many variations. One featured firefighters tackling a blaze by dousing the smoke; another, told to an elderly German with sciatic pain radiating down to a toe, featured a cat. As Still treated the fifth lumbar the man protested that the pain was not in his back but in his leg. "If your foot stepped on a cat's tail," Still smiled genially, "you would hear the noise at the other end of the cat, wouldn't you?"[33] A variant of this story compared methods to stop the noise: "Don't cut the head off (surgery); don't give it opiates (medicine); just take the foot off the cat's tail." Osteopathy was almost too simple. "No metaphysics. No great scenery in it," Joe Sullivan remarked. "Just common sense."[34] Cause and effect took the mystery out of the healing art and was something both doctor and patient could understand.

Walking about while speaking, standing motionless for emphasis, Still directed his remarks to one person or section after another so it seemed like he addressed everyone individually.[35] He spoke of a healing revolution standing before the people, one he hoped would result in anatomy ("one of the most important studies") being taught in all schools and colleges.[36] As he approached the end of his message he started down the aisle, still talking, his words gradually dying away as he passed through the door.[37]

It took time to change ingrained beliefs. It was hard for people raised to depend upon drugs as the only method for combating pain and sickness to be told that the body already contains everything the word "remedy" signifies. It was difficult for a society where the authority of science was rarely challenged to be told that within the body exists a greater science, one only dimly comprehended, "a science and truth of God, grafted into man's make-up and his very life."[38] The osteopathic idea had to grow in everyone's mind, just as it had grown in the mind of the founder. Dr. C. C. Moore of New York, a physician for forty-five years, wrote his wife while undergoing treatment for sciatica:

> I am 'out of the world' now and in a land full of cripples. They come from every nation and every way to this center of Osteopathy to be treated,

> to get rid of their pains, lame legs, etc. And it is strange to say that the most of them do really get relief, and never swallow a dose of medicine. Soon they are feeling better, and lay aside their crutches and canes, and go alone, to the marvel of the onlooker. I have to confess that it is not a little surprising to a man who has been so subject to giving medicine for every ache and pain we have – well, I don't altogether comprehend it, and sit in wonderment over all and say over and over again, 'How can these things be,' unless there is something at the bottom of it that goes farther and reaches deeper than any system of healing yet known to the doctors the world over.[39]

Cures were the talk of the town and none was more talked about than the case of Samuel McConnell, a sixty-five-year-old lumber merchant from Council Bluffs, Iowa. In July 1894 McConnell fell while alighting from a street car and sustained what his doctor initially thought was a simple ankle sprain, but when the ankle recovered and he began to walk again the knee began to swell. Another physician diagnosed "sub-acute traumatic synovitis" and bandaged the joint, but over the next fortnight the knee continued to worsen, so McConnell traveled to Chicago to consult leading surgeon John McKinloch, who recommended hospitalization for two months. "They boiled it, burned it with red hot needles and blistered it," McConnell related, "until my knee looked like a piece of raw meat." After the leg healed they set it in plaster and, against medical advice, he returned home. There, at the suggestion of his nurse, he obtained another opinion from Dr. Fenger, a well-known Council Bluffs joint specialist. Fenger said it was the worst case of sub-acute traumatic synovitis he had ever seen and told McConnell that if he expected to use his knee again he should give up his business and travel to Wiesbaden, Germany, for massage and baths.

This McConnell did not do. His health declined, his business collapsed, and friends encouraged him to pursue seemingly the only option left: amputation. He amended his will and, in April 1895, boarded a train to Chicago for the operation. En route, though, the conductor advised that before having his leg cut off McConnell should divert to Kirksville and give Dr. Still a try. He changed trains at Ottumwa.

Still's examination and treatment took all of three minutes. The cause of the problem, he said, lay not in the knee but in the hip, and after adjusting the offending joint informed the lumberman he was cured. Unable to take this in, McConnell asked if his leg needed amputating and was told no, of course not. "Do you think you can really help me?" he persisted. Then, suddenly livid in the belief he was being duped, he turned on Still. "Do you think that I came way down here to be made a fool of and to be told there is nothing wrong with me," he yelled. "I'll have you know. . . ." Of what followed all that is recorded is that his words were as strong as his feelings. Surprised by the torrent of abuse, Still told the patient that "if he did not like the job he could 'clear out of there' as far as his legs would carry him."

During the exchange the lumberman had risen to his feet and, suddenly realizing he was standing without pain, stepped into the corridor and strode off to the Wabash depot to wire his wife that he was well. The story goes that Mrs. McConnell thought it bad enough that Sam had gone to have his leg sawn off, but now he had lost his mind as well, and she telegraphed the infirmary to find out what had gone wrong.[40] McConnell caught the first train home and after further treatment and exercises to strengthen muscles wasted from disuse made a slow but full recovery. "My cure is only one of hundreds Dr. Still is making," he told the *Kirksville Democrat* in gratitude. "The scores of doctors I consulted previous to this diagnosed my injury as that of the knee, and you can judge my surprise when I found my hip was injured instead."[41]

Quick results made headlines, but it was often the chronic cases, those requiring painstaking treatment over months or longer, that perhaps provided greater testimony to the healing power of a normal nerve and blood supply. Restoring the physiology of chronically malfunctioning organs, normalizing derangements rendered almost permanent by years of neglect, or increasing the range of motion of joints hampered by chronically contracted muscles, fibrous thickenings and shortened ligaments could be a long, laborious process. Even after correcting the lesions it might take months or longer for the tissues to regain strength and function. "Nature, like the mills of the Gods," Still said, "grinds slow but exceeding well."[42] He instructed his operators,

> Nature does not jump from the abnormal back to the normal. Step by step she retraces herself; that is why it takes time for the chronic cases to recover. See that your patients understand this.[43]

Cure could never be guaranteed. Some patients were beyond help, but treatment occasionally yielded results that no one, not even the infirmary staff, had believed possible.

The case of Lorna Shelton was a lesson to all. After falling from a swing at age five, injuring her head, neck and spine, she suffered a progressive deterioration of vision. By the time she came to the infirmary twenty-three years later she was blind in one eye and could barely distinguish light from dark with the other. Student operator Charles Hazzard corrected prominent lesions of the first two cervical vertebrae and others in the neck and upper back, aiming to free the sympathetic nerves controlling the circulation of the eyes and optic nerves and, very slowly, Lorna's sight began to improve. By stages she was able to see a handkerchief protruding from Hazzard's coat pocket, distinguish the color of his suit, read large print, see the outline of a house and, after two years of treatment, discern people passing along the road.[44]

Diagnosis and prognosis were often complicated by prior medical intervention. Some patients arrived in a deplorable condition, irreparably damaged, rendered lame or incontinent by surgery that might have been averted by timely osteopathic treatment. Others complained of a myriad signs and symptoms caused by the drugs they had been prescribed: dry mouths, swollen gums, aching joints; faces pale from arsenic, pupils dilated by belladonna, hips and jaws stiff from mercury, and these patients often required a lengthy period of detoxification. "Our work here is principally to overcome the effects of medicine," Still lectured in Memorial Hall:

> Nine-tenths of the cases that come here, while they are wrenched and strained in many places in the body, have to be treated first by turning on the nerves of the excretory organs of the system, for the purpose of cleaning the dirty house in which their soul dwells. What do we find? We find the liver not acting right, we find the lungs affected; we find stones in the gall-bladder. We go a little further down to the renal nerves, veins, arteries; they are out of order. We go down to the water bladder, and there find more evidence of the thoughtless stupidity of man, in the form of bladder stones. By taking medicine many have converted the liver into a bank of cinnabar. A few doses of calomel, and out go the

> teeth. Any person in the audience has the privilege of saying I am wrong if I state anything that is not correct.[45]

His indignation was born of unlimited wonder at the wisdom of the living human body and "the sheer ignorant, irresponsible interference"[46] of loading it with "poisons that the hand of ignorance is ever ready to pour down the throat of credulity." He quoted Corinthians: "Know ye not that ye are the temple of God? If any man defile the temple of God, him shall God destroy; for this temple of God is holy, which temple ye are."[47] Still told patients who had been taking medication for months or years that they were suffering from a compound disease – the original one and another caused by the drugs.[48]

Such was the case of thirty-five year old Hugh H. Gravett. Ten years earlier, while bending to lift the lower end of a boxed organ onto a wagon, the top end slipped off the tailgate and gave him a severe twist. Something popped between his shoulders and he passed out. They carried him into the house and the doctor who was called diagnosed heart failure. Since then he had been taking drugs for his heart, stomach and bowels, and sedatives to help him sleep. Eventually his health began to fail, and when he was given only a short time to live his wife insisted he try osteopathy. In December 1895, against the advice and protest of his relatives, he travelled to Kirksville.

The consultation was so unorthodox that Gravett was initially mistrustful. Still entered the room and said immediately, "Young man, sit on the table with your back to me." No good morning, no questions. "Remove all your clothing down to your birthday suit. Bend your head forward and backward, to the right and to the left. Bend your body forward and backward slowly. Turn it to the right and to the left. Stand up. Walk forward from and back to me. Bend forward as far as you can bend forward. As far as you can, turn the entire body to the right, and then to the left. Sit down on the table." Going through these motions Gravett was thinking what a damn fool he was and wishing he had listened to the folks back home. Then, very gently, Still placed his hand on the fourth and fifth thoracic vertebrae and the corresponding ribs on the left, and they were so sensitive that he jumped off the table.

With the aid of charts and a skeleton Still explained the cause of the problem, rapidly gaining Gravett's confidence by describing what was wrong better than he could have done himself. Still told him he had no heart disease and the other symptoms were the effects of long term medication. He explained that before normalizing such an irritable joint it was first necessary to calm the nerves, otherwise the adjustment would not hold, and this might take weeks or longer.[49] He said it would be six months before Gravett saw any pronounced change and maybe a year before the parts gained sufficient strength to keep them in place.

Gravett protested that with a wife and baby to support he could not remain in Kirksville that long. Still considered this for a moment, then made him an offer: a new class was starting in January 1896 and he could enter it while undergoing treatment. If he felt no better at the end of six months he could just pay the infirmary bill and have his tuition fees refunded. Gravett thought that fair enough.

Treatment was always an opportunity for education and for Gravett it was a lesson on the heart. It does not pull or push, Still said, it merely gives the blood its initial impulse, and since the heart forms just one part of the circulatory tree its functioning will be affected by any disturbance anywhere in the system. He warned that the doctor who learns no more than "to just listen to the patient's heart and tell him how bad it is crippled isn't going to do much for the patient with any kind of heart trouble. But the doctor who learns to assist nature in keeping the fluids and forces moving to and from it on time will be able to rescue many consigned to the scrap heap." "And," Gravett said, "he did just that for me."[50]

16

THE FIGHT FOR TRUTH

"The Fight for Truth," Still proclaimed in the February 1896 *Journal of Osteopathy*. "Osteopathy's Battle against Legalized Ignorance and Stupidity."[1] The thirty-ninth session of the Missouri General Assembly was not due to convene for another year, but he was already preparing for the contest – and this time he would not lose. He declared he was not waging "a war for conquest, popularity or power," but "an aggressive campaign for love, truth and humanity."[2] He demanded not only equality with medicine but also a change in the law to prevent the regulars from using the legal system, under the pretext of protecting the people, to defend their own interests:

> The medicine men of America ask legal protection. They ask the legislatures to prohibit and punish by fine and imprisonment any and all treatments of disease but the old Bangwell system of pukes, purges, blisters, hypodermic syringes and poor man's plasters. They want the exclusive right to practice until the patient's money is gone; then they advise the mountains or Florida.[3]

Still planned a campaign on two fronts. First, to demonstrate, by sheer force of results, that osteopathy merited legal sanction. He instructed his graduates to adopt the motto *To Excel* and focus exclusively on trying to relieve suffering, reasoning that with enough public support "the protected pill peddlers" would be unable to prevent osteopathy being recognized.[4] Second, to raise the standard of education to enable his students to pass the state medical board examinations in all subjects "except those branches in which *treatment* is concerned" – osteopathic principles and practice replacing materia medica – and thereby give the lawmakers no logical reason to deny ASO graduates the right to practice.[5]

He asserted that he welcomed strict legislation, but only if it applied equally to dishonest or incompetent medical doctors.[6] "I know there are men in all communities claiming to be physicians, even panoplied with diplomas and certificates of registration," he charged, "who know no more about the use of drugs nor the treatment of diseases than a goat does of a problem in Euclid."[7] He challenged anyone who regarded his comments unfair to spend a few weeks in Kirksville to see the pitiable condition of some patients, poisoned by drugs and maimed by surgery, "living monuments of the malpractice of legally chartered schools of medicine."[8]

Still persuaded William Smith to return from Kansas City to develop a new curriculum and head new anatomy and surgery departments. They extended the course from eighteen months to two years (four six-month terms with no vacations except a brief holiday at Christmas), added extra anatomy and physiology, created new classes in urinalysis, microscopy, minor surgery, poisons, symptomatology, obstetrics and women's diseases, and built a new amphitheater for viewing dissection. They imposed new entry requirements ("over 20 and under 45 years of age, strictly temperate, of good moral character, good native ability, and at least a good common school education")[9] and, after careful consideration, Still decided to refuse anyone who had previously studied medicine, for he had found that doctors found it difficult to shake off their training and tended to adversely affect the other students.[10]

An exception to this rule was made for his brother Thomas, an MD for forty years. In May 1896, perhaps inspired by Mary and Fred's visit to Lapanza, Tom traveled from California to visit the infirmary. The brothers had not seen each other for thirty-three years and by chance an old acquaintance of theirs from Baldwin, the Reverend James Hall, happened to arrive at the same time. Hall had suffered knee trouble for thirteen years since being kicked by a horse and was hobbling along on crutches. After infirmary hours the three strolled over to one of the treatment rooms. "Tom here knows nothing about osteopathy," Still told the minister, "but I can show him enough of it in five minutes to fix you." Following his brother's instructions, Tom took hold of the injured limb and made a correction that immediately enabled Hall to walk unsupported. "It would be hard to say who was the most surprised, Dr. Thomas or Rev. Mr. Hall," the *Kirksville Journal* reported. "He [Hall] left Kirksville Monday morning a pretty happy man and a firm convert of the new healing science." Tom enrolled as a student.[11]

The May class, the third since September, swelled the year's intake to over one hundred students. During the same period patient numbers doubled to an average of four to five hundred and, with the new building already nearing capacity, Still commissioned the erection of a massive new 50- by 80-foot north wing. In July, with the work still in progress, staff and faculty arrived one morning to find their usual entrance blocked by twenty laborers excavating

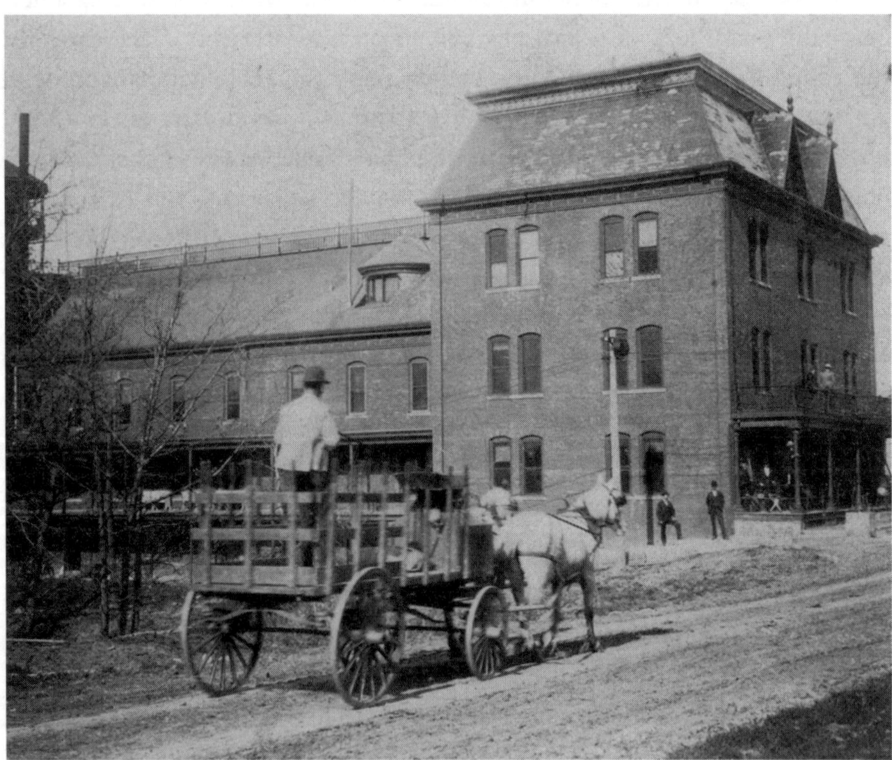

The A. T. Still Infirmary.

foundations for a similar south wing. Still had told no one of his plans and when asked what was going on replied unhelpfully that he was looking for the thimble janitor John Colbert's wife had lost.[12] The additions were designed to accommodate five hundred students and one thousand patients.

Worried about the cost – a staggering $80,000 – and the founder's judgment, Charley, Harry and Henry Patterson persuaded the more diplomatic Arthur Hildreth to tell Still the work should stop. To no avail. Hildreth returned "with temper and feathers much bedraggled," refusing to report what was said.[13] Still issued a written statement:

> There was a meeting of the busy-bodies of the American School of Osteopathy August 24, 1896, in which the President's mental balance was to be looked into. To them there had appeared many and grave signs of active insanity. . . . Breasts heaved and hearts sighed for the lost mind. Proof was undoubtedly conclusive.[14]

He said his business was his own and his actions never preceded his conclusions; he was paying the bills and he did not need their advice.

The medical men, meanwhile, making their own preparations for the coming legislative session, redoubled their efforts to undermine osteopathy. A St. Louis medical journal declared its intention to "expose Still if it took all summer,"[15] while individual MDs concocted a wealth of choice pejoratives, branding osteopaths (amongst other things) "quackish parasites" and their practice "the double rectified quintessence of humbuggery."[16] Still took scant notice. "When a man has a truth," he responded, "abuse does him good. I wouldn't take one thousand dollars for the caw, caw of crows that have croaked at me; they simply act as manure to enrich my life-work."[17] Since the regulars ("look wise, talk wise, theorize") had made no attempt to understand his science, he retorted, their "opinion about osteopathy is like my opinion about Chinese grammar."[18]

The medics retaliated by accusing osteopathy of being "unscientific" and of failing to provide statistical evidence – "scientific proof" – of its efficacy. Still turned the accusation back upon them, declaring that since medicine treated effects and not causes it had no right to call *itself* scientific.[19] "Physicians have taken the wrong road," he asserted:

> In their untiring search for 'scientific poisons' they have wholly ignored the practical truths which the Infinite has plainly written in every part of his handiwork, the human body. Medical researches have resulted in a vast scrap pile of 'knowledge' which is about as useful as would be a library of statistics regarding the number, shape and peculiarities of the shingles on the roofs of New York City. As pertinently admitted by an eminent doctor in the New York Medical Record, 'physicians know everything that can be known except how to cure disease.'[20]

He also challenged the suitability of a materialist philosophy for research on the living being:

> Medical writers have piled up volumes on the chemistry of disease and its specifics, and experimenters have analyzed almost every atom of the known universe, and studied the minutiae of the effects of bodily disorder, to the total neglect of the broader and more important phenomena of animal life. In their long and fruitless search of the outside world for specific poisons that would drive their 'devils of disease' from the human body they have totally ignored that great engine of life itself, and failed to recognize the presence of native forces which the Creator placed within the mechanism for its own government.[21]

Studies of drug efficacy failed to take into account Pasteur's finding that susceptibility to disease depends upon the condition of the "terrain," Virchow's conclusion that abnormal physiology can be reversed by restoring normal fluid circulation, not to mention the osteopathic principles of cause and effect and nature's innate drive to express health.

When these "broader and more important phenomena of animal life" were taken into account every case became a unique problem for the doctor to solve, with improvement dependent upon the patient's capacity for recovery and the practitioner's skill in identifying and removing the cause. Osteopathic treatment did not always cure, but neither a worn out machine nor a poor operator disproved the correctness of the approach. "We know what we can do," Still declared dismissively, quoting (or perhaps inventing) a medical statistic.

"For instance in broncho-pneumonia 46 die out of every 100 cases. I say with Osteopathy none has to die. Therefore we have no statistics."[22]

Nevertheless vague figures did emerge. The *Journal of Osteopathy* reported that 40% of infirmary patients had been "restored to fairly good health," and thousands previously resigned to a life of suffering had "found great relief."[23] Still himself estimated that 75% were "greatly benefited" and 50% were "sent home well."[24] Secretary Henry Patterson kept (slightly) more careful records:

> Asthma: 80% cured, 15% benefited, 5% no change.
> Nervous disease, spasms and epilepsy: 80% cured.
> Paralysis and consumption: 75-76% cured.[25]

A skeptical patient, George Harwood of Tarkio, Missouri, conducted his own survey. A sufferer of "spinal trouble of five years duration, retarded circulation and severe trouble with my head which at that time made me nearly wild," he had consulted leading physicians in St. Joseph, Kansas City, Chicago and elsewhere without benefit, and arrived at the infirmary determined to expose Still as "a quack and his science of Osteopathy a humbug." Harwood interviewed 109 patients currently undergoing treatment. 61% had "some kind of spinal complaint," he recorded, the rest a catalogue of woes including hip, arm and leg problems, heart disease, insanity, blindness, deafness, indigestion, and "bowel complaint in its varied forms," with the average course of treatment "a fraction less than five weeks." The results surprised him. "I found ten percent who called themselves cured and were just ready to start for home. Ninety-five percent readily admitted they had been materially benefited." And one final statistic. "Eighty-two percent could not sing their praise of osteopathy loud enough." Though not entirely cured – a sore back and occasional head pain remained – Harwood himself was very much improved. "To Dr. Still I owe an apology," he wrote on departing. "I believe now that [he] has discovered the grandest method of treating all kinds of diseases of any man of this or any other century."[26]

In July 1896 Still was sitting on his back porch, an anatomy text on his lap and a skeleton by his side, explaining something to freshman Asa Willard, when Mary came out to tell him that a distinguished visitor was waiting for him in the parlor. As Still rose to go in a young girl on crutches, a charity patient he wanted

Asa to treat, rounded the corner. Still was soon on his knees, a hand on the girl's back, completely absorbed, and after discussing her condition at length asked Asa to accompany him to the infirmary to demonstrate something related to her case. From the window Mary saw them setting off across the street and had to call him back.[27]

Few Americans were as influential as the visitor's husband, former Ohio governor Joseph B. Foraker, running for senator in the November elections. Julia Foraker had come across an American School of Osteopathy pamphlet and, clutching at straws, brought her five-year-old son Arthur to be examined. Specialists believed the boy, born a blue baby and diagnosed with valvular disease of the heart, was unlikely to survive past his seventh year.

Still recommended a lengthy course of treatment, and for the next two years Mrs. Foraker made repeated visits to Kirksville. During this period she founded the Sojourner's Club, a women-only meeting place for visitors to mingle with locals. Though primarily a social center, the club had the unanticipated benefit of providing a safe haven for discussing a class of medical conditions little mentioned openly: "women's complaints."

For the past year Still had been studying gynecological problems assiduously and regarded the work his "most valuable revelation yet."[28] He listed a host of conditions that had responded positively to osteopathic treatment: "abnormal discharges, ulcers, tumors, variations from [the normal position of the uterus], cancers, wounds caused in childbirth by forceps, retained monthlies, prolapse, sterility, menopause, inversion, procidentia, etc."[29] In treating all diseases of the "womb and its appendages" he had found that normal pelvic alignment was fundamental. A strained sacroiliac joint might irritate the lumbar or sacral nerves to produce back, sciatic or coccygeal pain, or affect the bladder, ovaries, uterus and supporting ligaments to precipitate menstrual and other problems.[30]

He had also begun teaching an osteopathic approach to childbirth. In fulfillment of the ASO charter's pledge "to improve our present system of obstetrics," his method aimed for shorter labor, less pain, and fewer injuries to both mother and baby. In 1895 he converted a twelve-room cottage on Fifth Street, just northeast of the infirmary, into a maternity hospital.

Still insisted that if childbirth was conducted "in strict conformity to nature,"[31] all normally formed women should be entitled to a reasonably easy delivery, without instruments or injury, within two to four hours of labor.[32] He criticized the regular system, complaining that although over ninety percent of births happened normally, books on obstetrics were "full of deformities," leading the student to believe he "must have a car load of tools to be successful as an obstetrician."[33] He particularly detested forceps. In a lifetime of general practice he had never owned a pair nor, he claimed, lost a single baby[34] – and woe betide any operator he caught using them.

After graduating in 1896 Washington Conner worked for five years in the school's obstetrical department, and one night was asked to show a group of students how to deliver a baby. Morning came without success so he called Charley and when he, too, failed they called Bill Smith, who finally delivered the child with forceps. As Conner returned to the school he saw Still sitting on the steps. "I understand you used the tongs on a baby this morning," the founder said accusingly. Conner tried to explain that it was a "case of inertia" and that they had no other option. Still exploded, telling him the inertia was all in his head and if he allowed forceps to be used again he would be out of a job. Conner asked what he should have done. "Call me," Still replied. "I can deliver them without tongs." But how, the graduate asked? The answer was perplexing. When more power is needed, Still said, "turn in the ovarian artery."

"When we learn the meaning of the above phrase," Conner wrote in his 1928 booklet *The Mechanics of Labor, Taught by Andrew Taylor Still, M.D.*, "the teacher who speaks of the uterine contraction will be in a class with the scientist who teaches that the earth is flat."[35] Conner explained that Still's obstetrical approach relied upon four basic principles.

First, a month or six weeks before labor is expected, treat the mother to generally loosen the muscles and joints of the lumbar and lower thoracic regions.

Second, "wait until the fullness of time."[36] Labor should never be hurried nor the waters broken prematurely, for the baby depends upon the amniotic fluid to turn into the right position for delivery.[37]

Third, "a new power plant." The "power plant" – the expulsive force – is not muscular but hydraulic, since the stretched uterine muscle is incapable of generating sufficient force to push out the baby.[38] Still taught that when true labor begins and more force is needed, apply a principle used by the hydraulic engineer: "Turn in more water when you want to have the press lift the load."

Hence his instruction to "turn in the ovarian artery." This meant stimulating "the nerves to that artery so that more blood will flow into the uterine sinuses, or close the outlet through the veins by stimulating them." More blood, more force. The "power plant" had a second component: the broad ligaments of the uterus. Conner noted that during the first stage of labor the cervix sits high in the pelvic cavity and during the second stage draws down towards the pelvic outlet, and argued that the only structures capable of pulling it down are the broad ligaments. "Why is muscle tissue put into the broad ligaments?" he inscribed in one copy of his booklet. "Elastic tissue is never put into a guy rope."[39] He believed that when sufficient hydraulic pressure develops, the broad ligaments contract to enable the baby's head to engage.[40]

Fourth, "eliminating resistance." Still's basic law of obstetrics was, "straighten the birth canal."[41] He had observed that all mammals instinctively adopt the correct position to achieve this – humans included, if left to their own devices, as he had seen among the Shawnee, who gave birth in a squatting position. Do not place the woman flat on her back, he cautioned, for in this position the weight of the gravid uterus will compress its own nerve supply and, since the birth canal will be more tortuous, more force will be needed to expel the baby. And, critically, since the baby's head will be directed through the cervix at an obtuse angle towards the posterior part of the vagina, laceration will be more likely at both the cervical os and the perineum. Still provided the homely analogy of a farmer trying to drive a wagon through a gate: to avoid tearing down the gateposts a straight approach is better than a crooked one, and the wagon will pass through easiest at a right angle. If the driver knows how to direct the wagon properly, he said, the gate is amply large in most women. He told his operators to place the mother in the same position as the Indian women but, instead of squatting, lying in bed inclined at an angle of thirty to forty-five degrees. This would allow the uterus to fall forward, taking pressure off the nerves, and present the baby's head at ninety degrees to the outlet. "Now it is your duty to prevent rupture of the perineum," he taught:

> [Take] a position at the patient's right side, and with the patient in the position above described a slight amount of work with the fingers will prevent any laceration. Place the fingers of the left hand firmly about

> two inches above the symphysis and push the soft parts down. With the thumb of the right hand against one of the tuberosities of the ischium and the fingers against the other tuberosity support the perineum with the ulnar border of the hand pressing the tissues strongly against the bones until the head passes over. This allows the stretching of the parts to take place at the sides of the vagina and prevents laceration. If you follow this law of Nature, laceration may occur in one out of a thousand cases, and you will be to blame for that one.[42]

He insisted that instruments were only necessary in extreme cases of pelvic deformity, as he demonstrated when the staff got into difficulties with a small mother and a large baby. "Do you think an architect would build a ship and after it was completed be unable to launch it," Still said, removing his coat. "If not, why then should the Divine Architect, the Master Builder of the universe create a baby and then be unable to deliver it?" He took a fetal skull in his hands and explained how to reduce its size for passage through the birth canal no matter how small the outlet. The baby was soon out and crying.

It took Conner years to fully grasp Still's principles, but eventually he learned to consistently deliver babies without forceps or tearing the mother, and after three decades specializing in obstetrics concluded that ninety percent of difficult labors arise because of measures taken to hasten the delivery. "I think many of those false pains are stimulated into true pains," he stated, "and a long tedious hard labor is the result, ending in a forceps delivery, a lacerated mother and perhaps a dead or maimed baby."[43] He urged his colleagues to "keep the faith" and adhere to the call of the ASO charter to teach a better system of obstetrics. "Now, in order for you to become Osteopaths you must be born again," he exhorted. "You must get all those old allopathic ideas out of your system. That will be hard for you to do, but you will never get anywhere until you do."[44]

Julia Foraker took a keen interest in the infirmary's obstetrical and gynecological work. "If Dr. A. T. Still had discovered nothing new in medical science but what he has done for woman," she wrote,

> his name would go down the ages as the greatest physician of any age and one of the historical benefactors of the race. His system has made

> it possible for woman to escape most of the ills which she has been supposed traditionally to be condemned to suffer; he has made it possible for her to approach maternity in calm tranquility, having assurance that the pains will be almost entirely overcome; and he has demonstrated that women need not spend their lives nursing functional derangements without finding succor. Who before has done so much in medicine?[45]

Arthur, too, was responding well to treatment. "The child is so much improved that everybody who knows them is delighted," the *Cincinnati Commercial Tribune* reported, "but no one so much as Mrs. Foraker herself, who is enthusiastic over the cures she has seen, and moreover she has Dr. Still's promise that he will eventually cure her boy."[46] With the Missouri legislative session less than six months away, such a high profile endorsement could not have been timelier.

In September 1896 Julia Foraker returned to Ohio to help with her husband's senatorial campaign, pledging to have him visit Kirksville as part of his electoral tour. She kept her promise, and on October 11 Charley, his brother-in-law Clarence Rider, Turner Hulett and Still's brother Tom caught the train to Moberly to escort the Forakers to the home of osteopathy.[47]

The former Ohio governor's visit coincided with an interesting case at the infirmary. David Clark, a twenty-seven-year-old farmer from Promise City, Iowa, had come to Kirksville the previous year for treatment of vertebrae and ribs injured in a fall from a tree. After being restored to health in three weeks he decided to quit farming and study osteopathy, but on selling his land and returning home with the money he was robbed and severely beaten, leaving him with almost unendurable head and neck pain. When he told his doctors he wanted to return to Kirksville they swore out a complaint stating that "a man suffering so much pain might easily become demented and run amuck," and had him admitted to the Iowa State Insane Asylum.

Once there he was powerless. They bound his neck with straps and plasters, kept him under strict surveillance, and administered up to seventeen doses of medicine a day. They vetted letters to friends and family, preventing the possibility of outside help, and to disabuse the notion that osteopathy might help subjected him to a brutal mock treatment. Clark realized that his only hope of getting out was to feign recovery, a ploy that eventually worked. On being released his father took him by carriage to a local osteopath and on the way back he slept soundly for the first time in months. In October, after another fortnight's treatment at the infirmary, he was well. Three months later he enrolled as a student.[48]

Clark had been sane all along, but Still had successfully treated a handful of confirmed mental cases. One was Kirksville farmer Lee Dye, brought to the infirmary six weeks after being knocked unconscious while felling a tree, suffering from severe muscle contractions, atrophy of all four limbs, and an acute mental imbalance marked by giggling, crying and a "wild and idiotic" expression. Still removed a neck brace, corrected a displaced vertebra pressing on the spinal cord and Dye's system immediately relaxed. In time he made a full recovery, both physical and mental.[49]

Another case was a violent man named Sims, "laboring under a dangerous form of insanity, brought from Hannibal guarded by his father and brother." Barely half an hour after having a lesion between the first and second cervical vertebrae corrected the patient's "mental fury" subsided. Afterwards Still asked Sims how he had felt when insane. The man replied that he knew he was "off base," with an irrepressible urge to commit some hideous crime, feeling it would be funny to stab and shoot and chop off people's heads. Sims returned home with no further inclination to violence.[50] These cases inspired Foraker to invite Still to visit some of Ohio's state insane asylums, but he declined, saying he knew too little about the subject.[51]

Herman, currently practicing in Hamilton, Ohio, accompanied the Forakers back to Cincinnati.[52] With Arthur requiring further treatment and Hildreth leaving to join Harry's busy Evanston practice, Julia purchased Hildreth's house close to the infirmary on the road formerly called Brown Avenue, now renamed Osteopathy Street.

In November 1896 Joseph B. Foraker was elected U.S. Senator, and his Republican stablemate William McKinley was elected the twenty-fifth president of the United States. In Missouri, as Still predicted, William J. Stone was consigned to political oblivion. The state's new governor, Lawrence "Lon" V. Stephens was a firm supporter of osteopathy, he and his wife having been infirmary patients.[53] The signs were auspicious for the osteopathic bill to be debated by the Missouri General Assembly in the New Year.

17

A BIG JOLLIFICATION

Three weeks after the November elections came surprising news: the state of Vermont had passed a bill to legalize osteopathy.

This unlikely occurrence followed a chain of events that began the previous year when infirmary patient A. C. Mills, an influential St. Louis clothing manufacturer, invited student operator George Helmer to accompany him to his vacation home in Chelsea, Vermont, to continue treatment over the summer. Mills induced others to take treatment from the student, including the young son of Orange County clerk Curtis Emery, whom he cured of asthma. The case attracted much public attention and Helmer left at the end of the summer promising to come back the following year.

He duly returned in June 1896, accompanied by classmate Charles Corbin, to an enthusiastic reception. Word had spread that cures made the previous year had been permanent and, despite Chelsea being fourteen miles from the nearest railroad station, the town was soon "crowded to overflowing" with patients, many from neighboring states. Alarmed at this development, a group of local physicians drove to Stafford, Vermont, to lodge a complaint with State Attorney Hon. Daniel Hyde alleging that "Dr. Helmer was imposing upon, humbugging and defrauding many feeble-minded people," and treating ladies with impropriety.

Hyde called for an immediate investigation. To his surprise this revealed not only no substance to the allegations but also that the "feeble-minded people" included many of his friends. Outraged by the action of the MDs, a group of Chelsea women led by Curtis Emery's wife demonstrated their support for the two osteopaths by feting them with an "outdoor tea and reception" on the town's North Common, attended by one hundred and fifty patients, friends and guests. "The intelligent and smiling faces and the hearty handshakes and expressions of good will and thankfulness that were extended to Dr. Helmer and his assistants," a local paper chronicled, "would convince the most skeptical that Osteopathy was not a humbug but was a scientific method of treating ills that flesh is heir to, and, though comparatively a new science, it bids fair to bring about a revolution in the treatment of disease." The "fine supper" culminated in a rousing performance by the Chelsea Military Band and amid a number of speeches was read a message from State Attorney Hyde congratulating the community for supporting a science capable of doing so much good for mankind.[1]

The medics responded by drafting a bill, to introduce before the Vermont State Legislature at the end of September, to prohibit osteopathy. They were outmaneuvered. On the fifteenth of that month Helmer moved his office to the state capital, Montpelier, and within a short time could count among his patients Lieutenant-Governor Nelson Fisk, ex-Governor William Dillingham and others of influence, who collectively took up his cause. Dillingham introduced a bill to *legalize* osteopathy.

Dillingham's measure was referred to the public health committee, who called for evidence of results and summoned witnesses to a public hearing. When the chairman asked for those cured or benefited by osteopathy to rise, over two hundred people stood up and medical examinations on a sample of cases verified their testimonies as "overwhelmingly convincing," but the committee contained several physicians and they refused to report the bill. However, on the last day of the legislative session, November 24, the president of the Senate suspended the rules to hurry through important matters and called up Dillingham's bill. An hour and fifteen minutes later the measure had been passed by House and Senate, and was formally signed into law by Governor Josiah Grout, making Vermont the first state to recognize osteopathy.[2]

When the news reached Kirksville the town erupted in spontaneous celebration. Students, patients and townspeople crowded into Memorial Hall to hear Still deliver a philosophical talk, but what would stick in their minds was how unusually well-dressed he appeared. Blanche had insisted he wear a clean shirt for such a historic occasion, so he took one from the closet and put it on over the two he was already wearing.[3]

With the Missouri contest imminent, well-meaning friends urged Still to adopt a more conciliatory approach and include materia medica in the curriculum to help sway the lawmakers. "I care nothing for pleasing legislatures," he responded dismissively, "by taking to them large bundles of blind useless rubbish."[4] Instead he had Judge Andrew Ellison draft a bill to amend Section 688, Article 1, Chapter 110, of the 1889 revised Statutes of Missouri, Medicine, Surgery and Dentistry, to grant osteopathy legal recognition, and asked Arthur Hildreth to return from Chicago to lobby support for the measure. On 1 January 1897 Hildreth traveled to Jefferson City to spend the rest of the month frequenting the State Capitol, joined intermittently by ASO secretary Henry Patterson.[5]

Hildreth had grown in stature since the defeat of the first bill, more confident in his role and, with the great strides made by osteopathy, more justified in demanding recognition. This time he resolved to speak to every member of the House and Senate, physicians included, to detail the principles of Still's science and explain why a law was necessary: to give osteopaths a legal right to practice and, by forcing the closure of diploma mills, assure the public that all were properly qualified.

First on Hildreth's list was Osage County representative Dr. Alonzo Tubbs, who had fought vehemently against osteopathy two years earlier. The two had never spoken in person, but Hildreth felt that despite his antagonism Tubbs was a man who always did what he believed right. "You voted against our bill in 1895," Hildreth told him, "but we want to introduce another in this session and I was in hopes we might talk this matter over and come to some understanding." Tubbs replied that the previous bill was "a vicious measure," for it would have given osteopaths exclusive rights to "bloodless surgery" and might even have prohibited MDs from setting broken bones, and if the new one was similar he would oppose it. But, he added, "If you will introduce a decent bill I will vote for it, because I believe your profession should have the same right to kill people as we do." Hildreth invited him to read the final draft and together they drew up a joint amendment to the effect that the measure would not interfere with the rights of licensed physicians of any other system. Tubbs became a personal friend who fought as vigorously for the new bill as he had against the old one.

Ten days before the session opened came wholly unexpected news: North Dakota had approved osteopathy. The story was extraordinary. The measure had not only been presented and argued by a woman – in itself remarkable at the time – but she had single-handedly taken on and beaten a powerful delegation of doctors and the state's Board of Health.

A year earlier Helen de Lendrecie discovered a lump in her left breast and, diagnosed with cancer, underwent a radical mastectomy. In September 1896, to her horror, she found a lump in the other breast and a Chicago specialist advised further surgery as her only hope. A few weeks after the initial operation she had come across an article about osteopathy that made the startling assertion that "an obstructed blood vessel will often cause cancer," so before submitting to the knife for a second time she boarded a train for Kirksville. Still identified and corrected displaced ribs, and with further treatment over the next six weeks the tumor gradually shrank until by 12 December it was no longer detectable.

Before returning home de Lendrecie made Still a bargain: if he would promise to establish an osteopathic institution in Fargo, she would endeavor to have osteopathy legalized in North Dakota. "If you have influence enough to make my science a legal matter in your state," he replied, "I will certainly do as you request."[6] De Lendrecie traveled to the State Capitol, Bismarck, and after a campaign of education was granted permission to present a senate bill.

On the floor of the chamber she declared that she was acting solely out of personal gratitude; she had come neither to fight against medicine nor to plead osteopathy's cause as a lobbyist or paid agent. She related her own story, outlined the theory of osteopathy, and told of having witnessed cures of "asthma, heart disease, quick consumption, hip disease, spinal curvature, rheumatism, kidney and liver troubles, withered limbs, paralysis, insanity and blindness." She spoke of the Vermont law, the improving health of Senator Foraker's son, and of osteopathy's prestige in Illinois,[7] following its endorsement there by eminent surgical textbook author Dr. E. H. Pratt, who Harry had treated in Chicago.[8] She stated that seventeen Fargo residents were currently undergoing treatment either in Kirksville or at Ed Pickler's Northern Institute of Osteopathy in Minneapolis, and presented a petition in support of her measure signed by forty-three businessmen. The Senate voted 22 to 5 in her favor.

Legislative procedure decreed that before being debated in the second chamber the bill required reporting by the House Medical Committee. Its members, largely physicians, responded bitterly and personally. A Dr. Wheeler savaged Pickler's character, branded Pratt a "faddist," and asserted that osteopathy, in common with any other method of healing, should come under the control of the State Medical Board. A Dr. Smythe then declared, among other derogatory remarks, that any osteopath who killed a patient should be hung. All but one member voted against reporting the bill. The following morning de Lendrecie's supporters advised that her cause was hopeless and suggested she try again at the next legislative session.

She would not let the matter rest. Inspired by the example of Still's early struggles, she succeeded in having the bill called out of the general order and the Speaker, friendly to her cause, allowed her to address the House on February 15.

The Senate adjourned and all trooped into the House to listen. The public galleries were filled to capacity as de Lendrecie was escorted to the speaker's stand to deliver what one North Dakota daily called "the most persuasive and effective address ever heard in the state." In her introductory remarks she asserted that her plea was none of the medical men's business but a matter between osteopathy and the people of North Dakota. She stated that she had not even mentioned the medical profession in the Senate and had not intended to do so before the House, but since they had thrown down the gauntlet she would pick it up.

In plain but respectful language she reviewed the arguments against her bill. She pointed out that in the Senate no physician had said a word about sickness or cures; they had merely boasted of their renowned colleges and magnificent protection of the public. She revealed that Dr. Wheeler, who had spoken so disparagingly of Drs. Pratt and Pickler, had had an old Native American medicine woman from Neche, a small town near the Canadian border, arrested five times for not having passed the State Board examinations and practicing medicine without a license. The woman was tried before a court, but when the jury learned that her patients had got better after medicine had failed she was acquitted. The "monopoly of the medical profession is the most gigantic combine of this or any other age," de Lendrecie charged:

> It is more autocratic than the Czar of Russia, and just as despotic. Its ramifications extend into every village and cross road in the state, and the Standard Oil trust sinks into insignificance when compared to this monstrous evil which defiantly lifts its head and says, 'I am dictator of North Dakota,' and if you rebel it puts on a patronizing air and tells you the combine is in the interest of the public. Against every other bill you can claim exemption, but against the physicians bill you have none. One dollar a mile, and power to take from you the bed on which you lay. Now, do you imagine these laws were enacted in the interest of the public?

She asserted the people's constitutional right to select any method of treatment on its merits, without the medical profession having oppressive laws enacted to restrict all but their own system. "As she warmed up to the subject," the *Journal of Osteopathy* gloated, "it was apparent that the supposed defeat was being turned into a brilliant victory, and when she sat down amid deafening applause, all the plug-hatted and gold-spectacled medicos in Christendom could not have prevented the passage of the Osteopathic bill. The doctors, who had felt so secure only a short hour before, now sat mute and bewildered, as though glued to their seats." The bill passed 43 to 16, and on the same day was signed into law by Governor Frederick A. Briggs.[9]

In Missouri ten days later, 25 February, Hildreth's measure passed 101 to 16 in the House, and, on 3 March, 26 to 3 (three MDs) in the Senate. After their momentous victory Hildreth and Henry Patterson remained overnight in Jefferson City, and the following morning, Thursday, 4 March 1897, walked to the governor's mansion on Madison Street to witness, at almost the same moment that William McKinley swore the oath of office as President of the United States, Lon Stephens sign the document that made osteopathy legal in Missouri.[10] "The system, method or science of treating disease of the human body, commonly known as Osteopathy," it stated, "is hereby declared not to be the practice of medicine and surgery within the meaning of Article 1, Chapter 110 of the Revised Statutes of Missouri of 1889 and not subject to the provisions of said article." It entitled only graduates of legally chartered osteopathic schools to practice in the state, forced the closure of diploma mills, and gave osteopaths equal rights to medical doctors.[11]

That afternoon Hildreth and Patterson returned home to a rapturous reception. Hundreds of students, patients and townspeople led by the ASO band joined a triumphal march to the Wabash depot, and as the train drew up to the platform the crowd surged forward to greet the returning heroes. When they appeared on the steps of the rear carriage the band struck up, the air filled with hats and wild cheering, and the pair were seized and carried, Hildreth on William Smith's shoulders, to a waiting carriage. The procession marched around the square and on to Still's home, with flags, handkerchiefs, hats, umbrellas, "and everything waveable" waving from doors and windows along the route. The students chanted,

> Rah! Rah! Rah! Missouri passed the bill.
> For A. T. Still. Goodbye pill.
> We are the people of Kirksville. Rah! Rah! Rah!

Still, Hildreth and Patterson delivered short speeches, and the following day, Saturday, was declared a "big jollification."

The morning was ushered in by the firing of cannons and scores of gunshots: 101 for the members who voted for the bill in the House, 26 for those in the Senate, and a dozen for the twelve MDs who supported the bill. Still fired ten rounds for Governor Stephens, and ten more were fired for him. At 2 o'clock the alarm whistles of the light and water works pierced the air, factory sirens screamed, church and fire station bells pealed, firecrackers exploded, and the cacophony was completed by the barking of dogs and the hammering of a dozen anvils. Citizens adorned houses and stores with decorations, businesses closed, and the entire town packed into Memorial Hall to congratulate Still in his hour of triumph.

Tumultuous applause delayed his speech for several minutes. When the cheering finally subsided he expressed his thanks to the House, the Senate, and the state's "broad-minded and sensible" governor. A telegram from Lon Stephens, offering congratulations on the "deserved victory," was read out and the pen he used to sign the bill, acquired by Hildreth and Patterson, was presented to Still, who said he would use it to sign diplomas. Rhapsodic speeches continued for five hours.

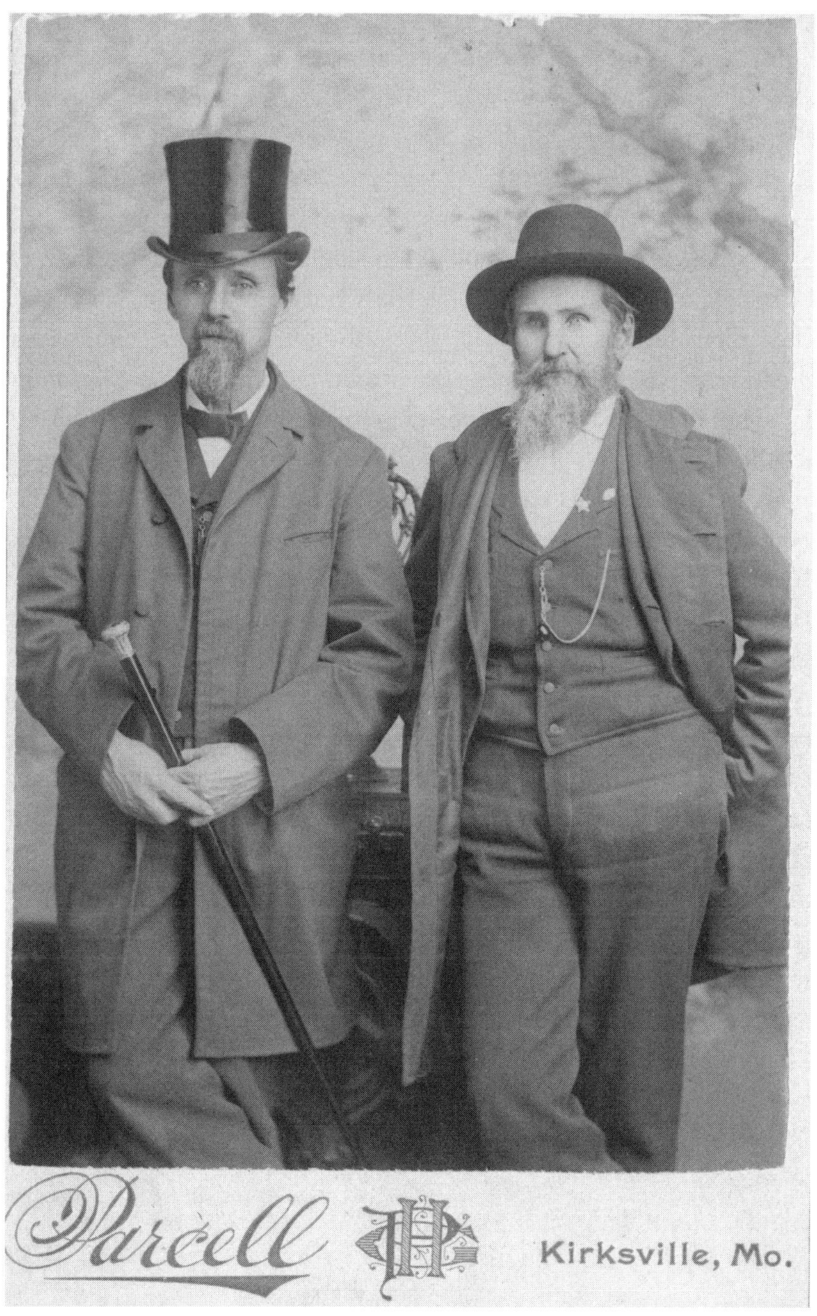

Andrew and Edward Still, 4 March 1897.

During the rejoicing Still was press-ganged into a clothing store and fitted up with a Prince Albert suit and silk top hat. Even worse, he told some students afterwards, they made him wear a stiff collar and necktie. He was led into a photographic studio to record the memorable occasion, but remained forever ashamed of the picture. The suit – the only new one anyone ever saw him wear – was destined to languish in his closet, but the top hat did not even make it home. On his way back he met a black minister and it found a new owner.[12]

The celebrations rolled on into the early hours. At half past midnight two hundred torch bearers gathered at the Wabash depot to welcome Helen de Lendrecie from North Dakota and, notwithstanding the hour, gave her a rousing escort to her hotel led by the ASO band in full uniform.[13]

Still himself made no noisy pronouncements. For him the celebrations were bittersweet. The previous day, Friday, he had called at Julia Foraker's house, temporarily occupied by her friends Colonel and Mrs. A. L. Conger of Akron, Ohio,[14] looking visibly shaken. "I have had some very bad news this morning," he said, removing from his pocket a letter notifying him of the death, on 2 March, of his old comrade James Abbott in De Soto, Kansas.[15]

They had last seen each other the previous August on Still's sixty-eighth birthday. On that occasion Abbott had delivered a nostalgic speech in Memorial Hall, recalling the struggle to free Kansas and their conversation on the banks of the Kaw River about the doubtful merits and indiscriminate use of drugs.[16] A set of photographs taken that day, presented by Still to Julia Foraker, hung on the living room wall tied together with red, white and blue ribbons. The images depicted Still, his brother Tom, and Abbott. Still's eyes filled with tears as he took his cane and turned Abbott's photograph to the wall. "It is hard to bear this separation," he said, turning it back again. "That was one of the best friends I ever had. He was the first man who put into my head the idea of osteopathy."[17]

Abbott was buried on the same day that the practice was legalized in Missouri.

18

WHY, HE COULD BE RICH

Legislation gave osteopathy respectability and Still new status as a public figure. He was loved by the community, fawned upon by the rich and famous, and the little Midwestern town he had adopted as his home bathed in his reflected glory. "The spirit that prevailed in Kirksville, that great outward manifestation of exaltation within, I shall never forget," one student wrote. "It existed everywhere, not only in the college itself, but was on the lips of the citizenry, and the dominating topic of the town."[1]

The infirmary additions, completed in January, proved timely, as in the wake of the Missouri law came a surge of new patients and prospective students. Before addressing this problem Still had a promise to honor. At the end of March 1897 he traveled to North Dakota to help Helen de Lendrecie establish the Fargo Institute of Osteopathy. He remained seven weeks, treated patients who flocked from all parts of the state, and left the practice in the charge of graduate E. B. Morris.[2]

Much happened while Still was away. The medical profession, determined to prevent the spread of osteopathic legislation, mobilized State Boards of Health, State Medical Societies and National Associations in organized attacks against osteopathy. With individual practitioners virtually powerless to combat "this almost numberless and well disciplined force," as a matter of urgency ASO students and graduates met in Kirksville on April 19 to form a national organization. The American Association for the Advancement of Osteopathy (AAAO) had two objectives: to promote the science of osteopathy and to protect its members against medical persecution. Still occupied no official position but was elected in absentia to "the exalted dignity of honorary member."[3]

Arthur Hildreth, meantime, was also working to counter the renewed aggression. After the victory celebrations he returned to Chicago and there received a visit from colleague Al Boyles, who practiced in Bloomfield, Illinois, accompanied by an attorney. The medics had introduced a bill in the Illinois legislature to prohibit osteopathy and Boyles insisted that Hildreth act immediately to oppose the measure.

Hildreth hired a prominent lawyer and they traveled together to the State Capitol, Springfield. As soon as the hearing began it became apparent that the bill stood no chance of being passed. The House Public Health Committee – containing, surprisingly, only two physicians – adjudged that the MDs were seeking to secure a monopoly and wasted no time in killing the measure. On his lawyer's advice Hildreth seized the opportunity to introduce an osteopathic bill, framed similarly to the one passed in Missouri, and for the duration of the legislative session commuted to Springfield to spend two days a week speaking to members of the General Assembly. The measure passed comfortably in both houses but, as with the first Missouri bill, failed to be signed into law after vigorous medical lobbying persuaded Governor John R. Tanner to exercise his power of veto.

In the middle of the Illinois campaign Hon. Thomas F. Carroll, postmaster of Grand Rapids, Michigan, arrived at Hildreth's practice complaining that he did not have time to travel to Chicago every week for treatment. "I am going to Lansing," he declared, "[to] get a law so I can have an osteopathic physician of my own in Grand Rapids." The deadline for introducing new bills to the Michigan Legislature had already passed, but Carroll learned that Senator Charles W. Moore of Detroit, inspired by an article about the improvement of Senator Foraker's son in *Munsey's Magazine*, had already introduced a "skeleton bill" (a bill by title only) to have osteopathy recognized. Carroll used his influence to arrange a joint hearing before the House and Senate Health Committees, and asked Hildreth to accompany him to the State Capitol.

The joint committee (containing only one MD and one homeopath) overwhelmingly supported the measure. The only member to vote against was the chairman, Senator David Preston, who acted aloof and obstructive. The previous day, Preston told Carroll, they had passed a stringent medical practice act designed to stamp out all unrecognized systems, therefore to recommend the osteopathic measure would appear inconsistent. But the senator threw a lifeline: he was to chair a meeting of the Health Committee that evening and he invited Carroll and Hildreth to attend for a hearing.

They convened at seven. "I am going after you with a sharp stick," Preston immediately set the tone. "Dr. Hildreth, what would you do with a case of peritonitis?" Hildreth calmly turned the situation to his advantage. "Senator Preston," he returned, "what is peritonitis?" The attack ground to an abrupt halt. "Oh hell," the senator admitted lamely, "I don't know." Hildreth proceeded to describe the condition (inflammation of the abdominal lining) and the osteopathic approach to its treatment. "Senator Preston, which sounds more reasonable?" he spoke confidently. "We can put our hands on the spine of a patient and affect the nerves which control the circulation to a given area. It is circulation alone upon which a reduction in fever is dependent. By manipulation, or changing the position of a patient, we can change the action of the nerves that control the circulation in the inflamed area. In this way we also bring fresh blood to the area to replace that which has deteriorated. Is not this more reasonable than expecting two or three drops of medicine in a spoonful of water taken into the system through the mouth to locate the spot of inflammation?" By degrees the senator's belligerence turned to interest and then to fascination, and after the hearing he had Hildreth and Carroll explain osteopathy until they left to catch their train. "I like you both," he said as they departed. "You are good fellows and I will see what I can do."

When the bill came before the legislature Senator Preston spoke on osteopathy's behalf. The measure passed unopposed in the House, 24 to 1 in the Senate and, on April 21, the signature of Governor Hazen S. Pingree made Michigan the fourth state to recognize osteopathy.[4]

Still returned to Kirksville the third week in May. To help cope with the new influx of patients and students he persuaded Harry, Hildreth and their colleague Charles Hazzard to return from Chicago. They passed the practice on to Joe Sullivan and reported to the ASO on May 23.[5] To bolster the school's credentials Still equipped a new laboratory with compound microscopes, expanded the curriculum, and strengthened the faculty. He appointed Hazzard, a philosophy graduate of Northwestern University, Chicago, histology lecturer and, later that year, chair of Principles of Osteopathy; Carl McConnell clinic operator and later Professor of Osteopathic Practice; D. M. Desmond, a Harvard graduate, physiology lecturer; and Charley's brother-in-law Clarence Rider assistant in anatomy. Mary's nephew C. M. T. "Turner" Hulett, graduated the previous year, became the school's first dean. Since the new law required graduates to have attended a course of twenty months of study, early students who did not meet this criterion were urged to return for extra classes. And, as an expedient, on June 22 the Board of Trustees passed a motion that Still, his sons, Ed, and others, many of them in teaching positions, be unconditionally granted new DO diplomas.[6]

The medical men meanwhile, seeking new angles of attack, turned to allies in the press. At the end of May the St. Louis *Chronicle* assigned cub reporter Henry Stanhope Bunting to write a syndicated article on osteopathy. Briefed on the "bone-setting coterie which tied its faith to bone carpentering," he was dispatched to Kirksville with instructions to expose the fraud.

Before calling at the ASO Bunting decided to gauge public opinion by interviewing a cross-section of the townspeople. He expected cynicism, but to his surprise found no one who considered osteopathy a scam or a fad. Nobody even shrugged their shoulders; they evidently believed in the system and loved and respected its founder. The hotel proprietor praised Still as a benefactor, stores and banks gave nothing but endorsements, and the master of the train depot told of scores arriving on beds and leaving happy and well. Drug stores reported that Dr. Still cured without medicines, medical doctors put in a surprisingly good word, and health was said to be the chief resource of the evidently prosperous little town. The reporter finally called on an undertaker, but even he complained that business was depressingly quiet.

Bunting headed to the infirmary. There were patients everywhere and when they learned he was a reporter they hailed him, eager to talk. These people were neither gullible nor ignorant; some knew a great deal about medicine and had tried to learn all they could about their ailments. "Their stories were almost incredible," Bunting recounted. "The blind had come to see. The halt walked. Epilepsy had been banished. Fevers were aborted in a few hours. One patient who had been brought from an insane asylum was endowed with sense in a few weeks and he straightaway enrolled as a student. Goiters, nervous prostration, and the whole catalogue of woman's ills had been banished for all except those who still put their trust in old-time medicines." And all this was apparently achieved by no more than an intelligent direction of the body's fluids and forces. It was certainly not faith healing; the students learned anatomy, physiology, symptomatology and pathology in greater detail than the standard required of a surgeon. Bunting interviewed Charley and other faculty members, but continued to possess only a limited conception of how osteopathy worked and the one person he had not yet met was its founder.

Still was evasive when it came to journalists. After two fruitless days trying to collar him, Bunting was advised that his best chance was to get up very early and wait in the "Old Doctor's" back yard. (Everyone referred to him as the Old Doctor, he learned, to distinguish him from his sons, all Drs. Still.) The following morning Bunting rose at 3.30 and stationed himself by the smokehouse. An hour later Still emerged and seemed surprised to see the loitering stranger. Bunting, flustered, opened with a clumsy, "Do you use saltpeter in curing your side meats?" The doctor replied that he did not believe in drugs in any form; he relied only on natural smoke. Still invited him into the smokehouse, explained the curing process, and gave a tour of the meat he had ready for the winter. He pointed out a tree in the yard that he used to perform certain treatments and, after an hour's conversation, asked abruptly if he was talking to a newspaperman.

Bunting came clean about his assignment. Still pondered for a moment, said they should talk it over with his secretary and, notwithstanding the hour, they set off immediately up Jefferson Street, across the Wabash tracks, and directly to Henry Patterson's house. Still rapped on the door, entered, and Bunting followed into what turned out to be the bedroom. The Pattersons were still in bed and as Henry got hastily dressed Alice hid in embarrassment under the bedclothes. The three men went out onto the porch. Bunting learned that Dr. Still did not believe in advertising – he said he had nothing to advertise – and employed no form of persuasion to attract patients; the infirmary's success rested exclusively on results. Still moved on to "serious subjects" and, taking Bunting into his confidence, produced from his pocket "a very fine article on physiological therapeutics, which was strong and condensed." This he read aloud, striking the young reporter "most forcibly because of the wide field that he had covered in a very few words."

The *Chronicle* did not get the story they commissioned. Instead an article, "A Skeptic Investigating Osteopathy," appeared in the *Journal of Osteopathy*. "Perhaps the way a newspaper man was overwhelmed and forced to capitulate in spite of himself may have interest for the public," it began. "The issue of this battle is of more consequence than wars for the independence of states or the possession of territory." It concluded, in italics, "*Osteopathy is the opportunity of an epoch.*" Bunting returned to Kirksville the following year, as a student.[7]

In the midst of rapid change the one constant was the founder. With an aquiline nose, dusky skin finely wrinkled like a piece of old silk, and a humorous twinkle in eyes creased by laughter lines, Still appeared younger than his sixty-nine years. Changed little in manner or dress since his frontier days, he sported an open jacket, a blue army overcoat, an unbuttoned waistcoat held together by a heavy watch chain, and trousers or jeans tucked carelessly into knee high "Missouri mud boots," as he called them. Beneath a wide-brimmed black felt army hat feathery strands of iron-gray hair played against his high forehead, and under his gray beard gleamed a gold collar button, though rarely with a collar attached. He chewed tobacco or, when he occasionally managed to quit, ate chocolate. He walked around town with a characteristic forward-leaning gait, rising on his toes, resting on a staff six or seven feet long – perhaps a hickory stick he had whittled or planed in his workshop carved with hieroglyphs to symbolize some great truth he was always delighted to explain.[8]

The way he saw others transcended sex, race, rank, religion, manners or clothing; his respect was for genuineness, regardless of education or upbringing. He despised the superior attitude of some visitors towards the local residents. "When I see a town woman fail to speak to a farmer's wife and family when they meet," he wrote, "I pity the shoulders that carry such weak heads."[9] He detested condescension equally, rebuking anyone who touched their hat in deference with a gruff, "Don't tap your hat to me."

Wealth or social position engendered no special privileges. "The rich man and the washerwoman's child might be waiting for treatment," Nettie Bolles told. "If he could not treat both he would send the rich man away and treat the poor child. He said that the rich man could get other help and the poor child could not."[10]

For several weeks Still studiously avoided the fashionable son of a well-known Pennsylvania family who pompously insisted on receiving his personal attention. He was "very much of a chappy," a student related, "exceedingly well pleased with himself from both personal and intellectual standpoints." Late one afternoon Still arrived home to find the dandy waiting on his porch. The young man introduced himself, mentioned his father ("of whom you have doubtless heard") and asked for an examination. Still tried without success to fob him off with instructions to the infirmary, so finally instructed him to take a seat and describe his problem. "Well, Doctor," he said, "some have indicated that I have water on the brain." Still said nothing and ran his hands casually over his patient's head for a few minutes. "Huh," he uttered at last, "I don't see any evidence of brain whatever." Then, abruptly, he went into the house and closed the door.[11]

At the infirmary those who had money paid, but no one unable to pay was ever turned away. The poor were invariably treated without charge, and often given free board and lodging. No record remains of the untold sums Still gave away on the sly. He was forever sneaking around to the office for money to give to some impoverished person.[12] "My motto is *Help the needy, and deal justly with all,*" he stated. "I am not going to get rich or bust. I have made one rule in life; *reason first, justice and humanity all the time.*"[13] A principle he extended to rich and poor alike. When a wealthy Chicago patient sent a $1000 check in gratitude for services rendered, Still ordered Secretary Patterson to return $975 with a note, "My bill is $25."[14]

In these days of prosperity Still's closest companions remained those from his humbler days.[15] Now able to gratefully repay those who had given encouragement or even sympathy in his years of adversity, he might be seen surreptitiously and half-apologetically sneaking a crumpled ten dollar bill into a hand, "just for a bit of backy, John."[16] He had Patterson send regular checks of twenty-five dollars or more to a farmer's widow in Kansas in return for a kindness extended thirty years beforehand.[17] On visits to Baldwin he often took Carl McConnell for company and entrusted him with the purse. McConnell soon learned to purchase return tickets before leaving, for when they came back the purse was invariably empty, its contents distributed to some old friend. Being able to give in this way, Still said, was a "blessed privilege."[18]

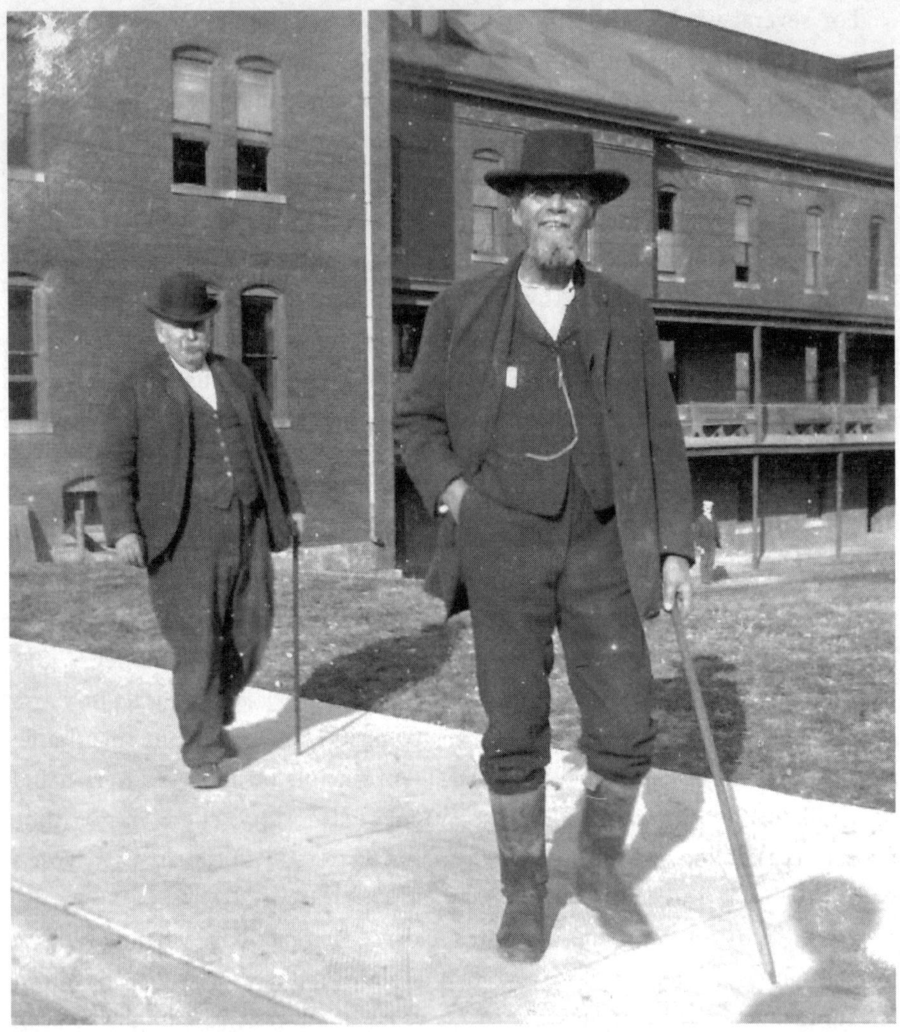

Still outside the infirmary with longtime friend Robert Harris, gunsmith.

He told his students he would rather have a much needed rest than their tuition fees,[19] and often accepted a personal note from a prospective matriculant unable to pay. All knew the curious ritual he performed with Charles Bandel, who arrived in Kirksville determined to study osteopathy but with practically no funds. On discovering just how little money the freshman possessed Still gave him enough to pay his room and board for the following week. At the same time every week, for the duration of the two-year course, he visited Bandel's meagerly furnished room, sat down to talk for a few minutes, and on leaving handed over a sum to pay the rent.[20] A few took advantage of his generosity, and many loans to unscrupulous acquaintances were never repaid.[21]

Some criticized his lack of entrepreneurial spirit. "Why, he could be rich," Still parodied, "but he has no business git to him."[22] He repeatedly resisted advice to patent osteopathy, insisting it was not for his own enrichment but for the benefit of mankind.[23] Besides, how could anyone claim ownership of the body's own remedies? "No man," he asserted, "has a patent right on any other man's privileges or nature's substances."[24] He detested the swindlers who tried to embroil him in financial schemes, urging him to form a closed corporation, and the sharpers who hung around the graduating classes "like buzzards over a dying hog," promising to make them rich by helping establish new schools and infirmaries.[25] Healing the sick should never form the basis of a money-making scheme.[26] Or, perhaps, anything else. "Whenever finance is your object," Still declared, "you are a thief and a liar."[27]

Many regarded him the incarnation of gentleness and kindness, the biggest hearted man on earth. "Now let me tell you something," he disabused any such notions. "I am as selfish as a wolf. I work and study hard from morning till night, year in and out, not for your happiness but for A. T. Still's. I love an honest toiler either of body and mind. I hate a liar, a thief, a hypocrite or a lazy person equally, they are all alike to me. I will help those who have an honest claim on my sympathy, and in a loving manner, as a man should help his fellow man."[28]

Eventually Mary became concerned that his generosity was getting out of hand and informed him that henceforth she would act as treasurer; he must hand over all monies received and she would give him what was to be paid out. "He who steals my purse steals trash," he was heard to comment, "but I guess I let go of my trash a little too easily sometimes. Mother says so, and she is right."[29] Of course he played on it. One morning, walking briskly past a group of students, he called over to say he was going home to see if Ma would give him a nickel to buy a paper.[30]

With hundreds of patients undergoing treatment it had long been impossible for the founder to supervise every case and to the displeasure of many a well-heeled patient he now saw only those he chose to. During the construction of the north wing a refined Boston lady insisted on being examined by Dr. Still and no one else, and only when told he was currently superintending the building work and not taking regular patients did she reluctantly agree to be seen by Arthur Hildreth instead. One hot humid day, as she waited for her appointment, a laborer in corduroy pants and a collarless blue flannel shirt ambled in from the construction site. He greeted her pleasantly, asked if she was waiting for treatment, and invited her to step into a vacant room.

The lady replied that she was perfectly satisfied with Dr. Hildreth's treatment and would wait. "All right," the workman said, a faint smile spreading under his beard, "if you prefer Dr. Hildreth to me, I have nothing to say." As he set off slowly down the hall the woman hastily beckoned the janitor to ask the identity of the impudent ragamuffin with the audacity to speak to her like that. "Why, don't you know him," John Colbert said, "that's Dr. Still." The woman stayed for several months (and went home cured) but Still never gave her another chance.[31]

Thekla Orschel from Livingston, Montana, was another accustomed to preferential treatment. For sixteen years she had suffered from a debilitating condition diagnosed variously as rheumatism, ganglion, "weeping sinew," and "tuberculosis manifesting as tendon tubercular synovitis." Her weight dropped from 150 to 103 pounds, her elbows and upper arms ached with intense pain, her wrist and finger joints were markedly swollen, and contractures drew the little and middle fingers almost to the palm. Despite the interested attention of leading doctors in many cities the problem continued to worsen until there came a worrying development: a small abscess the size of a pea appeared in the palm of one hand with red streaks of lymphangitis extending up the forearm. Her doctor drained the pus and suggested antiseptic poultices to retard septicemia, but did not know what further to do. A friend finally suggested Orschel consult a doctor in Kirksville, Missouri, who used no medicines but had a reputation for curing many stubborn ailments. Her husband Herman encouraged her to go and, despite lacking faith that it would help, she registered at the infirmary in May 1897.

Orschel was introduced to Still, escorted into a treatment room and subjected to a highly unusual examination. The doctor leaned against the door casing, cast his eyes vaguely towards her abdomen and sized her up with a peculiar, penetrating gaze. "Why do you look at me like that?" she challenged.

"I wondered whether you could look right through me." "Yes I can," the doctor replied. "I saw your liver, it looks awful and needs a good overhauling." She asked how he proposed to do that. Still said he would do nothing; the treatment would be given by one of his assistants.

Orschel asserted that she would be treated by him personally or consult a renowned specialist in New York instead. Still considered this for a moment and said he would speak to his secretary, Dr. Patterson, to decide the best course of action, and asked her to call at his house the following morning.

Next day Still informed Orschel that he would treat her for $100 a month, paid in advance. She protested that the advertised charge was $25. "That is correct," he acknowledged, "but you wanted Dr. A. T.'s personal attention and, of course, we charge more for it." This was untrue; he was calling her bluff. Orschel telegraphed her husband to ask whether to pay the extra or settle for one of his assistants. Herman told her to see Dr. Still even if he asked $500.

Still regarded what would now be called rheumatoid arthritis as a systemic problem associated with poor function of the "excretory system," with symptoms arising from the toxic effects of retained metabolites. Any joint from the skull to the coccyx might be responsible, especially those of the upper cervical vertebrae. Lesions here might cause congestion in the intricate venous plexus around the spinal cord, in the cerebellum, or – most importantly – in the brainstem, where the sympathetic, vagus and cardiac nerves originate.[32]

He began by addressing treatment to Orschel's liver, to detoxify it from years of medication. A month later the swellings showed no signs of change. She now had the upper hand and told Still that since she had trusted him, he would now trust her to pay not at the beginning but at the end of the second month. Still enjoyed a battle of wits. He told her to pay no more until he asked for it, then invited her to step onto some weighing scales. She had gained three pounds, the first increase in years.

After ten weeks the inflammation began to subside and after six months her almost useless hands regained normal form and function. "The gratitude I feel to Dr. A. T. Still is just as indescribable as the pity I feel for the M.D.s who meant so well with their thankful patient," Orschel wrote on returning home. "Perhaps Christ understood this method of healing to perfection, for he healed the paralytic, deaf and blind without medicine. So too does Dr. A. T. Still, only it takes a longer time with the latter gentleman."[33] The Orschel family became lasting friends.

Another wealthy patient was Ellen Barrett Ligon, of Okolona, Mississippi, an elocutionist of "rare culture and magnetic manners" chosen by the National Editorial Association to read the poem *Columbia Saluting the Nations* at Chicago's Columbian Exposition. Ligon arrived at the infirmary in October 1897 suffering from a progressive condition that had resisted all medical help. A bout of influenza seven years earlier had left her with "complicated nervous troubles," a jaundiced body she described as "a stack of bones covered with some yellow skin," and a heart that ran erratically, irregularly skipping beats or running at 140 a minute. For the past two years she had been able to digest little more than malted milk and raw egg whites.[34] Her uncle, grandfather and great-grandfather were all physicians and she had been raised to believe that any system not "regular" was quackery, but after reading a *Literary Digest* article about Charley's success with diphtheria in Red Wing her lawyer husband Greenwood, tired of doctors patching up symptoms, persuaded her to make the one thousand mile trip to Kirksville.

On her arrival Ligon was disappointed to learn that Dr. Still would not be able to treat her personally. For two weeks she waited patiently for an opportunity to speak to him, until one day she rounded the corner near his house and saw him talking to Julia Foraker, who made the introduction. Still took Ligon's arm and escorted her to his office. To her astonishment he asked no questions, made no examinations, yet seemed to know all at once everything that was wrong. "You know what happened to your eyes?" he said. She had not mentioned her eyes. "You had whooping cough and nearly jerked your head off. You did jerk your neck out of place, and that was what happened to your eyes." Neither had she mentioned the appalling attack of whooping cough at age eleven, since when she had needed to wear glasses.

Still instructed Ligon to lie on the treatment table. "Now, I have fixed your innominate bone," he said, correcting a sacroiliac joint, "and you won't feel any longer as if you were being poured out of a bottle. About nine out of ten sick women have slipped innominates."[35] He then asked her to accompany him to the dissection room to demonstrate the cause of her problem on a cadaver.

Ligon followed along in mounting dread of seeing the dead body. To her relief the room was being used by William Smith, but by the time they got back to Still's office her anxiety had precipitated an attack of hyperventilation. Still saw this and told her to unfasten her collar. He took the front of the left fifth rib in one hand and the back with the other, and gave a deft twist. "The rib is always wrong when you are short winded," he said. After that he passed her case over to Harry, who fixed "several dozen other things" and she returned home free of all symptoms. The experience was life-changing. Though in their late forties both she and husband Greenwood, who gave up his successful law practice, returned to Kirksville six weeks later to enroll as students.[36]

The dissection room had opened in summer 1897. Designed in the form of an amphitheater, it enabled students to view anatomical demonstrations in time-honored fashion. The ASO had difficulty procuring cadavers, though, as the medical profession did everything in its power to prevent it (and then accused osteopaths of being uneducated for lacking practice in dissection).[37] During the fall term a student approached William Smith with a possible solution to the problem.

The student's sister was married to a captain of the Chicago police at Dunning, Illinois, location of the Cook County Poor Farm, whose morgue supplied cadavers to medical schools. On November 13, Smith and anatomy assistant Clarence Rider (Charley's brother-in-law) traveled to Dunning to meet the police captain, who introduced them to the morgue's night watchman, Mr. Ulrich. Smith negotiated prices – $50 for males, $60 for females – and instructed Ulrich to hire an express man to collect from Chicago four trunks, built especially for transporting the bodies, containing surgical instruments, embalming fluid and packing paper. They arranged to meet outside the Poor Farm at midnight.

The two doctors arrived at the gate at the appointed time, drenched and dispirited after a two-mile walk from the end of the streetcar line in a steady drizzle. They were met by John Rowe, express wagon driver, and Ulrich, about whom they immediately began to feel uneasy. "His eyes were too close together," Rider noted, "his forehead was too low, he had a hard look in his cold blue eyes, and his conversation was uncouth and freely interspersed with profanity." Ulrich led them into a room containing thirteen dead bodies, twelve male and one female, all unclaimed and ready for the potter's field. If these were unsuitable, he offered helpfully, they could select what they wanted from the hospital's "killer ward." Smith made clear they had not come for freshly murdered specimens and quickly selected three males and the single female. Ulrich directed them to a derelict house nearby to embalm the bodies.

They heaved the four naked corpses onto Rowe's wagon, carried them into the tumbledown building, and laid them on the dusty floor of what had once been a parlor. In this forlorn place, with its collapsed staircase, unhinged doors and window shutters banging in the breeze, the two doctors undertook the messy process of preserving the cadavers under the dim light of Rowe's lantern. Two hours later Smith attached to the trunks shipping tags marked "books," addressed them to himself in Kirksville, and instructed Rowe to deliver them to the American Express office in Chicago first thing in the morning.

Filthy, sodden and reeking of formaldehyde, Smith and Rider returned to the city on the elevated railway. They checked into a hotel, took baths, ate breakfast, sent their soiled clothes to be cleaned, and slept till 1 p.m. On waking Smith sent for the noon edition of a Chicago newspaper, and was shocked to see emblazoned in large letters on the front page the headline: "BIG ROBBERY AT THE DUNNING MORGUE." A lurid story followed about how ghouls had smashed the door of the mortuary and made off with four dead bodies. The two doctors spent an unbearably anxious afternoon waiting for their train. When they arrived back in Kirksville the trunks were already waiting at the Wabash depot and Smith had them sent immediately to the ASO.

The Cook County Grand Jury offered $500 rewards for information leading to the arrests of the robbers and the wagon driver. In December Ulrich's girlfriend informed on Rowe, and a month later identified the thieves.

Smith and Rider were indicted of breaking into the morgue and, since by law a dead body possessed no monetary value, charged with stealing four sheets, value $1 each, in which they had supposedly wrapped the corpses (this was a fabrication; they had left the sheets on the mortuary slabs). Illinois governor John R. Tanner requisitioned his Missouri counterpart to surrender the criminals to stand trial. Lon Stephens summoned the pair to Jefferson City, but after hearing their version of events refused to comply with Tanner's request. "That bunch of politicians up there," he told the hapless doctors, "would want to put you in the penitentiary for life." The Missouri governor promised to use his influence to gain the ASO a fair quota of the state's unclaimed dead, and to preserve the reputation of the Dunning police captain Smith and Rider provided sworn statements attesting that he had nothing to do with the sale of the bodies. Ulrich was sentenced to a long stretch in the Joliet penitentiary.[38]

For Still the infirmary and school had become an immense burden. In November he jotted down a short composition entitled *Joy*:

> Joy is the reward for which all beings strive to obtain. Joy is that feeling that comes to a contented mind. Its effect is rest to soul and body. When

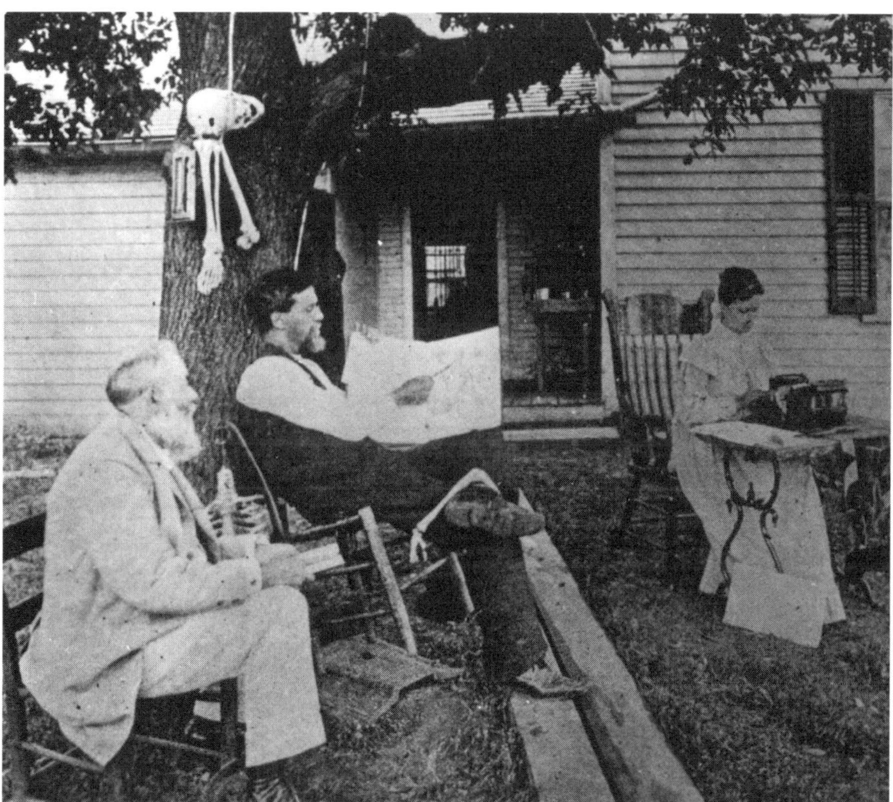

Col. A. L. Conger, Still and Annie Morris at the Morris farm, Millard, Missouri.

> a person is in possession of that precious gem, all is peace and love to man and beast, friend and foe. Joy comes often in a small way; it lasts but a short time then gives way to cares.[39]

At the end of January 1897 he penned another piece entitled *Blazes*:

> The once brilliant red blazes of life and ambition [are] now beginning to lose much of their charms to me. . . . Joy, like sugar, [feeds] the mind only for a time. The newest of the new soon grows old with me – I must quit the seas with my compass as a mental explorer and play with the babes and cats till my brain weighs more to the ounce and my heart weighs less to the pound.[40]

Mary and Blanche tried to protect him from an endless stream of callers. The infirmary staff constantly pestered him to work his magic on some stubborn case. New patients continually pressed for his personal attention,[41] and some even devised cunning schemes to waylay him. A favorite ploy was to watch where he left his hat and apprehend him when he returned to retrieve it. This rarely worked. Still had many hats and all looked alike. On entering the building he usually deposited the one he was wearing at the first convenient place and on leaving found another somewhere else.[42]

When the demands became oppressive a scared, hunted look came over him. At such times he might relax in his workshop,[43] walk self-absorbedly down the street,[44] or spend a few hours chatting with his old friend Father George Chappell at the priest's home or astride an old log in the woods.[45] When he wanted to get away completely he took the train to Millard's Station, the first stop south of Kirksville, and walked a mile down the dusty track to the farm of his old friends Sol and Annie Morris.[46] On summer days he took his horse and buggy, often stopping in the street to informally pick up a student for company.

The comfortable homestead, set between woods and fields, had well-fed animals, free-roaming chickens, a generously stocked barn and a heaping wood pile near the door. Still had first called there in 1877 to treat Annie, at that time a bedridden invalid. Inspired by her recovery, she taught herself anatomy and physiology, learned to type, and by stages became his secretary and amanuensis.

On the Morris farm Still worked out most of his philosophy, made plans for the school and infirmary, and wrote his *Journal* articles. Early sensing the importance of his work, Annie kept fragments of his writing, some of it dating as far back as 1885.

Still treated the property like a second home, a haven where he could write and study undisturbed. He visited almost every week, often staying for days at a time, and came and went as he pleased. On hand were skeletons, charts, and a library of medical and other books, and when an idea struck him Annie dropped everything to take down his dictation.[47] She possessed qualities he appreciated. "Am at 'Mother' Morris now and will stay until I get fat," he wrote Thekla Orschel. "She is good to me. And is a poor talker so I get to rest from gab."[48] For the past two years Annie had carefully transcribed some of his Memorial Hall lectures and suggested he prepare a book from them. With visitors continually asking to read his life story, he decided to combine the two ideas.

Nationally known writer John R. Musick, whose *Columbian Historical Novels* were admired by President McKinley,[49] helped compile the work. It was none other than Musick who in 1875, as co-editor of Kirksville newspaper *The Tattler,* had branded Still a "shameless humbug." When they became acquainted a year later, however, he found the bone doctor to be quite different to what he had been led to believe. During the seventies and eighties Still frequently called at the writer's law office on the square to talk politics, reminisce about army days, and tell humorous anecdotes about his peripatetic practice. Musick had found Still genial and kindhearted, if diffident, but continued to think him "peculiarly eccentric," the way "his brow was so often corrugated with thought and his form bent as if seeking into forbidden mysteries," and remained skeptical about the stories of cures.

While Musick was staying in a New York boarding house in 1889 a guest, on hearing that he hailed from Missouri, asked if he had heard of "that wonderful man, Dr. A. T. Still, the most remarkable man I ever met." She related how, in Hannibal, she had seen him perform "one of the most marvelous cures since Christ healed the leper," and asked how the doctor was regarded in Kirksville. Musick was taken aback, thinking the woman overly credulous, and replied that some thought Dr. Still crazy, the way he was always talking about bones and spinal cords and the like. "I don't believe you people in Kirksville appreciate what a genius you have in your town," the woman laughed. "People said Morse was crazy when he began to talk telegraphy; others that he was possessed of a devil, but he proved to be the wise man and they the fools. Dr. Still will some day break away the barriers of entrenched ignorance and prejudice and startle the world."[50]

In the intervening years Musick had grown to become one of Still's closest friends, staunchest supporters and an occasional contributor, under the sobriquet "M," to the *Journal of Osteopathy*. One of his lesser-known works, *Crutches for Sale*, dramatized the true story of a wealthy Montana rancher's daughter, injured in a riding accident and brought to Still after being pronounced incurable by an eminent Eastern specialist.[51] "The sight of a man running through the streets," Musick wrote:

> tears of joy streaming down his cheeks, offering to sell the crutches which his child had used for years, and thousands of hopeless cases restored to new life, everybody understood what that 'harmless old crank' had been doing all the years they were making him the butt of ridicule. When I recollect that all this hard study and scientific investigation was going on in our midst, in spite of the ridicule and opposition of scientific men, who entrenched in theories always oppose free investigation, I feel like exclaiming with Puck in Shakespeare's *Midsummer Night's Dream*, 'What fools these mortals be!'[52]

The *Autobiography of A. T. Still* was published in March 1898, and within a short time over two thousand copies had been "sold." A business venture it was not – he gave a free copy to every student and graduate. Freshman F. P. Millard, on only his second day in Kirksville, called to introduce himself and left with a complimentary copy inscribed, *I love you also. A. T. Still*. The student thought it unusually nice of someone he had never met before.[53]

19

MATTER

Still never stopped studying. Focusing exhaustively on some detail, approaching it from every angle, he shaped and squared and built what he learned into the edifice of his accumulated knowledge. The students were constantly surprised by his profound erudition, his ability to convey so much in a few words, and his success in cases that had puzzled others.[1]

They were awed by his mastery of anatomy. He would close his eyes and ask them to name a bone – any bone – and proceed to reel off its articulations, muscle attachments, nerve and blood supply. They tested him again and again, trying to catch him out, but without success. Equally impressive but less vaunted was his grasp of physiology. "He gave far more thought to this subject than to any other," Carl McConnell related. "The mechanism of an enzyme was to Dr. Still just as important, if not more so, as the locating and correction of a lesioned vertebra."[2]

But isolated facts occupied Still only transitorily.[3] His focus was ever on the whole, the body a "sum of vital unities," trillions of living beings each performing their specialized roles towards one common expression. "Every organ has a vote in a drop of urine," he lectured to one class. "If you get it so that every cell can come out and cast his vote, you have health. So in a drop of nasal secretion, so in ear wax."[4]

Faced with a new problem he applied himself single-mindedly to its solution, convinced it was to be found with the right search. Lost in a world of absorption, temporarily forgetting all else, he never rested day or night until he got to the bottom of it.[5] Joe Sullivan told of him regularly dropping in on his student lodgings, often before sunrise, to share his conclusions. Once, after a sleepless night mulling over an unusually difficult case, he called at 4.30 a.m. to report that he thought he had found the answer and, heedless of the hour, set off immediately to find the patient.[6]

Eager to share what he had learned Still would enter a class – freshmen or seniors, it made no difference – to tell them the new thing: an investigation he was making, an insight about some part of the body, an experimental treatment for a particular condition.[7] He would go on for days or months about his current topic, drawing analogies, suggestions or problems from incidents of the day, and these occasions were laden with gems for the student who listened closely. At first they might think he intended this one thing to supersede all his other teachings, but with familiarity they learned his true meaning: no part, however small, is insignificant. "If a thousand kinds of fluids exist in our bodies," he said, "a thousand uses require their help."[8] Nature does nothing in vain.

Still labored over obscure details. He observed that the omentum, the apron-like fold of peritoneum enclosing the intestines, was invariably abnormal in tuberculosis. He insisted that the medical books were incorrect in stating that the joint in the sternum between the manubrium and gladiolus ossifies in the adult.[9] He pondered the exquisite mechanism of the spinal cord's blood circulation, suggesting that lesions of the spine and ribs might interfere with it and impair the function of individual nerve tracts within the cord.[10] He proposed that a diminished supply of cerebrospinal fluid ("one of the highest known elements that are contained in the body") might adversely affect the entire nervous system and thereby reduce a person's general vitality.[11] He wondered what force enabled the blood to return from the capillary beds, where the pulse beat petered out, back to the venous system.

The school's acquisition of compound microscopes opened up new vistas, revealing to his eyes what he had previously only read about in books. He followed arteries and veins as they repeatedly branched and narrowed, "until the lenses of the most powerful microscopes seemed to exhaust their ability to perceive the termination."[12] He observed the lymphatic system, draining even the minutest recesses, each vessel served by infinitesimally small nerves. He saw "millions of nerves by which all organs and parts are supplied with the elements of motion" and, at the limit of magnification, "infinitely small fibers around which those fine nerve vines entwine. First like a bean entwining by way of the right, and then turn my microscope to the entwining of another set of nerves which is to the left universally as the hop." And, he noted, all nerves "go to and terminate in that great system, the fascia."[13]

The word *fascia*, in Still's usage, signified the ubiquitous connective tissues that unite every part of the body, at every level of scale, from the skin to the cell nucleus. The fascia "sheathes, permeates, divides and sub-divides every portion of animal bodies," he wrote, "surrounding and penetrating every muscle and all its fibers – every artery, and every fiber and principle thereunto belonging, and grows more wonderful as your eye is turned on the venous system with its great company of lymphatics." He beheld the fascia's complexity. "It is almost a network of nerves, cells and tubes, running to and from it; it is crossed and filled with, no doubt, millions of nerve centers." Awed at its universality – its "omnipresence" – he veered towards the religious, lauding the "great power with which the fascia is endowed" and glorifying it as "the material man, and the dwelling place of his spiritual being."[14] He went as far as to declare, "the soul of man with all the streams of pure living water seems to dwell in the fascia of his body."[15]

Driving this extravagant language was what he had learned from *Cellular Pathology*. Virchow laid great emphasis upon the "often very abundant mass of matter which lies between the cells."[16] He even described this intercellular substance as a "matrix"[17] – a word usually reserved for the uterus, the "mother" of the fetus – for here, he concluded, gestate "by far the greater number of new-formations which arise in the body in accordance with the same law which regulates embryonic development."[18] By "new-formations" Virchow meant benign and malignant tumors, and the various swellings and tumefactions produced by inflammatory processes. "The fascia proves itself to be the probable matrix of life and death,"[19] Still echoed. "By its action we live and by its failure we shrink, or swell, and die."[20] For in this fertile soil, "diseases germinate and develop the seeds of sickness and death."[21]

Since cells depend entirely upon the fluid-filled intercellular substance – the internal equivalent of Pasteur's *terrain* – to supply oxygen and nutrients and remove metabolic wastes, Still taught that unimpeded arterial, venous and

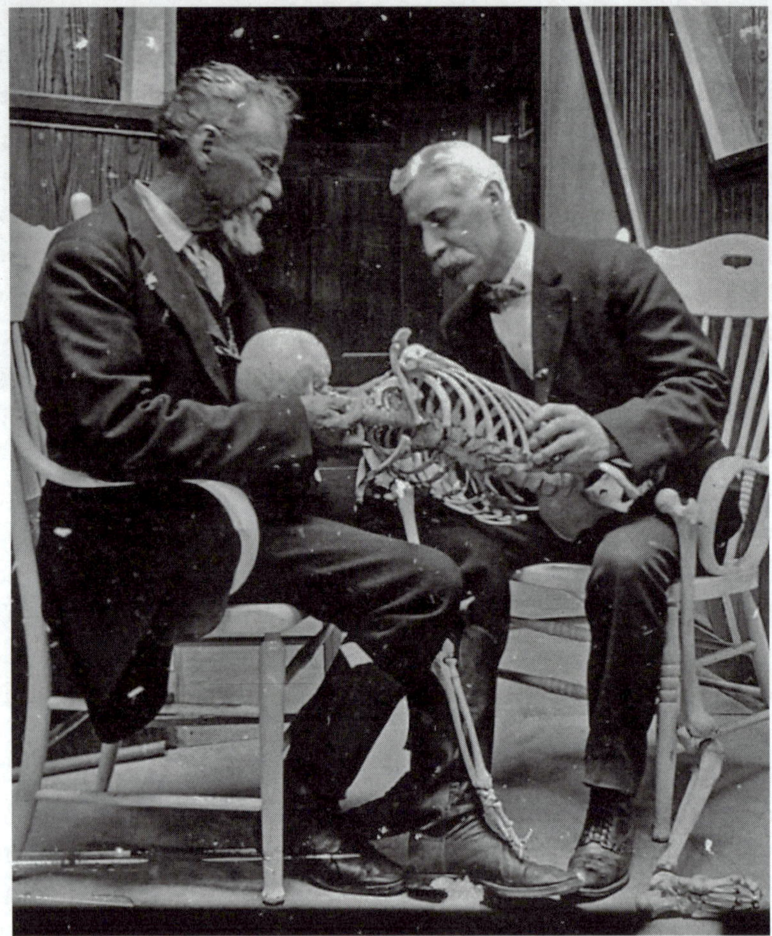

Still with graduate F. G. Cluett.

lymphatic flow is essential. He continually stressed that the body's circulating fluids must be free to remove "dead substances before they ferment in lymphatics and cellular system."[22]

Any mechanical disorder, however small, could be a potent cause of disease. Any slip, strain or bruise of the spine or ribs might disturb the circulation of an organ, gland or other structure, leading to fascial congestion and tumefaction, and suitable conditions for microbes to breed or growths to develop. "What we meet with in all disease," Still paraphrased Virchow, "is dead blood, stagnant lymph, and albumen in a semi-vital or dead and decomposing condition all through the lymphatics and other parts of the body, brain, lungs, kidneys, liver and fascia. The whole system is loaded with a confused mass of blood that is mixed with much or little unhealthy substances."[23]

Successful treatment demanded the restoration of normal physiology, and that, in turn, relied upon an intimate knowledge of the body structure. "We want you to thoroughly understand anatomy so that it will come to you as quick as 'ouches' to a Dutchman's mouth when he gets his finger hurt," Still lectured. "It ought to be second nature. It should be as indelibly fixed as passing the hat is on the minister's mind."[24] He insisted his students know accurately "the form of each bone, how and where it articulates with others, how it is joined by ligaments, what blood vessels, nerves and muscles cross or range with it lengthwise" – and even that they know which nerves supply "each minute cell, fascia, gland and blood vessel."[25] Some displacements of vertebrae and ribs might be so miniscule, he warned, that "an old operator has to use all his caution or he will fail to observe one, and many times is at a loss to know why his patient gets no better."[26]

The principle of cause and effect must be applied at all times. "Do you ever suspect renal or bladder trouble," he asked when teaching urology:

> without first learning from your patient that there is soreness and tenderness in the region of the kidneys along the spine? By this knowledge you are invited to explore the spine for the purpose of ascertaining whether it is normal or not. If by your intimate acquaintance with a normal spine you should detect in this region an abnormality in form, you are then admonished to look out for diseases of kidneys or bladder as a result of the discovered displacement, or slight variation from normal, causing a disturbance of the renal nerves. If this variation is not worthy of your attention, your mind is surely too crude to observe those fine beginnings that lead to death.[27]

Experience had taught Still that "the nerve at the anterior end of the eighth rib on the left controls tension in the intestinal and stomach walls," and that the head of the tenth rib on the left must articulate normally for "the solids of the body [to be] kept in soluble form until needed for building, instead of being pathologically deposited as calculi or arthritic deposits."[28] Such statements could sound farfetched to the uninitiated, but Ellen Ligon witnessed for herself the effect of a displacement of the right tenth rib when her eleven-year-old daughter Lucile became sick with fever, high temperature and urinary urgency.

After four weeks of Harry's treatment the fever subsided, but urinalysis revealed a persistent excess of urates. Two months later the fever returned, a mild temperature in the morning rising to several degrees above normal in the evening, and her urine showed excess sugar and chlorides. Charley took over Lucile's treatment and corrected some spinal joints. Again the fever abated but her urine continued to worsen, turning cloudy and dark with a brick dust sediment, until uric acid sands became visible to the naked eye. When Still heard this from the laboratory chemist he called at the Ligons' home that afternoon.

Lucile's fourth lumbar was lesioned and radiating heat. These local variations in skin temperature, missed by an oral thermometer, indicated disturbed sympathetic nerve function and proved faithful guides for identifying lesions. Still routinely swept his hands over a patient's skin, back and front, down the midline and a little to each side, comparing left and right, feeling for hot or cold areas.[29]

After correcting the fourth lumbar he announced that a lesioned right tenth rib was irritating the nerves to the adrenal glands. "Now," he said, adjusting it, "the nervous system can take a message through, and the proper solvents for the renal salts will be made, and they will no longer be thrown down as precipitates. There may not be any further appearance of them, as the mechanism having been adjusted the cure will begin instantly." Two hours later, to the amazement of her mother who called the laboratory chemist and several others for verification, Lucile's urine had turned a clear light straw color. A week later the dark cloudy urine returned, but this setback served only to confirm Still's statements. Lucile had fallen, injuring the same rib, and once corrected her urine again reverted to normal, with no further trouble.[30]

Another important structure was the clavicle, for a lesioned joint at either end, Still taught, could have "serious and far reaching results." A displaced clavicle might interfere with the thoracic duct (the main lymphatic vessel) where it discharges into the left subclavian vein and thereby affect almost any region of the body; or, by direct pressure or nerve irritation, compromise venous drainage from the head and neck to potentiate a host of problems.[31] Still compared tonsillitis to a water barrel with the bunghole closed; the bung – a lesioned clavicle or contracted neck muscles – preventing the efficient return of blood from the head to the heart to produce congestion and inflammation. Instead of performing a tonsillectomy, he advised, simply open the bunghole.[32]

Tonsillitis could have other causes, too. Of all things that can produce unsuspected and extensive effects, Still told Ellen Ligon, the little hyoid bone heads the list. Contraction of any of its muscular attachments – to the floor of the mouth, tongue, epiglottis, larynx or pharynx – could predispose to tonsillitis, laryngitis, croup, coughs, gastric disturbances or, by interfering with the vagus nerve, even heart trouble. In demonstrating how to treat the hyoid he asked Ligon for a clean handkerchief, wrapped it around his forefinger, and asked her to open her mouth. "Now," he said, putting the finger far down her throat, "when you want to treat tonsils, sore throat, or ears for deafness, go down there with your finger, stretch the hyoid muscles, stretch the pillars of the fauces, go as far as the opening of the eustachian tube."[33]

A lesioned hyoid could have serious consequences, as one student learned on making a house call. He asked Bill Smith to accompany him and they arrived to find the patient, diagnosed as being in the last stages of tuberculosis, vomiting fresh blood. Smith made an examination and corroborated the diagnosis, but as they were leaving, the patient's wife, in tears, begged them to ask Dr. Still if he could do anything.

Still returned with the student, ran his fingers over the sick man, said he thought he could cure him, and performed "some sort of a jerk." That night the patient slept well and in the morning felt much better, and after two more treatments was well enough to return home. The man did not have tuberculosis, Still explained: "He had a hyoid bone that was displaced, and the digastric muscles on both sides were interfering with the salivary glands, so that the poor cuss wasn't digesting his food right, and the hemorrhages came from the relaxed state of the blood vessels in his throat." A real mechanical diagnosis, the student thought, jaw hanging. "Now, boy," Still counseled, "you always look for that condition when you have a case with hemorrhage and wasting away of tissue, then you can cure them if you keep studying anatomy all the time."[34]

A woman with longstanding oral inflammation had consulted specialists in Chicago and St. Louis without benefit. Still examined her mouth and neck, then corrected the temporomandibular joints, saying that improper articulation of the jawbone often disturbed the little sphenopalatine nerve ganglia controlling the blood supply to the region. After a treatment lasting no more than three minutes he told the patient's husband, "That is all, you may go home if you want to, your wife will get well." The man was astounded, thinking he had come to the biggest fake in the world, but within twenty-four hours she began to improve and two weeks later was fully recovered.[35]

Oculists had failed to help a woman in constant pain after being hit in the left eye by half a lemon. Still looked intently at the eyeball and noticed a slight irregularity in the bulge of the cornea. Surmising that the projectile had pushed the lens to one side, he placed the ball of his thumb against the eyeball, gave a gentle tap, and the lens sprang back into place.

One patient experienced agonizing attacks of pain in his left foot. He would be seen rocking back and forth for a few minutes, pale and sweating, clutching the extremity until the misery subsided. Still happened to witness one of these performances outside the infirmary. Leaning on his long staff, he observed the man for a minute or two, then got onto his knees, grasped the foot gently, looped a handkerchief around the big toe, and gave a yank and a twist. Afterwards he told a student his diagnosis: the little sesamoid bone within the tendon of the flexor hallucis brevis muscle had slipped sideways, causing the irritation.[36]

The body's complex interconnections often made diagnosis difficult. One time Still's own condition perplexed him. After falling onto his back on an icy flight of steps he developed a "disabling" heart complaint that persisted despite a number of treatments. Eventually Charley found a lesion at the third lumbar and told his father he believed the problem was somehow related. Correction of the joint did indeed resolve the issue, but the question was why? The answer emerged as Still's parable of the goat and the boulder:

> You know if a goat butts something that does not get out of the way, the next time it butts a little bit harder, and its tail flies up; and the next time harder still, and its heels fly up; and the next time so hard that all the hind end of the goat flies up – and that's what happened with my heart.

> Charley found the cause but I found out why it was the cause. The pup smelled the rat, but it took the old dog to scratch it out. So watch your diaphragm, not only for the attachment of the six lower ribs, but for the attachment to the lumbar vertebrae.

The explanation: the diaphragm, the fibro-muscular structure separating the thoracic and abdominal cavities, attaches down to the second and third lumbar vertebrae by two tendinous elongations called crura, one on each side. Left and right crus join to form an arch anterior to the spine, through which passes the aorta, the main artery from the heart. Still reasoned that the lesioned third lumbar had caused reflex diaphragmatic tension, constricting the aorta as it passed under the crural arch, thus making the heart work harder to force the blood past the obstruction.[37] Like any other muscle, he taught, the heart will enlarge to cope with the added work and such might be the beginning of heart disease.

What would medicine have done for such a case? Still explained by means of another analogy. Suppose an overloaded horse is climbing a hill. To make the ascent it must proceed slowly and, left to its own devices, might accomplish the task, but if spurred or whipped might collapse under the strain. "A horse needs strength instead of the spur to enable him to carry a heavy load," he said, "so a man needs the freedom of all parts of the machinery."[38] Heart stimuli, by increasing pulse rate and force of contraction, impose further strain on an already laboring organ; sedatives like opium and morphine cause sluggishness of the entire vascular system. "Osteopathy seeks to avoid all unnatural stupefying substances or stimulants," he declared:

> This method of reasoning should reach a man who is stupid enough to inject in the human body an opiate that would produce inaction of any organ. He would see at once that he had perverted the absolute cause that governs the circulation of blood to and from the heart. By retention of blood confusion is set up in the body, and you may expect fermentation of fluids followed by disease.[39]

The diaphragm was a potential cause of innumerable problems, in many cases by interfering with the aorta or other important structures that pass through it. Pressure upon the esophagus or vagus nerves might upset digestion and assimilation of food, and thereby impair general vitality. Pressure upon the vena cava might compromise venous return from the lower half of the body, leading to a host of abdominal and pelvic diseases "booked as causes unknown" by medicine. Lesions of any of the diaphragm's bony attachments to the spine or lower six ribs might cause irritation and contraction and, by restricting the breath, disturb gaseous exchange in the lungs. "An unhealthy condition of the diaphragm," Still pronounced, "is bound to be followed by many diseases."[40]

In fall 1898 he himself experienced an irregular heartbeat and blamed diaphragmatic tension. On November 6 he wrote Henry Patterson (who, invited by Senator Foraker, had resigned as ASO secretary to open a practice in Washington, D.C.): "I am better now. Found the ensiform [xiphoid] cartilage stove in and that let 6th & 7th ribs drop off sternum and fall under the spinous process, which shut off intercostal nerves and nerve supply to diaphragm which bothered aorta as it passed through diaphragm, causing palpitation of the heart."[41]

A condition with potentially serious consequences was obesity. The compression and weight of organs sagging into the pelvis might stretch the *mesentery*, the connective tissue membrane supporting the internal organs and carrying their nerve and blood supply. "In gastroptosis there is a pulling of the esophagus," Still said, "a pulling on an infinity of infinitesimal nerves and fascia, stretching the meso-throat, the meso-tongue, meso-heart, meso-lung, and all the mesos [connective tissue supports]. Every fish on that pole is bruised. A small boy with a fish on a stick knows enough to carry the stick sideways."[42] His meaning: in quadrupeds the internal organs hang from a horizontal spine; in man they hang more vertically, making stagnation and congestion more likely, with a host of possible effects. Mesenteric tension might irritate the splanchnic nerves (the sympathetic nerves to the gut) to disturb peristalsis and result in diarrhea, constipation and sometimes, in chronic cases, impacted fecal matter.[43] Or, by restricting blood circulation, it might cause kidney, stomach, pancreatic and other problems, including all manner of benign and malignant growths. "Cut off the splanchnic," he warned, "and you will be all tumors below."[44]

Prolapsed viscera formed the substance of many a lecture. Sagging of the sigmoid colon and rectum, from obesity, constipation, falls, jars, or even an act as simple as straining to lift a heavy object after a large meal, might

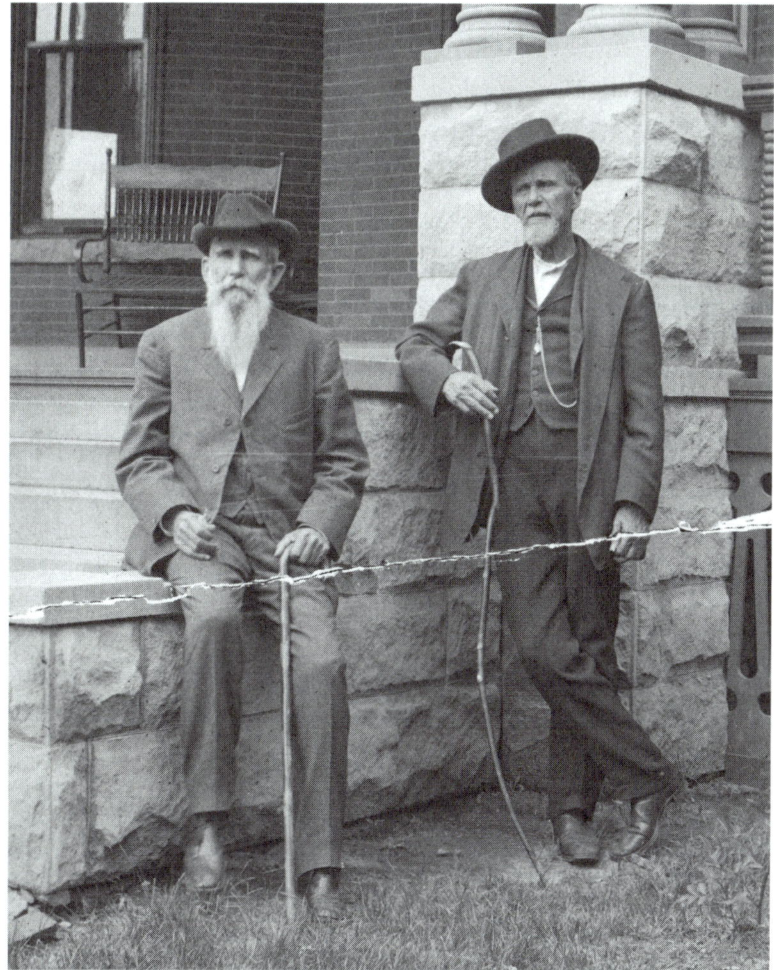

Still with cousin Abraham Still.

interfere with the hemorrhoidal arteries, veins and related nerves, and cause piles, inflammation, ulceration or cancer. The combination of prolapse and constipation was another consideration to bear in mind. The weight of retained feces could draw the cecum (the ascending colon) towards the pelvic floor and, through a combination of pressure and mesenteric tension, cause stasis of blood and lymph and many a case of appendicitis. "Lift the cecum, lift the cecum!" Still repeatedly admonished in the treatment room.[45]

In 1897 the *Journal of Osteopathy* conducted a survey of infirmary patients. Improvement or cure was reported in a wide range of conditions: chronic diarrhea, constipation, "neuralgia of the stomach," bronchitis, asthma, abscesses, eczema, epilepsy, diabetes, vertigo, loss of voice, visual disturbances.[46] Lewis Keyte of Elmer, Missouri, diagnosed by his doctor with heart disease and general debility, had suffered from "everything, pretty near" before coming to Kirksville. For ten years he had slept propped up with pillows, unable to lie flat, yet all his ailments had disappeared. "Yes sir, I am going home a well man," he said after six weeks of treatment. "I now feel like I couldn't wait to get home, I am so anxious to pitch in and go to work."[47] Methodist preacher Reverend Hoopingarner arrived with "no faith" in osteopathy, but after five treatments his back pain and nervousness had disappeared entirely, though his hemorrhoids remained troublesome.

Some hoped unrealistically for miracles. "Of course everybody cannot be cured," a Mrs. Ayres said. "I have met some dissatisfied people, but they have, almost without exception, been those who were impatient and would not devote sufficient time to give the treatment a fair trial."[48]

A few accused osteopathy of failing some patients. "Yes, who would not expect it," Still responded. "You are called to treat people who have been poisoned and diseased beyond the possibility of anything except a little temporary relief, or perhaps the osteopath is not able properly to apply the knowledge he should have before being granted a diploma. This reflects no more upon the science of osteopathy than the farmer who fails does upon the science of farming."[49] Prognosis depended upon myriad factors:

> We may have had a thousand cases of brain, heart, lung, liver, stomach, bowels and uterus previous to your entry, with no two affecting the system in the same way. . . . Thus you must expect nothing when you come, but to learn just what we think your disease is, and you must patiently give us time for a deliberate decision as to your disease and its cause. We will tell you of the probability of cure and about the length of time required for such. [We do] not feel satisfied to give you an answer in reference to your disease and its cause in anything like conjectures.[50]

Some cases were beyond help. In October 1897 thirty-nine year old North Dakota governor Frederick A. Briggs, signatory of the state's osteopathic law, registered at the infirmary with advanced tuberculosis. Two months later he joined a convalescent party organized by Colonel Conger, with Wash Conner as acting physician, to spend the winter in Phoenix, Arizona.[51] Briggs failed to rally and died at his home in Bismarck on 9 August 1898.[52] Still posted some *Information for Patients*:

> Some die and we cannot help it. We would save all if we could, but many come too late; disease has got in its work, and the case is without hope. One comes in the last stages of consumption, when the whole lung is a mass of ruin, and body dead in all its powers to sustain life.[53]

Three days before Briggs' death Still turned seventy. In his honor Memorial Hall was elaborately garlanded with flowers, evergreens and bunting for a musical and literary program, but a violent thunderstorm forced the organizers to postpone the event until 15 October.[54]

Julia Foraker, due to join her husband in Washington, delayed her departure to attend the rescheduled celebration. In delivering the opening address Judge Ellison congratulated the Old Doctor on his "past three score years and ten," conveyed the community's love and gratitude, and expressed pride in an impressive new courthouse built of Ohio blue sandstone, under construction on the square, a symbol of the prosperity Still had brought to the town. Ellison declared that one more thing was required to complete the work: a statue of Dr. Still to perpetuate his memory for having done so much to benefit humanity. It would come to pass, but not for another nineteen years.

Still's talk that evening was more of a sermon, its text the scriptural command Love One Another: *If we love one another, God dwelleth in us, and his love is perfected in us*.[55] It was obedience to this command, he said, that had prompted him to study the mysteries of man's organism and arrive at the conclusions upon which osteopathy was founded. "I love my fellow man," he addressed the audience, "because I see God in his face and in his form."[56]

Students afterwards inscribed the phrase in the technique room.[57]

20

WEEDS IN A FLOWER BED

Osteopathy's meteoric rise generated a host of unanticipated problems. Inexperienced graduates, with differing motives, scattered across the country to open practices and establish schools. In June 1895, directly after receiving their diplomas, Elmer and Helen Barber chartered the National School of Osteopathy in Baxter Springs, Kansas. In May 1896 George Burton opened the Pacific College of Osteopathy in Anaheim, California; a month later Ed Pickler the Northern Institute of Osteopathy in Minneapolis; in September 1897 Nettie Bolles the Western College of Osteopathy in Denver. More schools followed, some modeled on the founding school, others mere diploma mills.

In early 1897 Elmer Barber relocated his school to Kansas City, Missouri, where, in contravention of the new state law, he issued graduates practice licenses despite offering an abbreviated course. That August, William Smith (whom the Barbers had not met) visited the NSO under the alias G. H. B. Stewart, paid a $150 graduation fee, and returned, without attending a single class, with a diploma certifying completion of "the full course of study prescribed by the National School of Osteopathy." In one of the first actions taken by the newly-formed American Association for the Advancement of Osteopathy[1] the Missouri Attorney General, under Smith's affidavit, brought suit against Barber in the Kansas City Court of Appeals "to take away the corporate franchise of the respondent, because of an alleged abuse thereof." The court found Barber guilty of committing an unlawful act in issuing the diploma but, to the frustration of the AAAO, ruled that in the light of Smith's true identity and qualifications in both medicine and osteopathy the certificate had been issued in good faith and the gravity of the offense did not warrant revoking the school's charter.[2]

A greater problem, particularly in states where osteopathy remained unregulated, came from opportunists and fraudsters. "A score or more pseudo schools and probably as many individuals acting upon their own responsibility professed to turn out osteopathic physicians," Eamons R. Booth wrote in his 1905 *History of Osteopathy and Twentieth-Century Medical Practice*. "Schools were started without capital, equipment, brains, experience, or purpose, except to make money. Correspondence schools blatantly forced themselves upon the attention of the people by advertising. Private osteopathic practitioners, with an itching palm, took pupils and professed to teach them all about Osteopathy by teaching a few 'movements' and even issued books with cuts purporting to represent movements."[3] The last charge was directed at Elmer Barber, whose *Osteopathy: The New Science of Healing*, the first book on the subject, was published a year before Still's *Autobiography*. Barber not only lacked a proper understanding of osteopathy, but even had the temerity to challenge the founder's emphasis on adjusting bones, maintaining that the true cause of nearly all disease was nerve interference by muscle contraction.[4]

Even in Kirksville Still faced challenges. In June 1897 the disgraced Marcus Ward returned to town, opened an office on the southeast corner of Franklin and McPherson streets, and approached local businessmen with the proposal of establishing a new osteopathic school and infirmary in direct competition with the ASO. In the three years since his ignominious dismissal from the school the former lightning rod peddler had briefly studied homeopathy under Kirksville practitioner Dr. A. T. Noe before obtaining an esoteric qualification from the School of Finer Forces in New York and an MD degree from the Ohio Medical School in Cincinnati.[5] Businessman R. M. Brashear supplied Ward with the same plat of land he had offered Still three years earlier and became the venture's principal stockholder.

In November, as thirty-one students assembled for classes in temporary premises, an imposing three-story brick structure capped by a great white dome rose up on East Normal Street. The Columbian School of Osteopathy, its proprietor announced, aimed to revive "some of the lost sciences that were known, practiced and applied by the ancients in Athens over 2,000 years ago."

Ward held that these "original osteopaths" – namely "Zeno, Epicurus, Epictetus, Catelles, and others about ninety-five years B.C." – were not only skilled in bone-setting but also in the art of "Silent Diagnosis," a facility that obviated the need to know even a scrap of case history. Ward claimed to have been proficient in this "strange delicate something in the teaching and practice of osteopathy" since childhood, and he assured "real fame and fortune" to all in possession of the "wonderful secret."[6]

Even more extraordinary, Ward maintained that it was he, and not Still, who first discovered osteopathy. *True Osteopathy. Founded by Dr. M. L. Ward, August 2nd, 1862*,[7] the Columbian School's brochure proclaimed (he would have been thirteen at the time). Ward boasted (and lied) that he had cured over 700 patients after other osteopaths had failed to help, and that Still had once described him as "the greatest living Osteopath."[8] Such wild claims, coupled with his practice of intercepting prospective ASO students at the Wabash depot and poaching patients by offering free clinics, won Ward few friends. Still despised treachery and disloyalty,[9] and posted some general advice:

> Honor thyself that thy days may be long on earth. Now, brethren and sisters, the greatest honor a person can enjoy is to know that he has told the truth, every pop all day, every day each week. If you go into any business tell the truth. Don't lie and cheat in order to make gain. A man's heart may be full of wine, but one dirty lie will sour it and mar his joy. Don't say you were a pet student and got a special drill in all branches, and that you were the only object of admiration of all the professors. If you do tell such trash to strangers they will set you down as a fool, and not to be trusted. Your babe is as ugly as mine, and both are as green as a mess of boiled dandelion, so just be easy about your fine qualities. People will weigh you, and give you all the credit for good that you merit. The way of the righteous is easy, but the road of the untruthful brag is a way of thorns. Be honest and God will endorse all you do and say.[10]

Most irksome of all, Ward offered a regular two-year DO course with an optional third year in medicine and surgery for an MD degree. "Schools which pretend to teach medicine and osteopathy," Still fumed, "like the bat are neither bird nor beast. They are mongrel institutions, snares, set to capture the unwary and unthinking. Anyone who pays his money to such institutions gets knowledge of neither medicine nor osteopathy, but a smattering of each, enough to make a first class quack."[11] He left it to others to rubbish Ward's claim of being osteopathy's original discoverer.

Difficulties arose even within the ASO. When Nettie Bolles left for Denver in September 1897 Still had been unable to find a replacement anatomy lecturer and reluctantly appointed his nephew Summerfield S. Still, James's son, to the post. Summerfield promptly abused his position, writing a letter of recommendation on behalf of a student (referring to him by the title of "Doctor" and endorsing his competence to practice osteopathy in his home state despite having not yet progressed to treating patients), and was summarily fired by the ASO Board. "He is getting the reward that a hypocrite should inherit," Still jotted privately. "No light equals true honesty – I am sorry that S. S. had no pure manly sense, but a fool can not choose the time nor place of his birth."[12]

Summerfield and wife Ella moved to Des Moines, Iowa, to establish, a month later, the S. S. Still College of Osteopathy. They took with them Colonel Conger, appointing him secretary of the school and editor of a journal,[13] the *Cosmopolitan Osteopath*, whose first issue carried a vindictive article, "Advantages of Des Moines – Disadvantages of Kirksville," which contrasted the healthy climate and improved streets of the Iowa capital with the supposed squalor of Kirksville, a "hotbed for typhoid and malarial fever."[14] The S. S. Still College did at least aspire to a high educational standard – an increasing necessity because some states had begun to refuse practice licenses to osteopaths lacking equivalent training to MDs.

To address the issue of quality and uniformity in osteopathic teaching, representatives of the ASO, the S. S. Still School, the recently established Milwaukee Institute of Osteopathy, and the Northern, Western and Pacific institutions met in Kirksville on 28 June 1898 to form the Associated Colleges of Osteopathy. The ACO established strict membership criteria: minimum standards for curricula, a course length as stipulated under state law, entry and tuition fees of not less than $500, and a requirement to "teach Osteopathy pure and unmixed with any other system of healing."[15]

Both the ACO the AAAO worked strenuously to maintain professional standards, but neither organization had the power to prevent plagiarism. "As soon as osteopathy became established," E. R. Booth wrote, "imitators sprang up like weeds in a flower bed."[16] The first had appeared as early as November 1894 in the form of an "outgrowth" of osteopathy bearing the unlikely designation "Neuro Osteopathis."

The originator of this "science of bones and the electric forces of man,"[17] was homeopath A. T. Noe, relocated to Kirksville earlier that year from Craig, Nebraska. Noe knew scant more about osteopathy than having witnessed it cure a patient he had failed to help with homeopathy. Sixteen-year-old farmer's son Eddy Englehart, kicked in the side by a mare, was unable to digest food properly and had eaten nothing solid for two weeks. Fearing the teenager might die without more substantial treatment, Noe called at the ASO to ask for help. Still was away so Arthur Hildreth went to visit the patient instead. Hildreth knew Eddy well – they had lived on neighboring farms – and was shocked by the youth's emaciated appearance. An examination revealed painful lesions of the right fourth to sixth ribs and their adjoining vertebrae, disturbing the sympathetic nerves to the gut, and after their correction Eddy rapidly regained his appetite and went on to a full recovery.[18] Neuro Osteopathis vanished into oblivion, but it was a portent of things to come.

In early 1899 a Dr. Fulkerson opened an office on Kirksville's Franklin Street to practice "Endo-Pathy." Fulkerson claimed to have "developed and perfected" his method through "years of study, scientific research and experience" and, promising treatment "in harmony with the laws of nature," purported to rely on "a thorough knowledge of anatomy, physiology and psychophysiology" to improve blood circulation, correct "defective parts," and strengthen "weakened, imperfective functions."[19] It all sounded rather familiar. Endo-Pathy's end was nigh, but the next two decades saw the emergence of a plethora of derivative systems: naprapathy, mechano-therapy, spondylotherapy, zone therapy, and others. All borrowed wholesale from Still, but a new name had the advantage of circumventing the restrictions imposed by the progressive regulation of osteopathy.[20]

One copycat system would endure. In 1898 Daniel David Palmer, a magnetic healer from Davenport, Iowa, opened a school to teach "chiropractic," a method of treating disease by manual adjustment of the spine. Palmer professed to have stumbled upon his system by accident three years earlier when he restored the hearing of black janitor Harvey Lillard, almost deaf for seventeen years, by correcting (despite the tenuous anatomical relationship) his fourth thoracic vertebra.

Osteopaths cast a knowing eye over Palmer's "discovery." In summer 1893, after completing his first term at the ASO, student Obie Strothers opened a practice in Davenport, and that fall returned to Kirksville to resume his studies accompanied by a bearded, heavy-set man in his fifties going by the name of Palmer. Blanche remembered her father treating the visitor and inviting him to dinner at the house, a courtesy extended many patients at that time, while Arthur Hildreth recalled Palmer talking to and being treated by a number of students. Palmer strenuously denied visiting Kirksville or plagiarizing osteopathy, but in later years several Missouri chiropractors who visited Still's home attested to seeing the name D. D. Palmer entered in the guest book, dated sometime "in the early 1890s."[21]

Some maintained that Still might not have minded anyone copying him had they been true to his teachings, but heavy-handed mimics often injured patients and, by association, damaged osteopathy's reputation. "We have just cause for wrath," Josephine de France wrote, "when cheap imitators garble his principles and attempt to claim them under the other names which by ignorant and violent execution injure us."[22] Still merely commented, "All manipulators are not osteopaths, any more than all butchers are surgeons."[23] One graduate offered, by means of analogy, an anecdote about Mark Twain. The writer's wife, exasperated by his incessant swearing, rehearsed some of his more colorful phrases and surprised him with a rendition. "It's no use Mary," Twain responded, "you've got the right words, but you haven't got the right tune."[24]

Imitators, fakers and substandard schools were not the only problems occupying Still. The ASO was beginning to attract a different type of student, one motivated less by an inner calling to help the afflicted and more by a desire to earn a respectable living.[25] The mail brought letters from parents seeking advice on whether their sons or daughters should study osteopathy. "Yes, if they want to," he would reply. "I do not want a student to come and tell me they were persuaded to come by someone. If they coolly decide to make it a profession for life, I would say send them by all means."[26] The new type was evident in the classroom, as student Harry Vastine noted:

> As I listened to the great parables and bits of philosophy of Dr. Still, I tried to get back of this marvelous man, this superb scientist, and see through his eyes. Many of his hearers, however, by their flippant manner plainly indicated that he was talking above their heads. Many took his utterances as jokes. How I dwelt upon his philosophic statements, pithy and pointed, but revolutionary and convincing. To me he soon became the great master teacher that he was, soundly entrenched in immutable and unchangeable natural law.[27]

The greatest problem of all, for it threatened the very core of osteopathy, resulted from the drive to raise educational standards.

In February 1898 Still appointed to the faculty J. Martin Littlejohn, a Scot with qualifications in law, divinity and classical languages, and (although not a qualified doctor) a degree from Glasgow University's department of medicine. In failing health from longstanding neck and throat problems, Littlejohn had emigrated to America on doctor's advice and, after gaining a PhD (on the "Political Theory of the Schoolmen and Grotius") from Columbia University, New York, secured an appointment as president of Amity College, College Springs, Iowa. The previous year he had registered for treatment at the infirmary and on being restored to health accepted Still's invitation to chair a new physiology department.

Soon after Littlejohn's appointment Still converted the maternity hospital into the A. T. Still Surgical Sanitarium to enable the infirmary to accept more serious cases previously needing referral to distant hospitals.[28] Littlejohn's brother James, an MD from the University of Glasgow, joined William Smith in the surgical department, and a third Littlejohn brother, David, an MD from the Central Medical College, St. Joseph, Missouri, took charge of an up-to-the-minute x-ray department that boasted only the second Röntgen machine west of the Mississippi. All three brothers enrolled in classes to study osteopathy.

Smith, the Littlejohns and the other medically trained professors brought to the school a more intellectual, scientific atmosphere. The curriculum now included all subjects taught in regular medical schools except materia medica, with classes increasingly presented from the medical viewpoint. This bolstered osteopathy's credentials, but caused Still to become concerned that the faculty were placing too little emphasis on osteopathic fundamentals.

He disapproved of professors teaching the routine use of medical instruments, believing they blunted the students' confidence in their own judgment. He himself never used a stethoscope or a blood pressure machine, and particularly detested the thermometer, an instrument rare when he was a young doctor. Branding it a "pig-tail," he soundly berated anyone sissy enough to use one,[29] insisting that the eye and hand were "more useful in the sick room than any artificial appliances."[30] An osteopath should know by his refined sense of touch whether there was fever or not without sticking a pig-tail in the patient's mouth.[31]

Still also warned against overreliance on laboratory tests. The analysis of tissues and body fluids "may tell you how much the house is on fire," he cautioned, but it does "not always tell you what started the fire and what is keeping it burning."[32] Any physiological abnormalities ("whether the blood has microbes or hyenas in it")[33] should serve only as a preliminary step towards the real, mechanical diagnosis. He repeatedly stressed that in the early stages of disease laboratory tests might not show any discernible quantitative or qualitative changes, but the structural lesions predisposing to future problems could always be found by the trained hand.

Some students struggled to grasp his teachings. George W. Riley, despondent at his lack of progress, ran into Still while walking in the woods and confided to having doubts about osteopathy. "Well my boy," the Old Doctor said as they sat together on a log, "I can picture this science as the greatest contribution ever made to a suffering world, if only those who practice it adhere to its eternal truths." Riley asked what those truths were. "They are found in the spinal column with all of its intricate bony framework, plus the beautiful circulation of blood and lymph through the nerve centers of the spinal cord and throughout the whole body," Still answered:

> That's the one thing you must hammer home to your own satisfaction if you want to get the full concept of this thing called Osteopathy. Remember, if ever a time comes when you are discouraged with a patient,

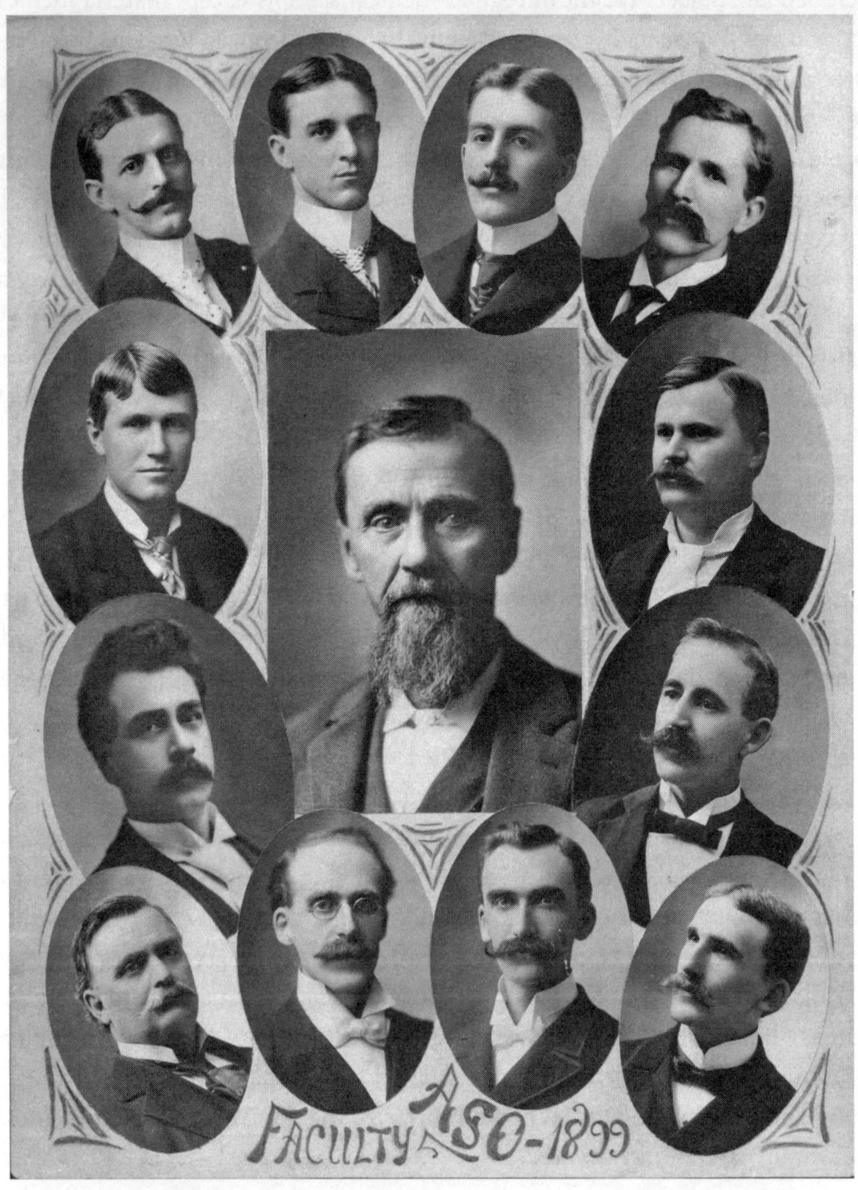

American School of Osteopathy faculty, 1899.
A. T. Still with (clockwise from top left) William Laughlin, Marion Clark, Carl McConnell, C. W. Proctor, Harry Still, Arthur Hildreth, David Littlejohn, James Littlejohn, J. Martin Littlejohn, Judge Andrew Ellison, William Smith, Charles Still.

> make up your mind the next time you see the patient that you resolve to locate the lesioned spinal anatomy. It will be there. It must be![34]

Getting the medically trained faculty to think osteopathically proved an immense challenge. J. Martin Littlejohn, despite having only just begun his osteopathic studies, was lecturing (contrary to the founder's emphasis on anatomy) that *physiology* was "the gateway by which this immense field of osteopathy is to be entered,"[35] leading students to focus more on effects than causes. "The greatest struggle of O. P.," Still scribbled privately, "is to get men to teach Opy from Harvard Yale or [illegible] who know nothing about the Philosophy nor anything belonging to our system. The school would be far better off without them."[36]

The use of standard medical texts did not help. On several occasions Still suspended classes for a day or two, concerned that the students were learning too much medical and too little osteopathic diagnosis.[37] Finally, in October 1898, he summoned the MDs on the faculty to a meeting and, without asking their opinion ("because they were not osteopaths to begin with"),[38] told them what he expected them to teach. To ensure they carried out his instructions he would enter classes unannounced, listen attentively for a few minutes, and either leave quietly or, more often than not, interrupt the lecture to make some quaint remark to indelibly fix the osteopathic principle.[39] These intrusions irritated the medics, but the osteopathically trained faculty advised the students to be very quiet and listen when the Old Doctor came in because he always said something that would be valuable when they entered practice.[40]

One day he crept into a classroom unnoticed and lay silently on a bench at the back, until he heard the lecturer advocate surgery for infected tonsils. "Tonsils were placed in the throat for a purpose," Still suddenly exploded, "and God didn't intend for them to be removed."[41] Another time he listened unimpressed as William Smith lectured on the quadratus lumborum muscle. "What's all that got to do with the practice of osteopathy?" he eventually broke in. Smith answered that if the muscle was contracted it would pull the twelfth rib down towards the pelvis on that side (to potentially irritate spinal nerves or, through ligamentous attachments, affect the diaphragm, and so on.) "Well," Still said, "why didn't you tell them that."[42]

During an anatomy class given by Will Laughlin he stole silently to the door, listened for a while, and strode in with his characteristic springy gait, rising on his toes.[43] Laughlin promptly stood aside. Still positioned himself behind the desk, leaning on his long staff, and looked at the class silently for a full minute. Then he smiled and broke into a chuckle. They chuckled back, looking for what was funny.

"Boys and girls," he said, "I'm going to draw you a pig." He took a piece of chalk and on the blackboard sketched a creature that initially resembled a pig, but soon acquired a long neck, two long legs and a fanlike tail. He turned to the class and let out another chuckle. Again they chuckled back uncertainly. Then his mood abruptly darkened. "How many of you diagnose that thing as a pig?" he demanded with apocalyptic sternness, making them jump. The tense silence that followed was punctuated by a sharp crack as he flung the chalk to the floor. He came to his point:

> You read in your textbooks that pneumonia is such and such and so and so. Maybe it is. But you look for yourselves, under osteopathic teachings, and see everything, not just what the book says. It is a turkey not a pig. You will never find it if you do not look for it, but if you look for it you will find it. If you treat that case according to what the book says you will get the result the book promises you, which is not much. If you treat what you find as osteopathic physicians you should be able to cure your case. That is the science of osteopathy. You take no man's word for it. You examine the body as an engineer, and the body itself shows you what to do, what needs to be done. If you go to consult different authorities you will get only confusion. They do not know what is right, or if any of their measures are right.[44]

It had been different at the beginning, when all had come under his personal supervision. The early students had felt part of a movement with the potential to benefit the whole of humanity. All-pervasive was an infectious enthusiasm, a sense of community, an air of adventure and responsibility. They witnessed Still demonstrate the truth of osteopathy; they had faith in the practice and they strove to emulate him. Even the faculty studied late into the night to perfect their knowledge.[45] "Yes, my friends," Joe Sullivan declared three decades later, "we were not averse to being called 'bone setters' in those days, as many of our folks are today. Some years later Osteopathy seemed to slow down in its general progress, coincidental with an era of high-hatters who wanted a wider field and more dignified cognomen."[46] As the turn of the century approached, the crusading spirit, the willing self-sacrifice in the face of collective difficulties, and the attitude of building for the future was receding.

As a medical undercurrent crept into the *Journal of Osteopathy*, Still circulated a plain instruction to all contributors to "Be Original." He wanted it "emphatically understood," he advised its then editor Henry Bunting, that the *Journal* should only publish accounts of personal investigations, with strictly no quotations from medical books. "When an Osteopath attempts to write," he said, "I suggest that he confines himself to what he knows to be facts, the results of his own experience, not a transcript of what old authors have said and quotations from papers."[47] Bunting did as he asked, and on 14 February 1899 Still sent him a note:

> The Journal is better now and suits me. I had about concluded to drop it out to stop needless waste of money. My School was chartered to teach Osteopathy only. Now it must foot its own expenses or go to the waste basket. I am willing to give it a reasonable time to do so. I think that can easily be done if there is any brains in running it. Do the best you can.[48]

Differences of opinion festered within the faculty. At the end of 1898 the balance of power shifted towards the medics when Still reluctantly released Arthur Hildreth to open a practice in St. Louis, and even more so at the beginning of the new year when Turner Hulett resigned the deanship and was replaced by J. Martin Littlejohn.

As if a portent of the impending crisis, at six-thirty in the evening on 27 April a devastating tornado hit Kirksville, cutting a swath of destruction three blocks wide, leveling two hundred homes and killing thirty-three people.[49] The dead included one ASO student, the wife of another, and the wife and mother of a third. In darkness and driving rain Charley, William Smith and David Littlejohn superintended a team of staff and students who, alongside the town's medical

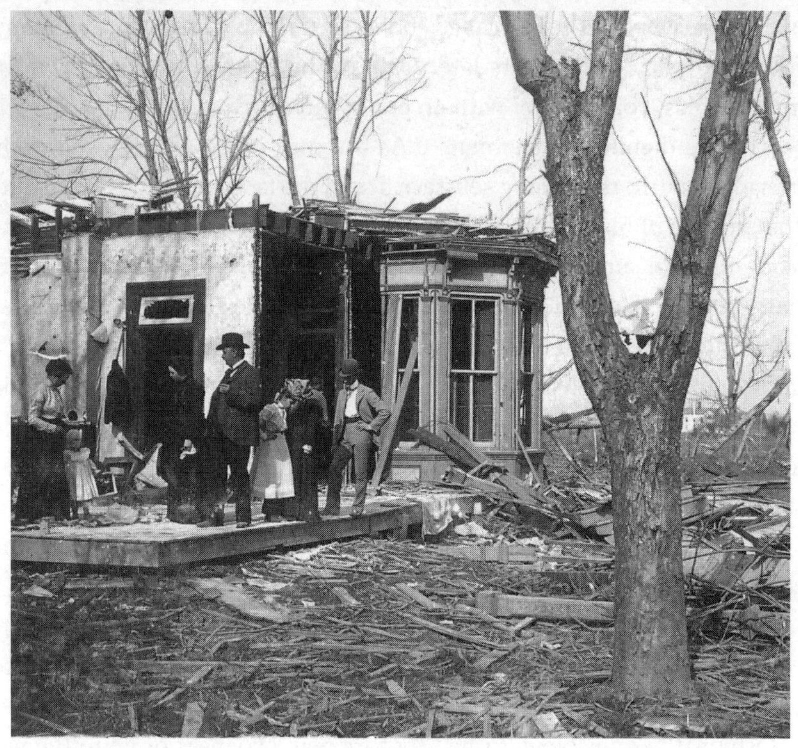

Thursday, April 27, 1899, at 6:20 p. m., a terriffic cyclone struck Kirksville, a town of about 10,000, in the northern part of Missouri, obliterating practically every thing in its path which lay from south to north across the eastern portion of the city.

The width of the storm proper varied as it passed through Kirksville from 300 yards to a half mile. About 200 residences were totally destroyed, leaving a thousand persons homeless.

The town is noted for its two great schools of ostœpathy. Here also is the North Missouri State Normal—the three schools named having about 2000 students. Following the storm, excursion trains were run bringing perhaps 10,000 people per day to the scene of the disaster.

Judge Andrew Ellison with the remains of his home after the tornado.

doctors, formed rescue and hospital corps, "hunting out unfortunates to set fractured bones, bandage the lacerated, and ease the pain of anguished hearts."[50] Still returned the tuition fees of students who had lost possessions.[51]

That summer's commencement exercises were set for 30 June. Since joining the faculty J. Martin Littlejohn had openly voiced an opinion that osteopathy should associate itself with the word *medicine*. In a speech at the previous summer's graduation ceremony he had argued that the word medicine, derived from the Latin "medicus, medicina and medeor, to heal," signified not merely a system of drug medication but more accurately, as defined by the *Encyclopedic Dictionary*, "a science and art directed first to the prevention of diseases, and secondly to their cure."[52] A definition well suited to osteopathy.

At the next graduation ceremony, held in Memorial Hall on 1 February 1899, he went a step further. Now ASO dean, Littlejohn prepared for the occasion a talk entitled, "Osteopathy in Line of Apostolic Succession to Medicine." Ill with a cold, his message was delivered instead by Bill Smith. "I think the time has come when Osteopathy must definitely declare the attitude it intends to assume in the field of science," Smith read aloud Littlejohn's words. "Medicine will ultimately be interpreted in the wider sense to include the whole art of healing and the laws upon which this practice is based, so that the Doctorate in Medicine will be the appropriate title of the Osteopath as well as the allopath."[53]

Littlejohn was tenacious in pursuing his goal. At the faculty meeting on March 22 he persuasively reminded his colleagues that the 1894 charter entitled the ASO to *confer such honors and degrees that are usually granted and conferred by reputable medical colleges*. "Whereas the title of Diplomate or Doctor of Osteopathy has never been conferred by any medical college," the minutes record, "it is hereby resolved that the faculty recommend to the Trustees the execution of the charter power of the School by hereafter conferring the Degree of Doctor of Medicine," and, "in recognition of Osteopathy as an Independent School of Medicine and system of healing as it is declared in Missouri and other states that have recognized Osteopathy . . . that the designation and the title shall be hereafter M.D. (Osteopathic)."[54]

On June 6, with the Littlejohn brothers due to graduate at the end of that month, J. Martin wrote to the Board of Trustees with a request: "I should like to receive the degree of M.D. (Osteopathic School), because I believe it is the right one . . . as a matter of policy for the recognition of osteopathy as an independent school of healing."[55] The request fell upon deaf ears. On 1 July 1899, a day after receiving their D.O. diplomas, J. Martin and James Littlejohn sailed to Britain for the summer.[56]

They left in their wake a ripple of discord. In that September's *Journal of Osteopathy* ex-dean Turner Hulett wrote of being told by an undergraduate, "D.O. does not mean anything. Our title ought to be M.D.O." To Hulett this was an affront. "In the minds of some of us D.O. stands for Dr. Still's work, and means just what that means," he responded. "Where did the student get the suggestion for any other idea? Why is there such an apparently eager desire to ring the changes on 'medicine'?" Hulett's article was appended with a message from Still himself: "We want no M.D.O. in our school – for the American School is strictly Osteopathic – and D.O. means just what it stands for, Diplomate in Osteopathy."[57]

The founder was missing the steadying hand of Arthur Hildreth. With over two hundred students due to matriculate that fall, bringing total enrolment to over seven hundred, Still urgently needed to safeguard the purity of the teaching. In August he asked Harry, who had spent much of the summer working in Hildreth's busy St. Louis practice, to convey Arthur a message: please return to the school. So desperately did Still want Hildreth back that he offered him a quarter share of both the property and income from the institution. Hildreth could not refuse, feeling he owed all his opportunities in life to Still. "If your father thinks he needs me," he told Harry, "I will go back."[58] For Hildreth it also meant resigning his position as that year's AAAO president, a post he had held barely a month, for faculty or board members of colleges were forbidden from holding office. "Owing to circumstances which I am unable to control," he stated in a letter to the *Journal*, "it has become necessary for me to leave St. Louis and again join the American School of Osteopathy."[59] Some poked fun at Hildreth's unstinting loyalty to Still, nicknaming him *Fidus Achates* after Aeneas's inseparable companion in Virgil's *Aeneid*.[60]

Moving to regain control of the school, Still ousted J. Martin Littlejohn from the deanship and installed Hildreth in his place. Still knew Hildreth could be trusted absolutely. They shared the conviction that the future of osteopathy depended upon it remaining a totally independent system, and that any deviation from its pure teachings would compromise clinical results and cheapen the profession.[61] (Hildreth's unshakable faith in osteopathy even merited comment from Still, who joked that Arthur would not give up treating until the patient had been dead three days.)[62]

Hildreth discontinued the Surgical Sanitarium and, purging the faculty of the medical influence, attempted to fill all teaching positions with osteopaths only.[63]

Smith and the Littlejohns, angered by Hildreth's appointment, complained that it was beneath their dignity to serve under the ex-farmer with no qualifications from a higher education establishment other than the ASO. They charged that he was too radical, too opposed to drugs, and too "ultra-osteopathic" – the very reasons Still appointed him. "It was very clear," Hildreth wrote, "that the objectors felt that a combination of 'old school' medicine and osteopathy would mean most."[64]

The aggrieved Scots wrote to the Board of Trustees (Still, his family, and Hildreth) stating their intent to resign if Dr. Hildreth was retained as dean. Most of the faculty, however, many of them early graduates – Carl McConnell, Ernest Proctor, Charles Hazzard, Turner Hulett, W. M. Clark and Will Laughlin – backed Hildreth and threatened to tender their own resignations if Smith and the Littlejohns remained. A majority of students felt the same way, leaving the Scots isolated.

Smith left immediately. Shortly afterwards a chalk inscription appeared on the bulletin board outside the infirmary. It read simply: *My three H---s.* The message bore Still's unmistakable handwriting and required little interpretation. The three Hs were Hildreth, Hulett and Hazzard, his best friends and most loyal supporters.[65]

"All is in good shape, School and Infirmary," Still wrote Thekla Orschel on December 14. "Dr. Smith is dropped out of the school. You will learn why when you come. We had too much boss and drugs to suit."[66] The Littlejohns held out until the Christmas vacation, and as the new century dawned Still wrote Orschel again, "All the old 'gods' are out of the school, and all is smoother now."[67]

In truth all was far from smooth.

21

MIND

When Ellen and Greenwood Ligon matriculated at the ASO in February 1898 they were accompanied by family friend Ernest E. Tucker for treatment at the infirmary. The twenty-one-year-old was eager to meet Dr. Still, his curiosity piqued by Ellen's description of osteopathy's founder as a great man, albeit with eccentricities, possessed of intriguing psychic abilities. Interested but skeptical, Tucker planned to test these alleged powers. He determined to call on Still and just stand there, say nothing, and see what the great man did.

Tucker climbed Still's front steps in three inches of snow, knocked on the front door and waited under a slanting morning sun. From the side of the house he heard the sound of another door opening and around the curve of the porch appeared a tall gray-bearded man, walking almost noiselessly, "his movement along the floor almost Indian in its smoothness, a bit tip-tilted as though on tiptoe."[1] Well versed in etiquette, Tucker was surprised; he had expected a gentleman of culture and manners, but instead encountered a simple direct man entirely devoid of veneer.

The plan went badly. As the young man stood there silently Still, perhaps sensing the challenge, gazed directly at him through uncleaned steel-rimmed spectacles and said nothing either. Suddenly gripped by self-consciousness, abashed at his good breeding, Tucker's composure faltered and he began to introduce himself. "What did you say anything for?" Still cut him short. "I would have told you all about yourself. You're from Dixie are you not?" (Dixie was his nickname for Ellen Ligon.) The visit was brief. Tucker engaged in some light, stilted conversation, and as he turned to go heard Still say, "Is the law of prophesy dead?"[2] Followed by, "In a couple of years you will be back here studying." The idea had not entered his head.

Tucker left in a welter of emotion – embarrassed, shaken up, yet oddly elated, and wondering how such simplicity could constitute greatness. "I felt a sudden sense of unreality," he wrote fifty-six years later, "a sudden sense of a reality greater than any I had known." As he stood face to face with this man who had cultivated nothing but his true self, to whom the refinements of society were alien, something resonated deep within and from that moment many things he had accepted as normal began to reverse themselves. "When anyone comes into contact with a revelation of such vast significance as Osteopathy," he continued, "he must do one of two things: close his mind, remain blind, deny; or else pour every ounce of his spare energy into it to give it the full measure of development possible."[3]

As predicted, Tucker enrolled as a student in 1900. By then Still had moved into an imposing twenty-eight-room residence overlooking the ASO on the west side of Osteopathy Street. He had offered Mary a choice: a new home or, his preference, a trip to Europe, knowing perfectly well which she would select. Raised in comfort, she had ventured West in the spirit of romance and ever since endured hardship, selflessly supporting her husband to enable him fulfill his dream. The impressive mansion was completed to her specification in March 1899.[4]

Still never felt comfortable there. Its contemporary design, modern conveniences and comforts, framed pictures, curtained doors and thick pile carpets offended his homely simplicity. A poem entitled *Soliloquy of Drew* appeared in the *Journal of Osteopathy*:

> Is this grand, highly finished house my home?
> No, never! I cannot call it home. I weep as I sit alone.

One of its three parlors housed a collection of gifts, and he gave conducted tours complete with their history. Among the exhibits was a seven-foot ebony staff with gold head and tassel commissioned by Mrs. Conger. Still walked to school with it a couple of times grinning like a schoolboy, but it was far too ostentatious for him.[5] So too was the house.

But I feel to say that I would be content to live as I did before,
In tent or log-house with thatched roof, sod walls, and dirt floor.
Now Ma has said, 'Listen to me; you must hang up your hat,
Comb your hair, black your boots, and things like that.
Because the minister might come at any hour of time,
And find you all covered with dirt, dust, feathers and slime.'[6]

His discomfort was displaced into acts of protest. He slept in a bunk and used the side door. When he slipped on the polished hardwood floor he put hob-nails in his boots. When he hurt himself on the newel post of the angled staircase he sawed off the offending corner. After "putting himself over" on the house, he told Ernest Tucker, he was able to live more naturally in it.

Tucker became as fascinated by the founder's personality and mode of thought as osteopathy itself, and became a student of both.[7]

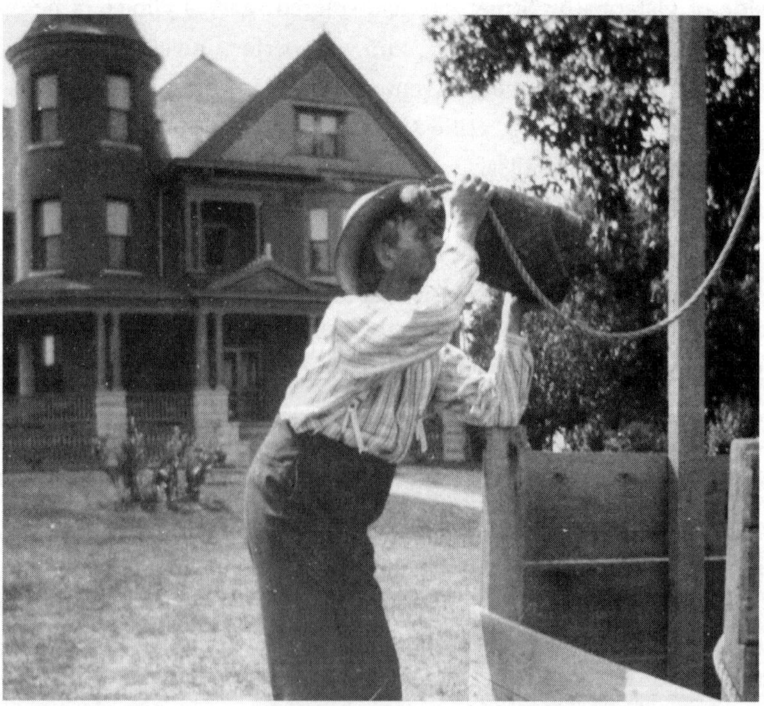

Still drinking from the well at his new home on Osteopathy Street.

Still obeyed no conventions, employed no arts or introductory maneuvers, engaged in no small talk or discussions of the weather. He seemed to address himself not to what you offered as yourself but to your essence, his clear eyes seeing past the camouflage, through you and far into the beyond.[8] All communication was on a human and profoundly intimate basis, and if you lacked the ability to tolerate this intimacy you barely seemed to exist to him and could feel uneasy in his presence. "The actual spirit of a man was all, the rest nothing," Tucker related:

> Now there are very few people whom I can allow to get past the intellectual guardians of my own spirit and so reach those intimacies. But Dr. Still seemed always to be there, never to find his way through, never to arrive; but to begin there and never be anywhere else. From this one may perhaps begin to understand the psychic powers of the man. A distilled essence of kindliness and sincerity that was as absolute as the law of gravitation – these were the telescopes with which he seemed to look past the camouflage into the natural consciousness of people; and into their bodies as well. . . . This, it seems to me, was the solute from which his thoughts and acts were precipitates. . . . It was a personality so selfless and so expanded that it achieved the nth degree and became impersonal.[9]

The student came to see Still as "a mind, somewhat wistful, looking, listening, feeling, thinking, trying to peer a little way into the Great Mysteries; just one small star in the heavens trying to see with its single small eye the meaning of the council of the stars."[10] A mind attuned not to the affairs of men but to the moral law written on the heart; a mind untrammeled by theory, assumption or tradition, molded and shaped by a quarter-century of learning from nature. The standard by which he judged others was absolute honesty,[11] an honesty without any underlying negative connotation of not being dishonest. Not "to do no wrong," but "never fail to do right, never fail to do or know everything a circumstance calls for." Being honest with others first demanded being honest with yourself, taking responsibility for right actions rather than merely falling into line with external rules.[12]

Since vowing in 1874 to investigate the assertion "all of God's work is perfect," the only flaw Still had been able to find in man's make-up was in his "power of reason."[13] The rational mind could override the moral law and lead a person down the path of error; this was the perennial struggle that Methodism strove to overcome. Man saw through a glass darkly, but at the ground of his being the perfection of nature remained. "Still's real philosophy could probably be summarized in a very few words," Tucker wrote. "How could a thing be, and not be perfect as of its class and degree of development? If it exists, it demonstrates; is final. It is not that he put this thought into words – that was not his métier – but his words circled around it like a rim around a hub; as though around some hidden center or source. It was intuitive, unconscious philosophy."[14]

The hub, the hidden center, was the spiritual: what man did not know and could only acknowledge, the unknown intelligence incomprehensibly blending and inspiring the material manifestations of *matter, mind and motion*. Still wrote: "First there is the material body; second the spiritual being; third a being of mind which is far superior to all vital motions and material forms, whose duty is to wisely manage this great engine of life."[15] Following Herbert Spencer's scheme, this "being of mind" had both Knowable and Unknowable aspects.

In Still's usage the word "mind" generally signified the Unknowable aspect – the body's inherent "wisdom of Deity." Every cell an individual sentient being, constantly adapting and harmonizing its function with trillions of others, "each organ and all other parts laboring together, seeming to know they are parts of a stupendous whole."[16] Still declared that "the body is full of the essence of mind and its action;"[17] the thigh bone is "perfect in its material and mental parts;"[18] and even that "there is much evidence that mind is imparted to the corpuscles of the blood."[19]

The objective nature of the mind troubled him little: "I cannot even think deep enough to reason on the subject."[20] The mind was a perpetual mystery – but to him no epiphenomenon of matter. Science had failed to resolve the mind into any known physical laws, localize it to any part of the brain, or demonstrate it to be electrical in nature.

The Knowable aspect of mind, the experiential part informed by the senses, was to Still simply the *subjective*. This multi-faceted faculty encompassed rational thought, feelings, emotions and a host of arcane powers. Though disparaged by the early scientists as a source of error, Still recognized the supreme importance of the mind to both doctor and patient. "It may be possible that we do not think often enough of man's dual nature," he stated, "and that his body is under his mind, and obeys its orders all the time."[21] At the very beginning of his medical career he learned that mental states can profoundly affect physiology.

Sometime in 1854 he traveled on horseback from Macon County to visit his family at the Wakarusa Mission, taking a friend for company. The cholera epidemic was at its height and everywhere they went the disease formed the main topic of conversation. In Kansas City they heard frightening stories of its prevalence on the riverboats and in the river towns all the way down to New Orleans. On the return journey, riding across the high prairie sixty miles from Kansas City, Still suddenly announced, for a prank, that he thought he was coming down with the disease. The effect was alarming. His friend turned deathly pale, with perspiration, nausea and all the signs of incipient cholera, and seemed close to collapse. Still tried to reassure his comrade that he was only joking, but without effect, and as he wondered what to do he suddenly remembered the childhood beatings meted out by his father and how, with the smarting of the leather strap, his anger rose and his body warmed:

> So I reached down and loosened my stirrup strap and began to lay it on him heavy. He paid no attention until I had struck him at least a half dozen strokes, then he looked at me and said, 'You hurt.' He was in his short sleeves and I continued to lay the strap across his back good and heavy until his anger was roused and he said, 'If you don't quit that I'll knock you off your horse.' Then I knew my medicine was taking effect and I was happy to know that my chum would not die there on the open prairie many miles from home.[22]

The power of the mind should never be underestimated. A doctor should choose his words carefully, for the patient might accept them as the final verdict on his condition. "What you say is weighty far beyond your concept," Still impressed on his students. "Should you find any hope for his recovery and make that your report, like a thrill of lightning dipped in the sea of love, his vitality dances with joy. But if should you be indiscreet enough in your report

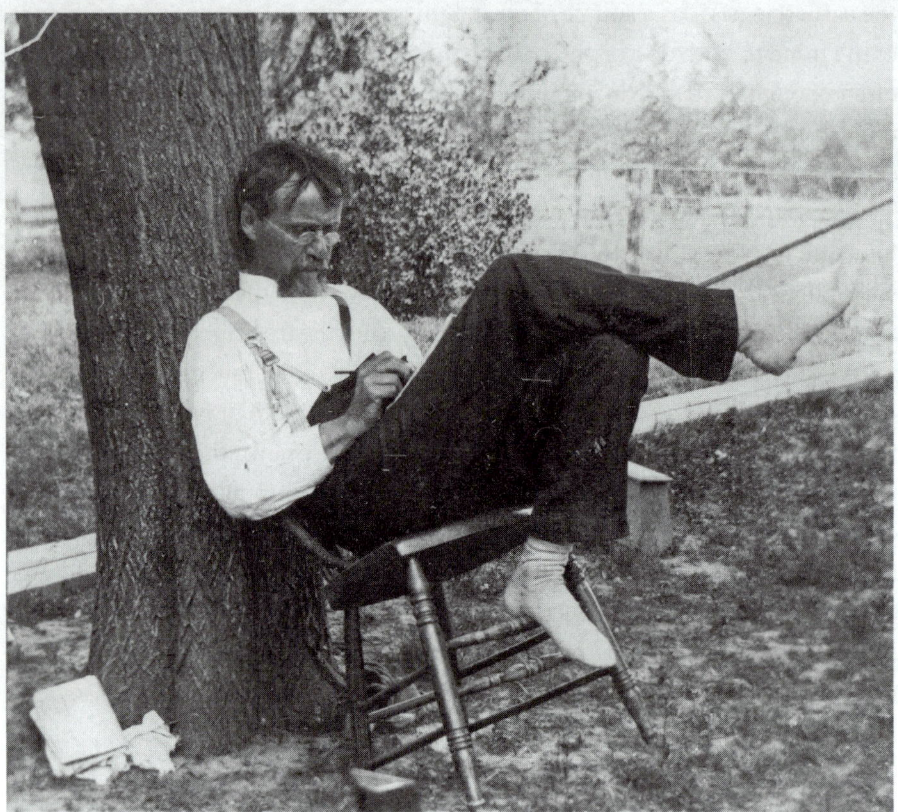

Still at the Morris Farm, Millard, Missouri.

to remove every ray of hope, you have chilled the vital energy, you have silenced it. Never tell a patient that he is in a bad fix, worse today than yesterday, or that he looks ill. More patients suffer and die from such imprudence and fright than the world has ever dreamed of."[23] By contrast, adopting a positive attitude and educating patients about their condition often hastened recovery. Above all, Still taught, the doctor's words must carry the weight of self-assurance. There was an unwritten law: for best results you must have the patient's trust, and to gain it you must have confidence in your own ability. Confidence, commitment and interest – or lack of it – is transmitted directly to the patient.

Cultivating the right mental attitude was only the beginning. The cognoscenti understood that Still's extraordinary results depended not only upon anatomical erudition and skilled hands, but also upon the development of latent mental faculties. The mind was a potent tool to hone for mastery of the art of osteopathy.

The first step was to perfect the art of visualization. Still insisted his students retain in their minds a "living picture" of every part of the body, as an artist would paint a face or a scene from memory.[24]

One morning before the clinic opened Ellen Ligon sat in the waiting room observing patients and trying to pinpoint their lesions, and when Still entered she asked him if he agreed with one of her diagnoses. He did not answer directly, but handed her a pencil and paper. "Draw me a picture of the fourth dorsal vertebra," he instructed. She was unable to. "Then draw me a picture of the fifth." She was unable to. "Do the transverse processes run directly across or at an angle and at what angle?" She did not know. He asked her to fetch a skeleton and on it showed the different planes of motion of each vertebra and other related things. "How dare you think you know anything about treating a human body," he said finally, "before you know how a human body is made."[25]

Arthur Hildreth asked Still to explain his thought process when assessing a new patient. "I never notice whether she is beautifully dressed and wears silks and diamonds or covered with homespun cloth," he replied. "I am listening to her story, and while listening I am seeing in my mind's eye the combinations of systems which go to make up the whole of that body structure." The bones, bound together by ligaments – "marvelous creations of strength" – maintaining the integrity of every joint from the toes to the base of the skull. The muscles, attaching to the bones in various ways; some covering ligaments, others beginning and ending in them, "placed to give needed protection to the framework and at the same time move the bony parts in such a marvelous way, with such harmony that it is hard for the mind of man to conceive of the perfection of their functions."

The arteries, conveying blood to every cell, bringing oxygen and nutrition for growth, repair and maintenance. "The mechanism whereby these materials are transferred from the blood stream into the vital living cells of the body is beyond description, almost beyond understanding." The veins, transporting wastes to the organs of elimination; the lymphatic system, protecting against harmful poisons and bacteria; the endocrine glands, each performing its special function in the service of the whole. The nervous system, "one of the most marvelous mechanisms ever created," voluntary and involuntary divisions acting in concert, motor and sensory nerves relaying messages to and from the brain, sympathetic and parasympathetic nerves regulating nutrition and adjusting blood flow to the moment to moment demands of each cell. "When you stop to consider how these two great systems are joined together," Still marveled, "you have, in my opinion, the most supreme example of the perfection of the work of the Divine Architect."[26]

Of paramount importance was the *way* Still visualized – from the perspective of the cell and its requirements for normal function. "He studied nature always from the inside, the heart, and as a subject, not an object;" Ernest Tucker related, "he looked from the creative angle."[27] Nature was unfailingly intelligent, dynamic, in constant flux. "He did not think by the book, but by the moving event, and that is just about all the difference in the world."[28] When Still was investigating a particular topic he would say he was "living in the liver" or "being a bone." To ascertain what was wrong with a sick baby he would feel himself inside of it. "He made himself en rapport with the body he studied, he tried to be that bone; he thought as a measle, he put himself inside of the spleen, or the trochanter major, to feel its operation as a part of the great unity of action and of logic and of life that was that body."[29] So conscientiously did Still train this power of visualization, Tucker noted, that "he saw conditions and processes as a whole, and by this ability could pick out the mechanical key to the disturbed function that the patient recognized only as discomfort or disease."[30]

One day, walking past a group of students chatting on his front porch, Still said without stopping, "Why don't you go have that fifth lumbar fixed, Asa?" Asa Willard was taken aback. During a baseball game a few days earlier the student had stepped into a hole while running backwards to catch a fly ball, and he asked the Old Doctor how he knew something was wrong. Still merely chuckled, "Always keep your eyes open, boy."[31]

Visualization was a mere scratching at the surface of the extraordinary powers of the mind. In the clinic Still strove to get his students to set aside theory, preconception and assumption, and adopt a receptive state of mind, calm but alert, open and unprejudiced to all impressions. They must develop the ability to take in everything at once, blend and harmonize with the patient, and become a participant in something greater. "Once in the operating rooms you are in a place where printed books are known no more forever," he counseled:

> Your own native ability, with nature's book, are all that command respect in this field of labor. Here you lay aside the long words, and use your mind in deep and silent earnestness; drink deep from the eternal fountain of reason, penetrate the forests of that law whose beauties are life and death. To know all of a bone in its entirety would close both ends of an eternity.
>
> Solemnity takes possession of the mind, a smile of love runs over the face, the ebbs and tides of the great ocean of reason, whose depths have never been fathomed, swell to your surging brain. You eat and drink; and as you stand in silent amazement, suns appear where you never saw a star, brilliant with the rays of God's wisdom, as displayed in man, and the laws of life, eternal in days, and as true as the mind of God Himself.[32]

Still noted that the most successful practitioners were often those without impressive scholastic qualifications,[33] and ventured the "immature suggestion" that the best were those who "worked for and obtained intuitive consciousness," those who learned to blend thinking with sensing, knowledge with intuition. "We should not be satisfied to know that we are right," he said, "but *feel* so, and act with energy to suit, and our successes will grow with time."[34]

Arthur Hildreth, who witnessed Still give many hundreds of treatments, regarded as the "most remarkable demonstration of his ability" the Old Doctor's treatment of an acutely sick man with a heart condition, virtually gasping for breath. Still approached the table and simply stood by the patient's side for minute or two, his facial expression changing "to one of sublime gravity," conveying the impression "that he was in the presence of God and he was appealing to Him to guide his fingers and his hands in order that he might be able to save this human life." The treatment itself was extremely simple. Still applied gentle but steady pressure at the junction of the left fourth and fifth ribs with the vertebrae where, Hildreth explained, "the little branches from the spinal nerves connected with the sympathetic cardiac plexus." As Still worked the patient's anxiety quieted, his breathing became easier and his distress ceased.[35]

For decades Still had striven to train the power of intuition, a faculty he believed all possess and, with practice, can polish to unlimited degrees of refinement. "I am something of what people call inspired," he declared on one occasion. "We Methodists call it 'intuitive.' The other classes have different names for it – clairvoyant and clairaudient."[36] Like his father before him, Still regarded intuition as a working of the Law of Providence, took it seriously, and acted on its promptings. While in Kansas, long before his mind-reading exploits on his itinerant circuit, he had often written Ed in Missouri describing what he had "seen" take place there and, reportedly, was almost invariably correct.[37] One student wrote that Dr. Still possessed "a distinct gift of intuition of the sort that quite baffles explanation. We speak of it as a sixth sense."[38] Still did not stop at six. "I love God," he said,

> because He can put the sight in your body, also hearing, and the sense of touch – in fact, the five senses, and about five hundred other kind of senses on top of them.[39]

Mind operated in skein after skein: a vast realm interwoven by thought, imagination, memory, intuition, clairvoyance and other psychic phenomena. Still treated all these faculties matter-of-factly and gathered them together under the heading *psychology*. He told Ellen Ligon he could see her aura and those of all patients, and could tell by its appearance whether a person was sick or well.[40] When the science department purchased its compound microscopes Judge Ellison joked that it was money thrown away, for Dr. Still's inner sight could do the job equally well.[41] When the school acquired the new x-ray machine, Still himself showed little enthusiasm for the device. "The x-ray, by increasing the vibrations, enables us to see under the surface what our eyes will not discover," he said. "Why can't we train our minds to do just that?"[42]

People said that Dr. Still was blessed by a mystic consciousness,[43] that he could see lucidly things that to the ordinary person were veiled in mystery.[44] "His diagnoses were not inferential hypotheses," student Addison Brewer wrote. "He *saw*."[45] Joe Sullivan told of calling on the Old Doctor for a second opinion on a patient, diagnosed with migraine but exhibiting worrying losses of consciousness. Still examined the man and stated that he had a tumor on the optic tract and would soon die. Two days later the man passed away and the autopsy revealed a "clean white tumor" in the precise spot he had indicated.[46] Henry Bunting related that Still was prone to "diagnose an obscure case now and then as by the flash of an inner light of consciousness, without even looking at the patient before him, without putting his hand to the patient's body or having heard a word of case history." But, he added, Still could sometimes fall prey to overconfidence. "There are traditions to the effect that he would sometimes rush into obvious blunder by this pell-mell hypothetical diagnosis, blunders which only considerations of sympathetic discipleship availed to keep from working to his instant discomfort."[47]

Tales of Still's psychic exploits circulated through the student body. Ed Pickler told of accompanying him to visit Charley in Red Wing. On arriving in Minneapolis they received a telegram asking them to return home urgently because a patient, the wife of a prominent figure, had become critically ill. They caught the first train back. During the journey, in the middle of a conversation about some point in anatomy ("about the only subject in which he was interested"), Still suddenly stopped. "That woman is better," he said. The incident so impressed Pickler that he made a note of the time, and on getting back to Kirksville learned that the patient had begun to rally at around that hour and was no longer in danger.[48]

Eliza Alderman, a patient from Macon, related her story. Gravely ill with puerperal fever after the birth of her sixth child, the alcohol prescribed by her doctor having no effect, she became vaguely aware of the Sunday school bell tolling and was struck by a desperate thought: if she died who would send her children there? She was wondering whether to telegraph Still when, she wrote, "this prayer came to me: Oh God, thou controlling principle that rules the universe, send someone to make me a mother for my children, and if the power and knowledge dwell in Uncle Drew Still let him come." That evening there was a knock on the door and her husband Wesley let in a visitor. It was Still, saying he had received a message. He had spent the weekend in Kansas and while returning home on the last Burlington train the name Wesley Alderman came to him, so he alighted at Macon. "He saved my life," Eliza wrote. "This is one prayer I have the proof of that was answered."[49]

A guest confided in the landlady of a Kirksville boarding house, and to no one else, an intention to consult Still. The two women resolved to apprehend him as he walked past the house, but when he approached they reacted too slowly and he walked so far up the street that they decided to wait for another opportunity. But then they saw him stop, turn around with a perplexed look, and come hurrying back. He climbed the steps and rang the bell. "There's somebody in this house that wants to see me," he said, "who is it?"[50]

Intuition merged with precognition. Still spoke of memory and prophecy:

> Prophecy is what can be seen by a cloudless mind. The events of the past and coming days must all be in sight of the eye of the mind. To prophesy well, you must see through two veils – one of the past and one of the future. If an event is to arise tomorrow, where is it now? Memory calls up the past; reason sees tomorrow. Thought is the action of the machinery of the upper story of life, fed by the nerves of sensation and nutrition, in which chamber only the corpuscles of life center – the arteries of reason to be woven into knowledge by the loom of the Infinite, which moves all there is of mind at one general move, putting that power into motion in all beings, forms, and worlds, a quality which is as plentiful as space. When you think you touch the cord that connects you to the Infinite.[501]

"The philosopher reasons that mentality is the highest attribute of life," he asserted. "Thus it has the power to rule and govern all below it."[52] He declared that "mind principle permeates the whole universe,"[53] and he believed that with the right training the universal mind can be accessed by human senses.

On 1 May 1898, during the Spanish-American War, Still foretold the victory of Commodore George Dewey over Rear Admiral Patricio Montojo at the Battle of Manila Bay, telling a number of acquaintances that he had seen sunken Spanish ships.[54] Then, on July 3, after marines captured Guantanamo Bay, Cuba, the Spanish fleet under Admiral Pascual Cervera attempted to break through the U.S. Navy blockade of Santiago. Still was chatting with a group of students when he suddenly put a hand up over his eyes. "A terrible battle is going on," he announced. "I see ships and hear cannon; there is great destruction." He had seen vessels dashed to pieces and submerged under water. Eager for authentic news he called at the Wabash depot at 5.30 the following morning to buy a newspaper, and on emerging from the station ran into a student. The report in the paper was wrong, Still told the undergraduate, for he had seen in his "mind's eye" one more Spanish vessel destroyed. He was proved correct; the initial report omitted the destruction of the cruiser Cristóbal Colón.[55]

Such tales generated a certain awe and respect, but on at least one occasion his powers of precognition aroused the suspicion of the authorities. After prophesying various fires, burglaries and other local events that later came to pass, the police kept him under surveillance to make sure he was not responsible.[56]

Anxious for Still's reputation and that of the school, friends advised him to be more circumspect about psychic matters, following the tarnishing of the Columbian School's name by Marcus Ward's association with the occult. ("This man was an out-and-out spiritualist," Charles Teall told, "and used to depend upon a rather obese old lady for his tough diagnoses. She would go into a trance and he would sit by her side and receive a message from some forgotten shade as to just what ailed the sufferer in question.")[57]

Still heeded the warning, for the time being at least, and took a dim view when student Rev. Mason Pressly organized extra-curricular classes in telepathy, clairvoyance and related spiritualistic phenomena. During a lecture to the group by William Smith, Still entered the classroom and, in no uncertain terms, admonished them that the spirits could neither treat their patients nor plow their corn.[58]

22
THE SOW RETURNING TO HER WALLOW

Still had regained control of the ASO, but not of the profession as a whole. The two governing bodies, the AAAO and ACO, on whose boards he had never sat, undermined his authority and weakened his leadership. Scattered schools lessened his influence. Osteopathic texts by raw graduates diluted his teachings.

In 1898 Carl McConnell issued his limited edition *Notes on Osteopathic Therapeutics* and Charles Hazzard published his *Principles of Osteopathy*, both comprising the substance of their lectures. That same year Elmer Barber, in his second book *Osteopathy Complete*, presumed to make the subject so simple that even a layman could practice it at home.[1] "Our readers can cure any acute disease in the head, almost instantly, by gently pulling on the head and rotating it in all directions," he maintained, "and any chronic complaint, except cancer, total deafness, or total blindness, by a continuation of the same method."[2] Barber's extravagant, misleading claims were gleefully seized upon by MDs and quoted to legislatures in attempts to discredit osteopathy.

Still had been reluctant to introduce his own text, believing it "a little premature," but after seeing graduates "who had not more than skimmed the surface of the science"[3] rush into print felt he could delay no longer. In November 1898 he announced he was preparing a book – not "a mere recipe for punching here or pressing a button there" but a "system of Independent Philosophy,"[4] a guide for the practitioner to work out for himself the appropriate treatment. The hastily prepared *Philosophy of Osteopathy* was published in late 1899.

By then another volume had appeared, Carl McConnell's compendious *Practice of Osteopathy*, a general textbook structured similarly to Sir William

Osler's *Practice of Medicine*. "It is about all taken from old medical authors," Still complained in a letter to Thekla Orschel. "It is a total failure to an Osteopath."[5] He added that his own book contained only what he had personally tested and proven to be true, with absolutely no quotations from medical books because he differed with them "on almost every important question."[6]

Directly after its release, though, he began planning a new, definitive volume, and had the unwritten work copyrighted at the Library of Congress on the first of December under the provisional title *Illustrated Practice of Osteopathy*.[7] He wrote Orschel again, "I began Jan. 1 – 1900 to write a text book for osteopathic Drs., with colored plates to illustrate all diseases. I will give [the] name of the disease, and show by Anatomical cuts just what the cause is and how to know you are right. The book will be as large as Gray's Anatomy with about 200 plates to show arteries, veins, nerves and so on."[8]

On the first day of the new century, meanwhile, Arthur Hildreth traveled to Columbus, Ohio, to contest a medical bill designed to prevent osteopaths practicing in the state. The Ohio State Board of Health sought powers to grant practice licenses only to applicants who had passed examinations in materia medica and medical therapeutics, and who possessed "a diploma from a reputable medical college in good standing as defined by the board" – criteria that no osteopath could meet. Instead of contesting the measure Hildreth introduced his own bill to regulate osteopathy independently of the medical board.

The medical bill was called up first and was passed by the House, but the Senate medical committee contained many members who supported osteopathy. Realizing that their measure stood to fail without some form of compromise, the MDs introduced an amendment: "This act shall not apply to any osteopath who holds a diploma from a legally chartered and regularly conducted school of Osteopathy in good standing as such, wherein the course of instruction requires at least four terms of five months each in four separate years." The amended bill came before the Senate on April 12 and was passed virtually unopposed. The legislature had been hoodwinked. No osteopathic school ran a four year course, therefore no graduate could meet the new requirements.

Hildreth's measure came before the House that evening. The MDs, having promised not to oppose it, now worked strenuously to have it withdrawn on account of their amendment. It was nevertheless introduced and passed with only three votes against (three MDs). The following day, Friday, as the osteopathic bill awaited its second reading, Ohio senator Joseph B. Foraker received a telegram at his Washington D.C. office signed by the president, secretary and treasurer of the Physicians' Municipal League of Cleveland:

> Eight thousand physicians in the state of Ohio will hold you responsible if the osteopathic bill, to be voted upon by the state Senate at ten o'clock Saturday morning, becomes a law.

Foraker was unaware the bill was pending. He replied:

> All this I greatly regret, because if I had been advised, I might possibly have helped to pass it, as I would gladly have done for the benefit of suffering humanity, who should somehow find release, as I did for my son, from some dependence on such bigotry, impudence, and plantation manners as your telegram manifests.[9]

Hildreth's bill did not become law. Pressure from lobbyists and delaying tactics by friends of the MDs resulted in it being irretrievably delayed, and the legislative session adjourned at noon on Monday with it still awaiting its turn. The medical bill was signed into law, enforced by the State Board, and no osteopath attempted to apply for a license under it.[10]

"If osteopathy has scientific merit and carries no bottles of poison that would produce death and destruction of human life," Still responded, "why should medical schools ask prohibitory legislation? Does an American have to say 'My Lord' may I think a little? Or will he say as he has said for one hundred years just passed, that all men are free and equal." The American people should be at liberty to choose the type of doctor they wanted without the "Czars of medicine" abusing the system by enlisting the aid of legislatures to stamp out osteopathy.[11]

On April 11, Blanche married ASO final year student George M. Laughlin. Her father approved of the match and took to calling his new in-law "Son George."[12] Still had disapproved her previous suitor, J. Martin Littlejohn, whose idea of romance was to lavish fun-loving, card-playing Blanche with a set of encyclopedias.[13] Littlejohn remained on the horizon, though. In May, four months after their ignominious departure from the ASO, the three Littlejohn brothers organized the American School of Osteopathic Medicine and Surgery in Chicago.[14]

At the beginning of May Still spent a week with Ed in Macon, and on his return mailed a letter to Thekla Orschel. He felt "stouter this year," he wrote, perhaps due to the sedentary nature of his "big summer job on the text book," and reported, "School is in good shape, people generally well."[15] But as the weather turned hot and humid a rumor reached Kirksville that the State Board of Health planned to introduce a bill to the Missouri legislature the following year to abolish the 1897 osteopathic law.

This cheerless news was tempered by a providential development. Representative Samuel M. Pickler of Adair County tended his resignation to run for Congress in that November's elections, and the local Republican Party invited Arthur Hildreth to stand as their candidate. Still urged him to accept, recognizing the benefit of having the osteopathic profession represented in the House. Hildreth vacillated, but finally agreed.[16] In advance of his campaign he relinquished the ASO deanship, and Still appointed his new son-in-law George Laughlin to the post.

Hildreth was duly elected Representative of Adair County and, at noon on 2 January 1901, proudly took his seat in the State Capitol, Jefferson City. That afternoon he called on outgoing governor Lon Stephens to pay his respects. Stephens had followed Hildreth's campaign with interest. "I would have felt that the people of your county had not indorsed my action in signing your osteopathic bill in the spring of 1897 should you not have been elected," he confided. "I congratulate you and your profession upon your election to our legislature and wish for you and your interests continued success."[17]

With Governor Alexander M. Dockery's inauguration set for 12 January, Hildreth made use of the ten day hiatus by introducing himself to other members, including one of the leaders of the House, Hon. Matthew Hall. Large, tall and distinguished, the Saline County representative had two physician brothers and had voted against the two previous osteopathic bills. "When a man does what he thinks best," Hildreth told him, "I never have any fault to find, whether or not he is voting for what I believe to be right." But, he added, he hoped Hall might feel differently towards their cause in any future vote. His candor immediately won Hall's trust. "Dr. Hildreth," he replied, "this House will not pass any legislation against you people." To Hildreth's surprise he further offered him a seat on the committee for the World's Fair Louisiana Purchase Exposition, to be held in St. Louis on the centenary of the great territorial acquisition.

Hildreth elected to sit on the Public Health committee and soon became privy to the State Board's plans. In the coming session of the General Assembly the twelve MDs in the House sought not only to repeal the 1897 osteopathic law but also take control of all aspects of medical education and practice within the state. They planned to create a board of seven examiners – three MDs, three homeopathic or eclectic physicians, and one osteopath – and they strongly urged

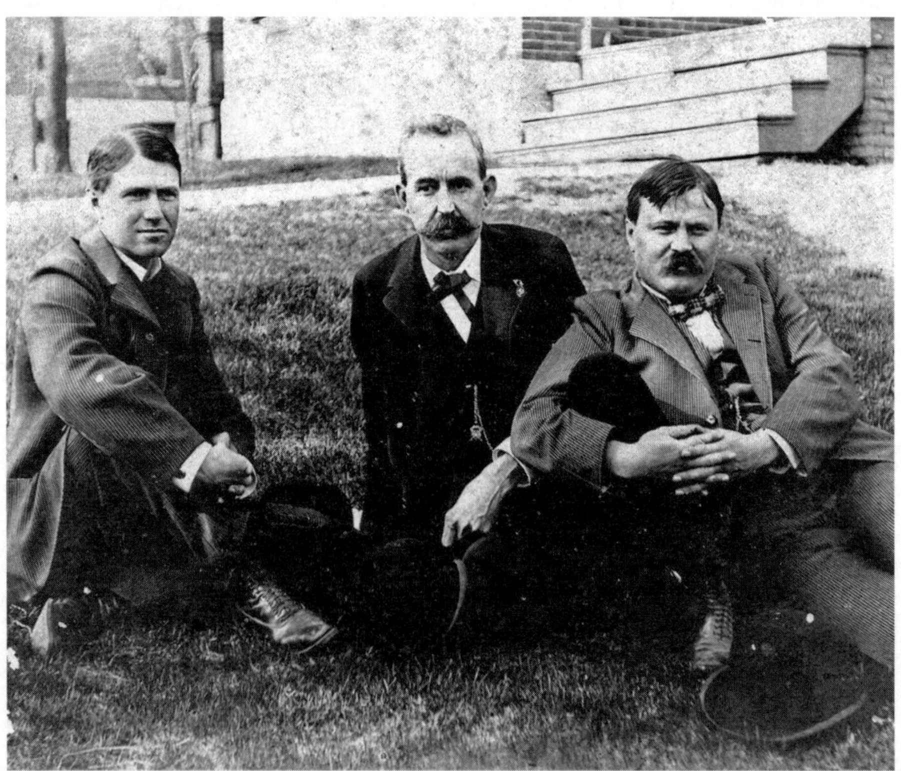

(left to right) Charles Still, Arthur Hildreth and Harry Still.

Hildreth to accept the proposal. The following weekend he traveled to Kirksville to consult Still, who instructed him not to accept it under any circumstances.

On returning to Jefferson City, Hildreth was sitting at his desk when Matthew Hall entered the room and proffered a document. "Write your amendment to this bill," he said. Hildreth recognized the immense favor being granted. The medical profession had chosen the Saline County man to introduce their measure – one potentially disastrous for osteopathy – and Hall, true to his word, wanted to make sure its wording was acceptable. He also prearranged with the Speaker of the House that when the medical bill was called up Hildreth would be recognized first.

Hildreth rose on cue and offered an amendment to the effect that nothing in the bill should interfere with the 1897 osteopathic law.

Eight hours of heated debate ensued. A profusion of amendments were offered in an attempt to overturn Hildreth's, but his was finally accepted. Some members, believing the MDs were seeking to benefit themselves rather than the public, even asked him how they should vote. "Vote whatever way you believe right," Hildreth said, "it will not affect us a particle if our amendment is accepted." The bill passed with seventy-one votes, five more than necessary. The following day, amidst ongoing arguments, the Senate also approved the measure and Governor Dockery signed it into law. This landmark ruling enabled Missouri osteopaths to practice independently of the State Board of Health.[18]

Legislative battles played out across the country. On 27 February 1901 the New York State Assembly convened in Albany to debate a bill to allow osteopaths practice licenses. The hearing drew much publicity due to the presence of Samuel L. Clemens, better known as the author Mark Twain, whose daughter Jean was being treated by George Helmer, relocated from Vermont to New York City. As a boy the novelist had lived in Hannibal, Missouri, and, according to Charley, was treated there by Still in the early 1880s.[19] Clemens had simply come to listen, but was persuaded to speak on behalf of osteopathy.[20]

Arguments against the bill were opened by Dr. Frank Van Vleet of the New York County Medical Society, who vilified osteopaths as charlatans and quacks, and branded Clemens a "funny man" who no one took seriously. Surgeon Robert Morris presented twelve hypothetical cases and suggested, with undisguised sarcasm, applying "the treatment advised by Elmer D. Barber in his book

Osteopathy Complete." Morris ridiculed neighboring Vermont for passing "such lax laws with regard to medical practice that it is now the garbage ground of the profession," and as a parting shot unwrapped a bundle to reveal a column of diseased vertebrae freshly dissected from a dead infant. Tossing the specimen onto the chairman's desk, he challenged "any one of these osteopaths to move a part of that bone the fraction of an inch." A crowd gathered around the table. "Now there are the gloves," he goaded, "come put them on and give us an exhibition of your professed skill."

For the opposing side Assemblyman Julius Seymour, author of the bill, delivered a preliminary speech, then attorney John T. Coleman introduced Clemens. A loud cheer erupted from the public galleries as the writer, an all-white outfit complementing his bushy white hair, stepped into the center of the well. "My general character was attacked a thousand times before you were born, sir," he bowed low to Van Vleet. "You have not succeeded in bringing to light more than half my iniquities, for which I am thankful." When laughter subsided he turned to Morris's gruesome specimen. "I was touched and distressed at that exhibition here of that part of a little child. I cannot take a child to pieces that way." Clemens asserted his constitutional right to do as he liked with his own body and declared that if New York failed to legalize osteopathy he would simply cross the state line into Vermont for treatment. "I might also call the doctor's attention to the fact," he added, "that the *garbage barrel,* as they call Vermont, is the healthiest state in the Union."[21]

The committee did not report the bill and osteopathy would remain illegal in New York until 1907. Still remained philosophical:

> There are many reasons why measures of justice are withheld from the masses by the few. . . . Nations often unjustly oppress their own subjects and extend their unjust tyranny over other nations because of the power of wealth and resources to enforce obedience to such demands. . . . The enemy has ruled so long that they think right is divine, and they will fight to the hour of death.[22]

In October 1900 the ASO's long-running battle with Elmer Barber's National School of Osteopathy ended in a Milan, Missouri, courtroom. Barber himself had initiated the proceeding, filing suit against the ASO for $100,000 damages after the *Journal of Osteopathy* accused him of running a diploma mill. The action backfired. At the close of the prosecution case Judge Ellison, on behalf of the ASO, raised a demurrer that the NSO's charter gave it no authority to conduct a school of osteopathy. The jury ruled in the ASO's favor and Barber was forced to close his institution.[23]

Marcus Ward's Columbian School of Osteopathy was also in trouble. In early 1901 a catalogue of problems – faculty resignations over unfulfilled contracts, students admitted on credit unable to settle their accounts, and others dissatisfied with the teaching transferring to the ASO – led stockholders to withdraw their support.[24] "C bursted financially," Still scribbled privately. "No stone is as heavy as dishonesty – that will take a man under some time, hands off. Ward pulls feb 10."[25] Ward left for California, never to return, while his students were allowed to complete their studies at the ASO for $24 cash or bankable note.[26]

Ward was gone, but he left a legacy. A new word entered the osteopathic lexicon: *mixer*. Mixers were osteopaths who combined drugs with their practice or employed *adjuncts* to treatment: electric vibrators, magnetism, Swedish movements, salt or medicated baths, to name a few. The trend angered Still, who repeatedly insisted that osteopathy was a system complete in itself. "I find the less we know of anatomical truths," he slammed the mixers, "the more we want adjuncts and a bottle of Mother Winslow's Soothing Syrup."[27]

To his exasperation some mixers were even professing to practice "medical osteopathy." J. Martin Littlejohn's "osteopathic medicine" was ambiguous enough, but this was a hideous oxymoron. Osteopathy and medicine "are so opposite," Still fumed, "that one might as well say white is black." He declared that any "half and half who pretends to be an osteopath and at the same time uses drugs wants the dollar and is neither an M.D. nor an osteopath."[28] To mix allopathic, homeopathic or herbal remedies signified base ignorance of osteopathic fundamentals. "No system of Allopathy, with its fatal drugs, should ever be permitted to enter our doors. No homeopathic practice, with its sugar-coated pills, must be allowed to stain or pollute our name. Osteopathy asks not the aid of anything else. It can paddle its own canoe."[29] In the public's mind medicine meant drugs, and only by keeping the two systems separate could people know what to expect when they chose an osteopath. Still wanted patients to know from beginning to end that they were coming to a different kind of doctor.

The medics, unsurprisingly, made much of the mixers. One of their journals predicted that within five years every osteopathic school would teach osteopathy and medicine combined. "We will acknowledge," Still conceded, "that there is danger of the sow returning to her wallow." He accused the mixers of being "weak," of having "less honor than a hyena," and charged that they would "administer morphine, whiskey, blisters or any other damnable drug if they could make one dollar or one cent" from it. He warned, prophetically, that the greatest threat to osteopathy came not from the medical profession but from "osteopathic-medical dummies" within their own ranks.[30]

On Saturday, 22 June 1901, Kirksville celebrated osteopathy's twenty-seventh anniversary with an enormous barbecue on Still's lawn. Trees were wound with ribbons in red and black (the school's colors), and linked by festoons of red, white and blue. From midnight till dawn "the slain carcasses of nine beeves and twenty sheep simmered and sizzled" over trenches filled with glowing beds of charcoal, lighting the hill with incandescence. Overnight giant thunderheads piled up in the western sky to shoot "bolts of lightning more beautiful than rockets," and as the heavens boomed and reverberated a sprinkling of rain settled the dust and cooled the sultry summer air.

The morning dawned clear with fluffy clouds. A big brass field gun resounded down the hill from the school and, at precisely 10 a.m., a parade headed by the ASO band began to snake its way from Baird's corner. Still rode with Mary in the leading carriage, tipping his hat to an enthusiastic crowd, and behind followed their sons, faculty, alumni, students, local dignitaries, and carriages from surrounding areas, with the rear brought up by the local company of the Missouri National Guard. The procession wound its way to the square, circled the impressive new courthouse, and returned via Pierce and Osteopathy streets to the school. Still, Hildreth and Judge Ellison delivered speeches from a platform erected in a natural amphitheater nearby and the whole town turned out to honor northeast Missouri's most celebrated citizen. It was resolved that henceforth June 22 should be known as Founder's Day.[31]

Ten days later Kirksville hosted the fifth annual AAAO convention. The profession had grown to two thousand practitioners, with another thousand being educated. The committee agreed to publish a new journal and change the organization's unwieldy title to the American Osteopathic Association. The Associated Colleges of Osteopathy, now comprising twelve institutions, held their meeting concurrently, but most of the three-day event was spent in bickering over the schools' differing business relations.

The ASO commencement exercises were held during the gathering. On a stiflingly hot evening Still stood on a low platform, "feet in slippers, no coat, one suspender, at least, held the trousers by a nail, shirt open at neck," cooling himself with a palm leaf fan.[32] He advised the graduating class to ignore politics and the medical men, and stick to what was important: cultivate their sense of touch, prune the osteopathic profession of all that was obsolete, and take an obligation to improve medicine for the health and happiness of all.[33]

Early in 1902 came encouraging news. The Ohio Supreme Court ruled that in the matter of the 1900 osteopathic bill the state's Board of Health had acted unconstitutionally in denying practice licenses to osteopaths who had not completed a four year course, for although no osteopathic school ran a course of that length, neither did any medical school. The new ruling allowed the introduction of another bill to establish an independent osteopathic board. In February, as Arthur Hildreth left for Columbus to fight the hardest legislative challenge of his life, Still delivered his students a plainspoken address:

> If we are to fight battles in defense of our country, pay taxes, build public buildings, schools, work out our road taxes, and do our full duty in all things that our government requires of its people, why in the name of reason and common sense can't we expect the government to say that you and I, this and that and every school of the healing art are to be equal in the sight of the law to one another? It doesn't step in and attempt to dictate to you or to me what religious principles we shall entertain or to what church we shall give our moral or financial support. But would all this be more unreasonable than the laws on the statute books of many a state conceived by an iniquitous medical fraternity that would dictate to the people how, when and where your child, my babe, ourselves, are to be treated when sick in body and sore afflicted. Think for a moment how they would curtail our God-given and man-fought-for rights. And

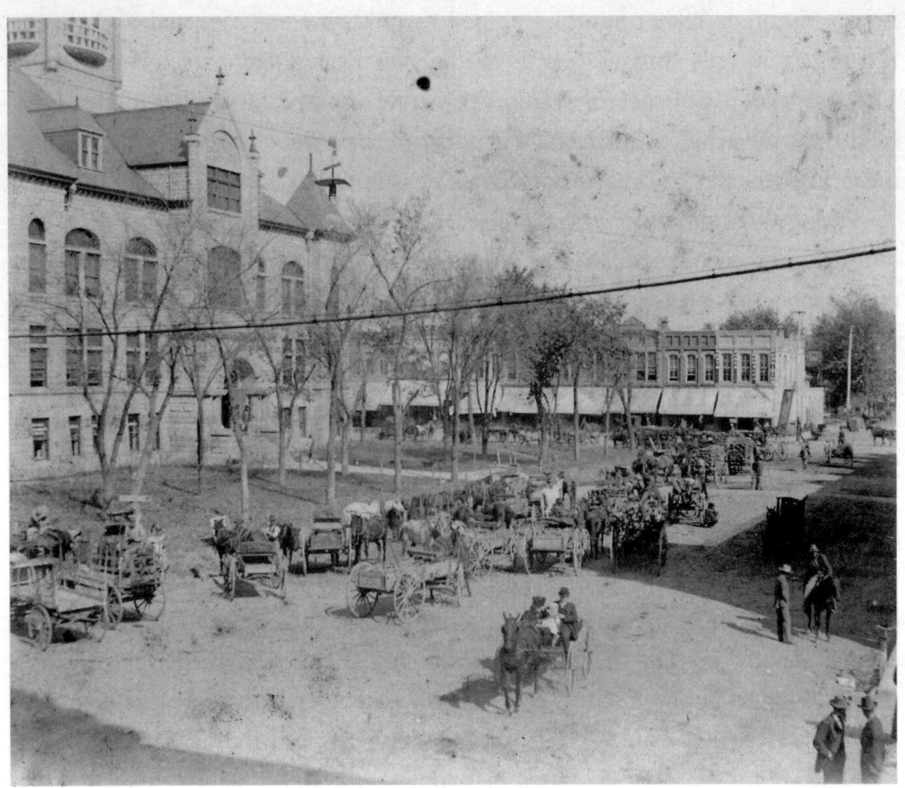

Kirksville's new courthouse on the public square.

> the saddest thing of all is that many of us have sat quietly by and haven't raised so much as a finger in protest.
>
> I want you to interest yourselves in politics to the extent of getting clean men in your state legislatures, irrespective of the party he may represent. Let a man's honor and abilities determine whether he is to get your support. In a few years we will have no red-nosed drug doctors meddling with our business or our profession, but in the meantime do your work in your profession and as American citizens and voters, to the best of your abilities and with ever a high standard of moral ethics as your guide.[34]

A majority in both House and Senate supported the osteopathic measure, but felt constrained by a powerful medical lobby. At the preliminary judiciary hearing Hildreth and colleagues M. F. Hulett and Mary Dyer faced a formidable group of forty physicians, including ex-presidents of the American Medical, Homeopathic and Eclectic associations. Bitter, intense and prejudiced, they accused the trio of ignorance, derided the osteopathic colleges, and disparaged their graduates as unqualified to practice. Most of the nine-member Judiciary Committee felt Hildreth's measure just, but some dared not support it. Five voted for, four against; an insufficient majority. It appeared that the bill had failed, but at the last minute a lawyer from Cleveland approached Hildreth with a compromise. "Let the medical board examine osteopathic physicians in the four subjects provided in their proposed bill," he suggested, "but with the provision that your profession to be given a committee from your own school to examine your own applicants in the other subjects taught in your colleges." It was a major concession. Having no osteopathic representation on the State Board would mean a loss of independence, but Hildreth finally accepted. The amended bill was passed on 21 April 1902, making osteopathy legal in Ohio.[35]

Still, too, was being forced into compromises. That August, at the AOA convention at the Hotel Pfister, Milwaukee, the education committee voted to extend osteopathic courses to three years of nine months each, to be implemented the following year. Still vehemently opposed the idea, regarding two years as sufficient and the inclusion of yet more medical subjects both unnecessary and damaging.[36] "We cannot afford to spend years on infant theories of the distant past when all that is useful in a thousand pages can be written in more intelligent form on a single sheet of foolscap," he asserted. "Our school wants long strides towards brevity in all branches. When a house is on fire who would stop to read how the city of Sodom burned and what kind of goat skins was used to tote water in to quench the fire?"[37]

He was also exasperated by the ACO, whose meeting was held concurrently. The organization's lax enforcement of educational standards and liberal attitude towards adjuncts had long troubled him, while membership of the ACO made it possible for schools to teach methods of which he disapproved while ostensibly having the support of the founding institution.[38] Two years earlier he had even published a "letter" to ASO students and graduates declaring that a diploma from Kirksville was more valuable than one from any other school.[39]

Still did not go to Milwaukee. Acting on his instructions, Hildreth tabled a motion recommending that the ACO be disbanded and the AOA be given the power to decide which schools met the accepted criteria. When the ACO objected, Charley tendered the parent school's resignation from the organization.[40]

Most Kirksville graduates approved of the move,[41] but it created much consternation among the other schools. "I regret the action very much," J. Martin Littlejohn complained from Chicago. "I know that Dr. A. T. Still opposed the A.C.O. from its inception, as I personally discussed the matter with him at the origin of the A.C.O. I told Dr. Still then I believed he was mistaken, and I still believe so." Littlejohn added that although he "respected" the founder, it did not mean that Still was "the only exponent of the science or that the A.S.O. is the only school of Osteopathy." Mason Pressly, secretary of the Philadelphia College of Osteopathy, described the episode as "an 'acute lesion' in Osteopathic comity."[42]

Amid ongoing recriminations Still made public his reasons for withdrawing: he could neither endorse the teaching of non-osteopathic material nor sanction questionable business practices. He detailed the ASO's position in nine "planks":

> 1. We are opposed to the use of drugs as remedial agencies.
> 2. We are opposed to vaccination.
> 3. We are opposed to the use of serums in the treatment of disease.
> 4. We realize that many cases require surgical treatment and, therefore, advocate it as a last resort. We believe many surgical operations are unnecessarily performed and that many operations can be avoided by osteopathic treatment.
> 5. The osteopath does not use electricity, x-radiance, hydrotherapy, but relies on osteopathic measures in the treatment of disease.
> 6. We have a friendly feeling for other non-drug, natural methods of healing, but we do not incorporate any other methods into our system. To cure disease the abnormal parts must be adjusted to the normal, therefore other methods that are entirely different in principle have no place in the osteopathic system.

7. We believe that our therapeutic house is just large enough for osteopaths and that when other methods are brought in, just that much osteopathy must move out.
8. Osteopathy is an independent system and can be applied to all conditions of disease except purely surgical cases.
9. We believe in sanitation and hygiene.[43]

That month, October 1902, Still's long-awaited "textbook" was finally published. The volume originally copyrighted as the *Illustrated Practice of Osteopathy* was more modest than planned, containing neither plates nor diagrams, and had passed through a series of proposed titles before appearing as *The Philosophy and Mechanical Principles of Osteopathy*.[44] The pressing need to maintain the purity of osteopathy had led to him spending more time in the school during the past two years than since the very beginning, but the book's publication was also delayed by the deaths of his faithful amanuensis Annie Morris on March 1 that year, and of his close friend John R. Musick the previous April. "I miss him more today than any man I know of," Still wrote in an emotional tribute to the writer who helped compile his two previous books. "I am now at a point that wise counsel is at a premium with me."[45]

In reviewing the book Still's nephew Turner Hulett worried that "people whose experiences are bound by the horizon of convention" might fail to "appreciate Dr. Still's grasp of the problems of organic life." Hulett's tone was almost apologetic. "To be properly understood and appreciated," he continued, "the peculiarities of his methods of thought and of expression, his abundant use of figure and illustration, and especially his impatience of elaborate discussion of minor points, if tending to prevent the reaching of the essential point in the shortest and quickest way, must be kept clearly in mind."[46] No up-to-date scientific terminology here. "His language is quite unique, a bit quaint, with overtones of the Scriptures, a bit laborious at times," Ernest Tucker enlarged. "Often it is difficult not to be amused to the point of quite missing the intensity of inquiry, the wistful courage of it."[47]

The poetic, almost religious, style was deliberate. The spiritual lay at the heart of osteopathy and, as in the Bible, spiritual truths were best expressed through metaphor and allegory. Carl McConnell urged all osteopaths – particularly the "few who do not seem to grasp the osteopathic philosophy" – to digest the timeless wisdom contained in the volume, to mull over the words and read between the lines, since "even after a careful reading of the book much will escape."[48]

McConnell's words reflected a growing apprehension among the faithful. Spreading through the profession was a question first posed at Milwaukee by Herbert Bernard, the childhood friend of Still's sons, now practicing in Detroit: "are you a lesion osteopath?" In the corridors of the Hotel Pfister, Bernard pleaded with his colleagues to "get back" and stick to basic principles, warning that by prescribing drugs and tying to "the osteopathic kite a tail made up of electrotherapeutics, hydrotherapy and a few adjunct knots," the public "might mistake the tail from the kite."[49]

ASO alumni rallied behind the founder's teachings. Arthur Hildreth criticized the growing number of graduates who, "after taking a course in osteopathy, think they are not competent until they take a course in medicine."[50] William Smith, returned from Europe and practicing in St. Louis, wrote, "And so today when I look around me and I see so many adjuncts to osteopathy, when I find this man using the colon tube, and the other man using the vibrator to treat the eyes, and a third using electric massage to fix up a patient's back, another man with a static apparatus to restore manhood and another with something to grow hair on bald heads, I ask you where in the name of common sense is osteopathy in all that?"[51] Smith asserted that he had stopped administering drugs because he had found something better. Joe Sullivan, despairing at the situation, declared bluntly, "there is something lacking in the osteopathy imbibed outside of Kirksville."[52]

In January 1903, as graduates of other schools veered off on tracks of their own, Henry Bunting's *Osteopathic Physician* published an article, "The Lesion Osteopath Is Too Narrow." Its author, influential Pacific School graduate Dain Tasker, preparing a book on osteopathic principles that would become a standard text for the next thirty years, argued that Still's principle of cause and effect was too limited. "This may be the sum of some people's osteopathy, but it is not mine," he opined. "I would really like to know how many men of five years active practice are willing to balance themselves on this two inch strip of a plank." Tasker asserted the right of all practitioners to employ any adjunct if they so wished.[53]

Still continued to work tirelessly on behalf of graduates practicing in Missouri. Though the 1901 bill entitled osteopaths to practice independently of the State Board, he felt that the law regulating osteopathy itself was poor. In 1903 he had Arthur Hildreth, newly re-elected to the Missouri House of Representatives, introduce a bill before the General Assembly to request the establishment of an independent osteopathic board to examine candidates in all subjects, issue practice licenses, give osteopaths the same rights as medical doctors with regard to infectious and contagious diseases, and entitle them to sign birth and death certificates. The measure passed with only five votes against and would become the model for uniform legislation across the Union. It also finally granted the ASO the right to obtain dissection material.[54]

Osteopathy had entered the mainstream. Accepted by the public and sanctioned by law, it faced increasing pressure to conform to the dominant political and economic values of American society, and with it moved ever further from its own distinctive philosophy and principles. Still was seventy-five and losing his grip on the profession he had founded.

In November 1903, in a mood of desperation, he pleaded for each state association to adopt rules to force the resignation of all "two-faced practitioners" and bar "all mixers and their ilk."[55]

23
MOTION

As the profession bickered amongst themselves, Still was never long distracted from his quest to penetrate the mysteries of health and disease, life and death.

He had studied anatomy more thoroughly than perhaps anyone before him. He had developed latent mental faculties until they became a normal and unconscious part of his way of being. He had worked with the living human body, normal and abnormal, to the point of absolute conviction that the principles he had elucidated were universal laws. "With me it is no longer a debatable question," he asserted now. "If I fail to get the results desired, I am frank to say that my ignorance is responsible for the failure and not the ability of the body to vindicate the intelligence of its architect and builder."[1] But the subject he had perhaps too narrowly called osteopathy did not begin and end with the body and mind; it extended to the spirit of life and the immutable Power behind the creation. "The osteopath finds here," Still gloried, "the field in which he can dwell forever."[2]

And dwell he did. He yearned to gain knowledge of the arcane power that animates living nature. Over the years he repeatedly scrawled the question *What is life?* on scraps of paper and dictated it to Annie Morris, who preserved his inconclusive musings.

Was life "a quality of matter,"[3] he asked, perhaps some kind of "finer matter that is invisible and that moves all that is visible to us?"[4] Or perhaps some kind of energy or force, related to or produced by electricity, distributed to all parts of the body by the nervous system? (Emil DuBois-Reymond had demonstrated that at death the nerves cease all electrical activity, no longer deflecting a magnetic needle.) "All [living creatures] must have, and cannot act without the highest known order of force (electricity)," Still reasoned. But how and where was the electricity generated? Did the movements of the heart act as a dynamo and the brain a storage battery? Electricity was not life itself, though, merely one of its manifestations. "We are now in the presence of the great questions," he asserted, and cited examples: by what force does the heart beat, the embryo grow, the organism maintain its existence? "One could easily say by vital force," he said, "as vitality is one of the secrets that has never been delivered to man from the bosom of nature." But to name it as such would clarify nothing.[5]

Still nevertheless rejected the scientific assumption that life emanates from matter, in favor of the diametrically opposite view. Man's "existence in form is the effect of life," he held, "the cause antedates him by mind and deed. With no conclusive evidence that man's existence is as old as cause, his life or spirit must be the cause of his form."[6] Perhaps, then, religion might hold the answer.

"When God formed Adam from the dust of the ground and blew the breath of life into his nostrils," he asked, "was that breath a substance or a principle?"[7] Still chose words carefully when dealing with important concepts (with the acknowledgment that words were imprecise tools, "only labels for thought, chosen to represent some quality belonging to the package manufactured in the mental work shop.")[8]

In theology the word *substance* denotes the divine nature or essence uniting the three Persons of the triune God – Father, Son and Holy Ghost. "Is [life] a substance?" Still probed. "If so, what are its attributes? Is this substance, life, above all elementary substances?"[9] (He even described man as "triune"[10] – his trinity that of matter, mind and motion.) The word *principle* denotes a fundamental truth, an ultimate cause, or a law of nature. If life is "an individualized principle of Nature," he argued, then "definite arrangements" must exist to allow this "living and separate personage" – this *soul* – to associate with the body.

Of substance or principle, Still favored the former: "Life surely is a very finely prepared substance which is the all-moving force of nature."[11] But religion brought him no closer to a definitive answer. He complained that a lifetime of listening to "the ravings and unsatisfactory assertions of the theologian" had "contributed nothing" to his understanding of the soul.[12] On the subject of life, he lamented, "we are in a sea of mysteries from start to finish."[13]

Beyond life lay the greatest mystery of all. "What is God?" he questioned again and again.[14] "Who or what is behind the curtain that veils the human eye and mind?" He listed names: Jehovah, the Unknowable, the All-Wise, the Shawnee's "Illnoywa Tapamala-qua."[15] Still did not ascribe to the Christian notion of God, an anthropomorphic Father in Heaven, a transcendental spirit present in every part of the universe yet separate from it; he favored a God similar to that of the American Indian, Creator and creation inseparable, the universe intelligent at all levels; God the whole, a "universal universe," and man a part, a "dependent universe."[16] But he did not proselytize; liberty demanded that all be free to decide for themselves "whether God be an individualized person or not."[17]

In truth no one knew – even the Bible stated that *No man hath seen God at any time*.[18] "The little which we do know of God," John Wesley had preached, "we do not gather from an inward impression, but gradually acquire from without. 'The invisible things of God,' if they are known at all, 'are known from the things that are made;' not from what God hath written in out hearts, but from what he hath written in all his works. Hence, then, from his works, particularly his works of creation, we are to learn the knowledge of God."[19] Still echoed, "When we have accumulated all the knowledge that the human mind can possibly acquire, it is acquaintance with the work of that Architect that constitutes the real knowledge of God. Outside that, all is silence."[20] He once told Ed Pickler:

> Every bone in the body, every muscle, nerve and blood vessel is continually telling you that they are parts of this great Creative Scheme, and when you study them intelligently and gain proper understanding of *them,* you are developing your spiritual understanding to the same extent. When I study anatomy, I not only develop understanding of the physical, but I unfold and enlarge my mental and spiritual qualities. Anything which tends to give us a better comprehension of the great creative power which fashioned us must necessarily make us appreciate the wonderful mind or spirit back of it. It has been said I am not an orthodox believer. Perhaps in some ways I am not, but no man lives

> who has a deeper seated, more implicit faith in the Power who created this human machine than I have, or a more exalted reverence for that Creator and his work.[21]

Still advised the clergy not to rely upon "theories" (doctrine, dogma, scripture) to support their assertion that *God's works prove His perfection,* but to read *Gray's Anatomy* and bring before their flocks a skeleton "to prove that God's wisdom is vindicated in that sacred relic." "Go on and on, Reverend Sir," he taunted, "until you know what man is. Take your text from the truths of nature; give us facts, and your sexton will not have to crack your congregation's heads together to keep them awake whilst thou talkest."[22]

To see God and nature as inseparable, and matter and spirit as two sides of one reality, led to a radically different worldview to that espoused by Western society. *The Philosophy and Mechanical Principles of Osteopathy* contained a chapter entitled "Biogen,"[23] a metaphoric scheme of the universe as a union of terrestrial forces and celestial wisdom:

> Life terrestrial has motion and power; the celestial bodies have knowledge or wisdom. Biogen is the lives of the two in united action, that give motion and growth to all things. The result is faultless perfection, because the earth-life shows in material forms the wisdom of the God of the celestial. Thus we say biogen or dual life, that life means eternal reciprocity that permeates all nature.[24]

And that faultless perfection, Still maintained, should extend to all phases of nature's cycle – including death. "We are in the universe therefore we are with God and help to compose that great all, and journey as it journeys. That great compound is eternal, so are we. We have lived, do live, and will live out the full number of the days of the universe."[25] So he believed, but for half a century he had yearned conclusive proof.

Ministers preached vehemently of living souls and dying souls, of the blessed and the damned, and of the soul's continued existence after death, but when Still asked for "certain knowledge" they merely repeated quotations from scripture and labeled him an unbeliever.[26] But unquestioning belief did not satisfy this truth seeker. "As belief and doubt are synonymous terms," he asserted, "the philosopher must take neither in this court of inquiry. If you only believe and don't know, you should go back to your anatomy class and stay until you know that the blood and nerve supply are perfect, and can again give God the credit for perfection."[27] Faith, in the popular sense of the word, did not satisfy Still either for it, too, implied not actually *knowing*. He favored the Apostle Paul's definition of faith as elaborated by John Wesley:

> [Faith is] a divine evidence and conviction . . . of things not seen – not visible, nor perceivable by sight or by any other of the external senses. It implies both a supernatural *evidence* of God and of the things of God, a kind of spiritual *light* exhibited to the soul, and a supernatural *sight* or perception thereof. . . . By this twofold operation of the Holy Spirit – having the eyes of our soul both *opened* and *enlightened* – we see things which the natural 'eye hath not seen, neither the ear heard.' We have a prospect of the invisible things of God. We see the *spiritual world*, which is all round about us, and yet no more discerned by our natural faculties than if it had no being; and we see the *eternal world*, piercing through the veil which hangs between time and eternity.[28]

Still regarded this veil to lie not only "round about us" but also within us. "I believe in the unlimited possibilities for the development of our spiritual and mental organizations, just as I do the physical," he told Ed Pickler. "You do not need a medium to get into communication with the Infinite. You have this infinity in yourself, and it is only a question of whether you will recognize and cultivate it. The door into the spiritual world is open. All you need to do is to search until you find it and walk in."[29]

In a talk entitled *Body and Soul of Man* he spoke of the scriptural stories of angels and visions, of prophets and seers, and of the transfiguration of Jesus on the mountain, witnessed by disciples Peter, James and John:

> And his face did shine as the sun, and his raiment was white as the light. And, behold, there appeared unto them Moses and Elias talking with him.[30]

Methodists were taught to regard this passage as "sacred evidence that Moses and Elias were not dead but were yet living," and Still argued that what was true then should remain true forever:

> When did God change His ways? There are plenty of people who testify in these later days, and there were plenty in the days of Moses and Elias. In this day all over America people are testifying that they have seen their departed friends. If they are mistaken it is no fault of yours. If it is true, worlds for the victory that they have gained. That was Christ's mission on earth. He was a medium. If Jesus was a medium through whom Moses and Elias did appear that is a triumphant victory. . . . If that is not a lie it is the most brilliant truth ever recorded . . . and if they were mistaken, it is a mistake, but I positively believe that they did appear. I have seen spirits too. The superstitious fear of such things should be overcome.

Still urged his listeners not to stop at anatomy and physiology but to go on and investigate the question *What is life?* If they could demonstrate that the spirits of the dead can communicate with the living it would prove that life is not an emanation of matter but an eternal soul, and he encouraged them to research the question by any means possible. "It matters not to me from what point knowledge comes," he said. "I would as soon take the truth from the old colored woman down here who does washing, as to take it from the Pope of Rome. It matters not into whose possession it falls. The truth of life beyond the grave is what we seek."

He declared it was the "duty" of the American School of Osteopathy to seek truth, and that no one should fear talking about unconventional matters. "The very foundation stone that is in this building is for liberty of thought," he proclaimed. "Liberty of thought! That is your right, and you are a coward if you do not use it." His position was clear. "Now you know how I stand on these subjects. No man living, in or out of the pulpit can give me this knowledge, but the dead can come and talk to me of the life beyond. You have my sentiments." He singled out a member of the audience. "If this man says he lives after death, I will say, 'come back, Bob, and tell us about it.'"[31]

Such talk made uneasy listening for the increasingly conservative ASO faculty. When Still invited a spiritualist to deliver a lecture in Memorial Hall they branded Spiritualism "disreputable," declared it "not respectable" to attend, and accused him of disgracing the school. They boycotted the event and went to a dog show instead.

Still's introductory talk that evening brimmed with indignation, his voice sweeping the audience like a scythe through grain, his hands, mimicking the same movement, rising high and curving down in unconscious cutting gestures. "I'm ashamed that none of the professors in this school are here," he spoke:

> I say it's not respectable to be an ignoramus on any subject. I'm ashamed they're not here tonight to come up a little nearer to the mystery of God, which is thought. Disreputable? This day is progressive. The same fellows who in 1874 thought me disreputable and a crazy crank, today say 'God bless you' because I was not ashamed of the psychic forces that operated through me for the good of mankind. It's the unpardonable sin to ignore that voice of God or of spirits trying to speak in or through you to man. By that psychic law I can answer any question you put to me about osteopathy. When you ask a question that you can't answer by your books, I'll answer it by this psychic power. Not a professor can ask me a question that I cannot answer scientifically by that psychic power. But let them answer a question I will put to them scientifically and I'll give them a better pair of breeches than I've got, and pay their way to a hundred dog shows.

Years ago, he said, his brothers were ashamed of him and his uncles avoided him. "I've been prayed to, and for, and been cursed up and down, backward and forward, because I said that man was immortal and I could prove it. . . . Am I disreputable or crazy? Have I disgraced them?" His voice, though not loud, assumed a "terrific" intensity. "Not a professor shall occupy a chair in this outfit who is ashamed to come up to the subject of psychology," he averred. "It is the origin of this business."[32]

This assertion inevitably raised curiosity. Did it mean that on that fateful June day in 1874 he really did receive assistance from on high? Student Charles Teall broached the subject while walking with Still south of town, and their conversation "turned into the channel of the psychic or unexplained source of help that has aided all great, original thinkers in times when the sought-for solution was elusive." Still offered no explanation, but stopped and spread his arms upward. "There is something," he said, "and it is the grandmother of osteopathy."[33]

In early 1903 Still announced that he intended visiting one or more Spiritualist camp meetings that year and report his findings. At the end of August he boarded a train for Clinton, Iowa, to attend the annual gathering of the Mississippi Valley Spiritualists Association, held on bluffs west of the river. "Let me say right here," he told the ASO student publication *The Bulletin of the Atlas and Axis Clubs*:

> I feel as a hungry child seeking the milk of its mother's breast. I am hungry mentally, absolutely hungry beyond description, to obtain a more thorough acquaintance with that substance or principle known as human life. This hunger has been with me many years. I have nothing so precious that I would not give to have it satisfied. I want an undebatable knowledge, a better acquaintance with life and whether it be a substance or a principle that contains the many attributes of mind, such as wisdom, memory, the powers of reason, and an unlimited number of other attributes. This short statement is to honestly acquaint you with my object in devoting all of my time far beyond a quarter of a century to the study of man, his life, his form and all his wisely adjusted parts, both mental and physical.[34]

"Dr. Still to Talk. Founder of School of Osteopathy in Clinton," the *Clinton Daily Herald* announced. "Kirksville Man will Deliver a Lecture in Mount Pleasant Park Thursday Morning [August 27]."[35] It must have reminded him of his itinerant days as, on the invitation of the organizers, he explained osteopathy, gave demonstrations of treatment and was besieged by patients, all of whom he treated without charge.

The meeting was marred by an acrimonious exchange with D. D. Palmer, founder of chiropractic, who attended annually and was distributing promotional leaflets to the crowd. "We recall vividly, even now, one Sunday at Clinton when father met A. T. Still on the Camp Grounds," Palmer's son B. J. wrote of the incident. "They got into a heated argument. . . . They were sitting on the lawn. They attracted quite a gathering because by this time both characters were well known." Still accused Palmer of stealing osteopathy and labeling it chiropractic, the altercation ensuing when D. D. denied the charge.[36]

On returning home Still gave his report. The lectures on man's spiritual nature were interesting, he said, but fell short of demonstrating the continuity of life after death. The seeing mediums had impressed him, though, their testimonies "confounding if not convincing." They named and described a number of his deceased friends, revealing when, where and how they died without a single mistake. "I have listened to the theologian," he summarized:

> He theorizes and stops. I have listened to the materialist. He philosophizes and fails. I have beheld the phenomena given through the spiritualist medium. His exhibits have been solace and comfort to my soul, believing that he gives much, if not conclusive proof, that the constructor who did build man's body still exists in a form of higher and finer substances, after leaving the old body, than before.[37]

Still's involvement with Spiritualism fuelled much speculation about his religious convictions. One patient asked him directly if he was a spiritualist. "What, me?" he replied with a quizzical smile. "Why I am a Methodist." Then he laughed, "At least Ma is."[38] Mary had attended Kirksville's First Methodist Church since 1876, but Still was no churchgoer. "I've taken many a shot at religion," he told Ernest Tucker privately (and with genuine sadness), "but never hit anything."[39]

Still could be mercilessly outspoken on the subject. "My opinion is that all so-called religions, from their remotest history," he wrote, "have been, are now, and always will be a curse to the whole human family in this and every other age." He did qualify his remarks, however; it was not religions per se that he objected to, but to what was done in their name: competing creeds and denominations engaging in wars for conquest or religious extension. The Holy Scriptures, he said, did not condone "blood, death, intolerance, hatred, war, widows, orphans, murderers, and all that stands for oppression, slavery, and immorality."[40] To sacrifice human lives in the name of God was a base corruption of Christ's teachings.[41]

Still could also be critical of Christian worship: "a lot of flattering words, forms and ceremonies" designed to appease an anthropomorphic God. "Has God such passions as man?" he asked. "If so he would be passionately fond of flattery. If God takes no flattery and man's deeds, good or bad, are all a just God will judge us by, we will have to change our worship from words to deeds."[42] "Still did not genuflect to the orthodox," Ernest Tucker noted. His God was not "the conventional kind, but was exceedingly vital, exceedingly real, and exceedingly there."[43]

"My religion – Love and Justice to all," Still asserted his position. "First, I love and adore all the works of nature. I love them because of their harmonious perfection."[44] He made clear what worship signified to him: "To respect to honor to treat [all beings] with civil reverence." To act in harmony with nature's laws. "Is it true that man does not only wish to be happy but wants to make others happy? It is true to the design of nature when we act our true selves. Then let us please God by going to sleep when we feel sleepy, cry when we feel sad, fight when we can not get reason to take effect, and stop oppression."[45]

Some ministers remonstrated solemnly on the supposed errors of his teaching, but Kirksville pastor F. W. Gee appreciated and even endorsed it: "The Old Doctor does not believe in sham, and cant, and hypocrisy. Sometimes he shocks super-sensitive people, but then a shock is good for some people to break up the adhesions in the gray matter they call their brain." Gee added, "I do not know of an individual who communes more with the Infinite than he. Some people preach and their preaching is excellent, if they would only practice what they preach, but the Old Doctor practices what he preaches. Some people pray for God to change his purposes and plans to suit their conscience, but the Doctor adapts himself to God's plan and credits Him with sense enough to run His own affairs."[46]

Reverend J. F. Harwood, too, approved of Still's viewpoint and invited him to deliver a lecture in the Kirksville Presbyterian Church on 25 October 1903 on the human soul. "You clothed with scientific truth the greatest theological question of all the ages and harmonized science with Holy Writ," Harwood wrote in a letter of thanks. "You are the first man in the world to do this."[47]

On November 11, Still traveled to Chicago to spend a few days with his friends the Orschels. He said he was tired of running a college and staying home all the time, and promised Mary to keep out of mischief provided Charley, "Son George" and business manager Warren Hamilton did not curtail his freedom.

With osteopathy now legal in twenty-three states[48] a visit from its founder was newsworthy – though what interested the city's press most was Still's

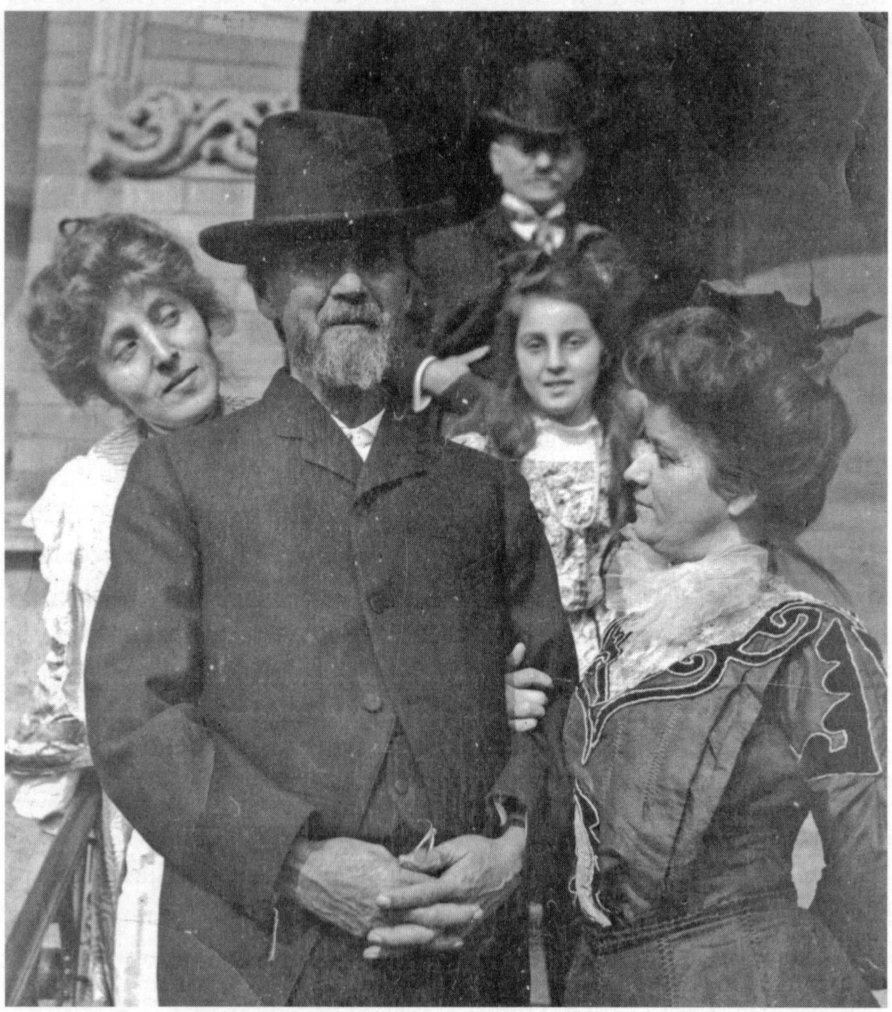

Still with the Orschel family in Chicago.

sartorial eccentricity and peculiar circadian rhythm. Styling him "a bitter enemy of the necktie," the *Chicago American* reported that despite being "worth at least $1,000,000" (a gross exaggeration) Dr. Still indulged the foibles of fashion no further than a paper collar; refused to wear boiled shirts, insisting that blue flannel was good enough; and – oddness personified – thought four in the morning the proper time to get up. The paper reveled in his refusal to attend a celebratory function planned by the Chicago Osteopathic Society because it clashed with his customary bedtime:

> 'Aha!' exclaimed several of the noted Osteopathists of Chicago when they heard of Dr. Still's presence. 'We will give him a banquet that will make Kirksville, Mo., appear like Kentland, Ind.'
>
> So they rushed off to prepare for it. They ordered the finest banquet in the land and – revoked the order.
>
> 'You are to be the guest of honor at a great banquet,' said a member of the committee which met him.
>
> 'Huh? queried Dr. Still, who is 76 years old. 'Banquet? When?'
>
> 'Tomorrow evening.'
>
> 'Not for me,' replied the physician. 'I am in bed at 8.30.'
>
> 'But doctor, this is. . . .'
>
> 'At 8.30,' repeated the doctor.

The banquet was cancelled, replaced by a reception at seven o'clock in the Auditorium Hotel. The guest of honor wore neither tie nor cuffs.[49]

The following year, 1904, the ASO commencement program was organized to mark the thirtieth anniversary of osteopathy's discovery. At precisely ten in the morning on Tuesday, June 22, Still stepped onto the platform in Memorial Hall garbed in a threadbare suit, high boots and a black alpaca coat worn at the elbows, to address the graduating class immaculately turned out in black gowns and starched white collars. "Ladies and Gentlemen, Students of the A.S.O.," he spoke:

> Thirty years ago today at this hour I got my first idea of Osteopathy. It is proper that we appear at any gathering, be it religious or social or

scientific, in appropriate dress. Today you see me in this torn coat. I appear as well dressed today as I did thirty years ago. Thirty years ago today I was in discussion with a brother asking the extent of the laws of God, of which man, a miniature representation of the universe, was the result. Man has matter organized. He has motion. And he has mind to control that work of architecture.

Notwithstanding my poverty I was satisfied with my life. I had been taught to pray, 'That thy angels watch over me while I sleep.' Should I make a mockery of that teaching? I told my brother I believed the angels returned as of old. My brother said, 'None but the wicked return.' I replied, 'Why, if God is no respecter of persons should the wicked only return?' Just then came a shock as if I was going into a paralysis. Whether it was an angel or a devil, I know not, and this language came to me as an impression, 'Will you carry our flag if we place it in your hands?' Then I took an obligation: I, A. T. Still, will stand by that flag as long as life shall last.

I lost four of my children by cerebrospinal meningitis. The preacher said, 'The Lord loveth whom he chasteneth.' Why did my children die? Did the Lord kill them because He loved me? No, no. Medical doctors ministered to them. It was no fault of the doctor, he was ignorant of the law. His ignorance made his efforts of no effect. Then I took up the study of the cause of these deaths. I studied life. I found in the human body the red, white and blue of our national flag. Red, the blood of life. Blue, the blood of the venous system. White, the connective tissue between the mortal and the immortal. The question came up: what can the spiritual influences do for you? I was told they were all false.

Notwithstanding the discouragement of so-called friends, I continued my investigation. I carried my medicine case with me, but as I discovered one by one that diseases could be treated by adjusting the body, the medicine was left off with each new discovery. For thirty long years I have been fighting this battle. The science is yet in its infancy, there is yet much to be learned. And when I make a mistake or reap a failure, I pray, 'O Lord God Almighty, pour a little more anatomy into my head.'

We commence with the dry bones of man. What is it that discriminates between qualities? Take up the subject of a single drop of blood. Follow

> it through the viscus, the blood vessels, into the heart, to the lung, again to the heart to be distributed. The Creator builds all parts according to knowledge absolute, not according to reason. Man makes blunders. God, the intelligent force, after forming man supplies him with the necessary intelligence for eternal success. It is impossible for God to make a blunder. The world is full of mysterious things that we do not understand, and why should anyone scoff at spiritual matters they do not understand? How many of you understand the wireless telegraphy? Then why should you doubt the wireless telegraphy to heaven? Thousands of people over the earth acclaim this method of communication with the wise ones on the other side; their numbers would surprise you. By mental telegraphy they can tell you the exact words

The transcript ends abruptly in mid-sentence. "Thirty years ago I took God for my champion," Still told a student afterwards, "my brother took medical theories for his. Can you imagine me regretting my decision?"[50]

The speech did not appear in July's *Journal of Osteopathy*, a conspicuous omission when four others by ASO professors were faithfully reproduced, and would remain unpublished. Perhaps it was deemed another disreputable episode, but those attuned to his economy of words and unique mode of expression would have recognized between the lines sources of knowledge more conventional than perhaps imagined.

Still retained from Methodism a belief in the direct guidance of a divine providence[51] and of angels as its special intermediaries. In his speech he alluded to a prayer, quoted by Wesley in his sermon *On good angels*, written by Bishop Thomas Ken:

> O may thy angels while I sleep,
> Around my bed their vigils keep:
> Their love angelical instil;
> Stop every avenue of ill.
>
> May they celestial joys rehearse,
> And thought to thought with me converse.[52]

Methodists believed that angels communed with man through dreams (and other means). They also believed that angels could appear in different guises. *Good* or *guardian* angels answered prayers, bore truth to man and intervened benevolently in human affairs.[53] *Evil* angels had devilish motives. "These skilful wrestlers espy the smallest slip we make, and avail themselves of it immediately," Wesley warned. "Indeed each of them 'walketh about as a roaring lion, seeking whom he may devour,' or whom he may 'beguile through his subtlety, as the serpent beguiled Eve.' Yea, and in order to do this the more effectually they transform themselves into angels of light." This is what Jim believed had happened to his brother in June 1874 and why he disowned Drew for nearly two decades.

To a select few Still revealed his own experience of that memorable June morning. "He pointed out to me the exact spot in which it suddenly came over him what it all meant," Ernest Tucker wrote,

> what it was in its entirety, this thing that had been coming to him piecemeal and growing up in him by degrees; and he said it was like a terrible blow on the back, a blow that sent him staggering and reeling. His 'spirits' had been revealing to him one item at a time, as is wise for the merely human kind, and by graduated stages, this vast insight into the conditions of human efficiency and disease; but when he all of a sudden saw the completed edifice ('suns and systems of planets ordered and wheeling in space where I never saw a star'). It was overwhelming in its suddenness and power and it affected him like a physical blow. He indeed described it as a blow from the hand of some powerful spirit, ordering him ahead.[54]

Addison Brewer added further detail. He wrote of Still's grief over his dead children, his disillusionment with materia medica and of being "alone in a moody state of mind pondering over this subject" when,

> he had the sensation of being struck by a fist between the shoulders. Straightening up he was made aware of the presence of three men from the unseen. They gave their names as Traliape, Trenagore and

> Lahemphanen. They stated that they were Egyptian philosophers and healers; that they had come to give him a new system of therapeutics. Of he would fight the medical doctors, they would 'clear the drift wood' out of his way.[55]

An unsigned 1902 composition typed on ASO notepaper, apparently the record of a séance, mentions two of the Egyptian spirits, albeit spelled differently. The piece bears Still's unmistakable style:

> 'On the twenty-second day of June, 1874, in the city of Eudora, Kansas, at ten o'clock in the morning, we entrusted you with a commission which you promised to honor and obey. We, as your spirit friends, on our side did then and there promise to hold up your arm and guide your head to a victorious charge on all the lines of the then existing medical theories of all schools. At the end of twenty-eight years we are proud to say that you have faithfully and honestly honored your obligation to us, during those long and wearisome years, and crowned the cause which you championed with a glorious victory in each and every engagement. We wish you to receive our thanks, Abram Still, Lea Hemphanum, Twalaape, and many, many thousands of our best and wisest angelic hosts. We then promised to hold up your arms and guide all moves in this combat to victory, and we will not abandon you or allow you to fall in the days of your declining or physical life. We will stand by you in the future as in the past.
>
> In order to leave something of a textbook as a guide for future generations, we have dictated a system of five divisions of the human body, beginning with the head, as follows, Head, Neck, Thorax, Abdomen, and Pelvis.'

The Philosophy and Mechanical Principles of Osteopathy is structured according to the same five divisions. The piece concludes with a commentary:

> Some of the angelic hosts have been behind me in all this fight. They have led me through the dark woods and danger's paths under the promise that they would see me through this intellectual fight. Often I

> have been sick to the very soul, but what I considered abuse has every time proven a blessing.[56]

"Spirits are all around you," Still once assured Ernest Tucker.[57] Their "quality of life is finer than ours, but they can take on enough matter to reflect appearances for accommodation's sake."[58]

The student listened to the Old Doctor's talk of angels and spirits with a mixture of skepticism and impressionability, and sometimes challenged him to have the spirits disclose facts unknown to science: "Still would throw his head back, squint his eyes, leaning on his long staff, slightly open his mouth like a person seeking a delicate sensation or a lost memory, and mumble something in the Indian tongue. 'They say so and so,' he would then translate."[59]

"What, for instance, is light?" Tucker probed on one occasion. Still assumed an attitude of intense listening. "Light follows in behind the bolt of the electric," he stated. "What is measles?" "It is a ferment." "How does it confer immunity?" "By the death of the mother tissue." Tucker asked if the spirits could reveal the nature of God. "God is a term by all living beings spoken mentally or vocally," Still said in a husky half-whisper, "signifying that I am going to lift myself above individual and personal limitations and thoughts, and rise to the broadest freedom of thought." As his voice trailed off he "came to" with a shake of his head, "as of a man emerging from deep water."[60] "Mumbo jumbo?" Tucker mused:

> Oh quite possibly. He could play games with the best of us. But not necessarily. It might have meant only that he thought in the Indian tongue – as well he might, having lived among them; or even that he thought certain thoughts better in their language, as again well he might. Or it may be true that his messages came from Indian 'guides.' One point to be considered here is that the Indian thought system differed widely from the white man's thought system. It may have been desirable to escape from the thought idioms of civilization in order to reach other horizons. This gave him a binocular vision, at least a double point of view. It is only one small step from this thinking to thinking of such thoughts as coming from spirits. Which does not mean that they could not actually have come from such spirits.

But Tucker acknowledged that, whatever the truth, "Dr. Still believed himself to be a psychic, and no honest portrayal of the man may ignore that fact."[61] One day Still showed him a tick-tack of fine flexible wire attached to his metal bedpost, fashioned so that the slightest disturbance would generate a tapping sound, "so the spirits can wake me if they want to talk to me." Maybe it failed to work, for the next day the contraption was gone.[62] Tucker remained undecided about whether the "spirits" were real or merely an emanation of Still's subconscious, but he could not fault the founder's method of investigation:

> He carried observation as far as it would go. Beyond that he followed reason as far as that could be made to go; and reason does see far beyond mere fact. Beyond reason he followed intuition, the voice of the subconscious whole, as far as that would speak. Now, whether the so-called psychic senses are merely intuition in some high distillate, or whether they are faculties next beyond intuitions, is anybody's guess at this time. But in all of these, from factual observation to psychic or 'spirit' messages, he checked up on them.[63]

From 11 to 15 July 1904 the eighth annual AOA Convention was held in St. Louis within the opulent grounds of the Louisiana Purchase Exposition, hosted by the city to celebrate the centennial of the great land acquisition.

Twelve hundred acres of woodland, thickets and swamps in Forest Park were cleared and turned into a grand landscape of waterways and gardens. Seventy-five miles of avenues and walkways connected fifteen hundred buildings; huge classically inspired exhibition "palaces" showcased the latest advances in science, art and industry; and a mile-long strip known as the "Pike" bustled with fairgrounds and sideshows. The "St. Louis World's Fair" attracted twenty million visitors between April and December.

Arthur Hildreth, a resident of the city since opening an ASO branch infirmary at the corner of Garrison Avenue and Morgan Street in spring 1903, had sat on the Fair's organizing committee and used his influence to have July 12 officially designated Osteopathy Day. It was a great honor for a system with such a short history and a reflection of the national status it now enjoyed.

The AOA established its headquarters at the Inside Inn, the only hotel within the Fair's grounds, and staged its lecture program in the ornate Missouri State Building. Still had spent a few days ill in bed and, though not fully recovered, caught an early train on Osteopathy Day. Charley ushered him through the gigantic rotunda of the Missouri building, beneath the frescoed soffit of its immense dome, and into the impressively muraled 1000-seat auditorium.

"The minute Dr. Still stepped into the door every person in the room was on his feet and the cheering that filled the air the next ten minutes was beyond description," Hildreth recorded. "It was a great ovation, a tribute to the man who had made one of the most remarkable discoveries of the nineteenth century. Such an outburst, such cheering, such enthusiasm; men threw their hats to the ceiling, howling lustily and continuously."[64]

When the noise died down Still delivered an impromptu speech to the capacity audience. Sixty-seven years had passed since he had last been in St. Louis, on the long journey to Missouri from Tennessee. At that time, he told the delegates, the city was "no bigger than a corn field," but had now grown to become "quite a village." A village large enough to host the third Olympic Games of the modern era, held during the Exposition. He spoke of his lifelong quest to prove the self-sufficiency of nature and, again admonishing the mixers, rallied the faithful to follow in his footsteps:

> Your head has often been talked to here; I shall talk to your hearts. I have long since been told that the works of God would prove His perfection. I have searched for the man that could prove that assertion was not correct. I have also searched for the theologian who could take that assertion and prove it. That assertion can only be proven by the thoroughbred, loyal, genuine osteopath, because he will start with the human skeleton and terminate with the soul of man. The union between life and matter, mind and motion is the proof of the perfection of the Divine Architect of the universe.[65]

Enraptured by the grandeur of the event, the *Osteopathic Physician* hailed it as the "Greatest Meeting In Our History." "Osteopathy's recognition came in the gleam and resplendent shimmer of myriad electric lights, in the rush and roar of cataracts," it effervesced, "in the spell of a great organ with its limpid, mystic, majestic melodies; in the impressive splendor of a great audience; in the public greeting and applause for the venerable man who gave their science birth, and in the joyous gratulations of about twelve hundred Osteopaths who had gathered from the four corners of the earth to do the occasion reverence." Differences of opinion were temporarily forgotten as the profession indulged in "a week of unalloyed fraternity."

But behind the camaraderie lurked festering discord. The parent school remained outside the Associated Colleges of Osteopathy, smaller ones were being swallowed up in a rash of mergers and closures, and new ones continued to appear, many of them substandard ventures that Charley and ASO business manager Warren Hamilton worked to close.[66] The previous year, when the ACO had voted for a uniform three-year course to be implemented in September 1904, Still had reluctantly agreed to conform, but had now changed his mind. "Talk to me about three years, two years, five years!" he addressed the audience. "Some heads will never make an osteopath if they are five hundred years at it. My first thousand graduates are a success, and all others are who have persevered at it." He feared that adding yet more medical content to the curriculum would serve only to further adulterate the pure osteopathic stream.

The convention closed with an alcohol-free banquet at the Inside Inn. "You must be prepared for straight truths if you want to read after me," Still declared in a plain-spoken farewell address:

> I want to go from this world with a clear conscience. I have commissioned myself to vindicate the works of the Great Architect, to show their perfection. My pen will never write that which I do not know to be true. I hate a coward, a liar, a thief, a lazy man. Wake up. I compromise with nothing; I consult with nothing but my own conscience.[67]

24

TO THINE OWN SELF BE TRUE

That osteopaths should choose to mix drugs with their practice at this time was ironic. Animal experiments were showing that all medicines caused physiological disruption and abnormal changes in body organs, and recognized authorities were openly admitting that they could no longer be considered to possess any curative value in themselves.

Sir William Osler, author of the standard text *Principles and Practice of Medicine*, citing the earlier experiments of the Paris and Vienna schools, declared, "There was but one conclusion to draw, that most drugs had no effect whatever on the disease for which they were administered." A generation earlier Still had been ridiculed for labeling medication "a system of blind guesswork," but now similar language was emanating from the hallowed halls of Oxford, England, where Canadian-born Osler spoke of "a popgun pharmacy, hitting now the malady and now the patient, the doctor himself not knowing which."[1] Osler wrote for the *Encyclopedia Americana*:

> The new school does not feel itself under obligation to give any medicine whatever, while a generation ago not only could few physicians have held their practice unless they did, but few would have thought it safe or scientific. Of course, there are still many cases where the patient or the patient's friends must be humored by administering medicine or alleged medicine where it is not really needed, and indeed often where the buoyancy of mind which is the real curative agent, can only be created by making him wait hopefully for the expected action of medicine; and

> some physicians still cannot unlearn their old training. But the change is great. The modern treatment of disease relies greatly on the old so-called natural methods, diet and exercise, bathing and massage – in other words, giving the natural forces the fullest scope by easy and thorough nutrition, increased flow of blood and removal of obstructions to the excretory systems or the circulation in the tissues.[2]

Dr. Frank Billings, in his inaugural address as 1903 president of the American Medical Association, painted an equally bleak picture:

> Our present methods of clinical observation enable us to do little more than name the disease. In the vast majority of the infectious diseases we are hopeless to apply a specific cure. Drugs, with the exception of quinine in malaria, and mercury in syphilis, are valueless as cures. The prevention and cure of most of the infectious diseases is a problem which scientific medicine must solve. What is true of the infectious diseases is also true of the afflictions of mankind due to chemical influences within the body. We know but little of diabetes, of the primary blood diseases, or of the various degenerative processes of age and disease. We hopefully look to chemistry to reveal to us the cause of these and other conditions. Experimental medicine must be the means of removing the ignorance which still embraces so many of the maladies which afflict mankind.[3]

As time-honored remedies fell into disuse some physicians turned to homeopathy, though the theory of the so-called "high potency" dilution (the smaller the dose, the greater the curative effect) remained unconvincing to many. In 1895 Rudolf Virchow, criticizing the system's lack of grounding in anatomy, derided the "mystique of the minimal dose" as a "plaything of blasé circles" and charged that homeopathy had "prolonged its sham life into the present" with "extremely little to show in the way of positive results."[4] ASO professor Michael A. Lane conceded that the system did at least accord with the Hippocratic dictum *first do no harm,* since with its "vanishing quantities of drugs" it could "literally do no harm,"[5] but unlike osteopathy it "did not cure patients whom the older school dismissed as incurables."[6]

Many doctors stopped prescribing medicines altogether, turning instead to advising on hygiene, disease prevention and the avoidance of bad habits. "As a matter of fact a cold is evidence of weakness," a former New York Commissioner of Health now announced sagely. "When you take cold it is pretty nearly a certainty that you have neglected yourself in some way. If you overwork and worry, if you lose sleep, if you neglect your meals, bolt your food, you are preparing for trouble. The nose and throat always carry the germs of influenza and pneumonia. Fortunately our powers of resistance are sufficient to guard against their attacks."[7] In 1905 the state's Board of Health declared that the best remedy for spinal meningitis, the disease that had claimed Still's children forty years earlier, was fresh air.[8]

But Still had discovered that finding health required more than fresh air. Thirty years of applying osteopathic principles had convinced him that no other system could hope to provide a lasting cure if the cause was anatomical. Normal cellular function demanded unobstructed blood circulation and this process was upset by osteopathic lesions, especially those that irritated spinal nerves at the intervertebral foramina. "Here, as nowhere else," he now declared, "would an apparently minor condition cause widespread results, and here I found most of the mechanical derangements that I knew must precede disease. I say most, because other mechanical lesions, such as contracted muscles, tumors causing sciatica, constipated colon causing varicocele, etc., do occur."[9]

As osteopathic knowledge began to diffuse into the medical arena MDs resolutely refused to give Still the credit. Dr. John Little Morris wrote in the April 1904 issue of the journal *Alkaloidal Clinic*:

> There are very few conditions confronting the specialist that will not be greatly benefited, and often cured, if the nerve centers associated with the distant organs can be stimulated at the same time that the lymphatic and venous circulations are awakened and the waste products carried off. It is a well-known fact easily demonstrable in any physicians office, that all chronic and most acute pathologic conditions are accompanied by more or less spinal tenderness.

This, he insisted, had medical provenance and was "not deduced from that nefarious class of quacks known as osteopaths, but from such physiologists as Foster, Landois and Starling."[10]

A year later Boston physician Joel E. Goldthwaite "discovered" that the sacroiliac joint can move and, when strained, cause back pain. The eponymous "Goldthwaite's disease" was no great revelation to osteopaths. Still had early concluded that the anatomy books were incorrect in stating that the sacroiliac joints are immovable.[11] For three decades he had corrected their lesions without fanfare, and for the past thirteen years ASO students had watched as he placed his hands over his sacrum and pelvis and twisted about to demonstrate their rocking motion.[12] Arthur Hildreth was moved to paraphrase Cherokee actor, author and broadcaster Will Rogers who, in a speech to the General Society of Mayflower Descendants, remarked, "Your ancestors may have come over in the Mayflower, but mine met them at the dock."[13]

Where medicine could rightfully claim new discoveries, though, was in the new discipline of bacteriology. When the first Nobel prizes were awarded in 1901 the leading contenders for Medicine or Physiology included many of its pioneers: Louis Pasteur, who proved that microbes are responsible for devastating epidemics, found a way to immunize birds against chicken cholera, and developed vaccines for human anthrax and rabies; the German physician Robert Koch, who demonstrated that the bacterium *Bacillus anthracis* is present in all cases of anthrax, *Vibrio cholerae* in human cholera and *Mycobacterium tuberculosis* in tuberculosis, and formulated a set of rules known as Koch's postulates to verify that specific microbes are responsible for each type of infection; Friedrich Loeffler, who isolated the causative agent of diphtheria, *Corynebacterium diphtheria*; and the Frenchmen Émile Roux and Alexandre Yersin, who cultured the bacillus and separated its injurious toxin. The Nobel committee finally settled upon Emil von Behring for finding an efficacious remedy for diphtheria – antitoxin – which, although it did not kill the bacterium, effectively neutralized its toxin.[14]

Subsequent winners were Ronald Ross for elucidating the mechanism of malaria transmission, Niels Ryberg Finsen for his treatment of lupus vulgaris and other diseases with concentrated light rays, and Ivan Petrovich Pavlov for his work on the physiology of digestion.

In March 1905, with no American having yet won in any of the five Nobel categories, the New York weekly *Independent Magazine* asked readers to nominate native scientists, authors and peace-makers worthy of the prizes, awarded annually on December 10. Still's followers believed his discovery overshadowed the achievements of all the previous winners and, as a general principle applicable to virtually all medical conditions, represented perhaps the greatest advance ever made in the treatment and prevention of disease. The *Journal of Osteopathy* suggested his name be put forward as a candidate, and over the summer his proponents circulated petitions and postal ballots to drum up support.

That May, Still, Charley and Blanche traveled to New York City to visit Harry, who had been practicing there for the past two years,[15] and in the founder's honor the New York Osteopathic Society organized a celebratory banquet at the fashionable St. Denis Hotel on the corner of East 11th Street and Broadway. Still cared little for "gabby gabs," as he called formal dinners,[16] and disapproved of lavish meals, styling them "slaughter pens of show and stupidity."[17] He believed that overeating ("the most idiotic stupidity of the present age") exerted pressure on nerve centers and major blood vessels in the chest and abdomen to commonly cause strokes, heart disease, hemorrhoids, and other complaints.[18] Tired from a day of sightseeing and in no mood for the repast, he left untouched the first course of soup and oysters and asked graduate Ralph Williams, sitting next to him, "Son, do you suppose the boy could bring me some bread and milk?" The head waiter, shocked but compliant, did as he requested while Blanche tried to ease her embarrassment by eating both his dinner and her own.

The incident reminded Williams of a passage from Shakespeare's *Hamlet*:

> This above all: to thine own self be true,
> And it must follow, as the night the day,
> Thou canst not then be false to any man.

Dr. Still "did not ignore the dictates of society," Williams noted, "they were simply nonexistent to him." Declining the meal was not inverted snobbery but an example of the Old Doctor being true to himself *all the time*. Entirely unembarrassed, not even amused at the situation, Still knew – guest of honor notwithstanding – that he was too tired to digest rich food.[19] "We should eat when we are hungry, drink when we are thirsty, sit close to the fire when we are cold, and wear spectacles when we are old," was his canon. "True we are made and it is true to the design of nature when we act our true selves."[20] He had planned to continue on to Boston and Washington, but did not feel up to it and returned home.[21]

Accidents, however, were beyond his control. In July, en route to the 1905 AOA Convention in Denver, the Santa Fe train in which he was traveling collided at 60 mph with a stationary freight train. "I was lying in the berth with my head towards the engine," Still recounted. "My head struck against the head-board of the berth and hurt my spine from the atlas to the eighth dorsal, and left all the ribs on my left side on a heavy strain, and the fifth and sixth were thrown out and above the articulation on the transverse processes." A few weeks later he developed a shaking palsy of the head, and on examining his neck found that "the facets on the upper surface of the lower cervical were shoved to the right on the under facets of the upper dorsal." He clamped a walking stick in a vice, rested the crook on the spinous process of the offending vertebra, and pulled himself back against it "with great force." He then had someone else adjust his ribs "as low down as the eighth" on the left side.[22] The tremor soon disappeared, but he never fully recovered from the injury.[23]

During the summer he received a communication from the *Independent Magazine*. Medicine or Physiology had drawn more interest than any other section of its poll and Still had received the most votes, many accompanied by letters "indicating great reverence and affection" and "gratitude for benefit derived from his treatment." The intrigued periodical asked him to contribute an article on his discoveries.

The November 9 issue carried a piece entitled "The Principles of Osteopathy," attributed to Still but actually compiled from several interviews by his newly-graduated grand-nephew George Still, Summerfield's son. The Old Doctor's words tumbled out unselfconsciously. He championed the perfection of nature, explained that normal cellular function demands freedom of vessels and nerves, and indulged a curious comparison of osteopathy and medicine: "Just as the 'osteons' or bones differentiate man from the jelly-fish, so is Osteopathy differentiated from the jelly-fish systems of therapeutics which, like the boneless ink-fishes, hide their weakness and stupidity in a cloud of long, meaningless words and outlandish symbols taken from the Greeks, Romans and Egyptians."

The following week the magazine published a scathing rebuttal by James J. Walsh, MD. "Here is absolute truth at last," the well-known medical author sneered, "ninety-five percent of all disease is due to a slip of the parts of the backbone." Categorizing osteopathy alongside Christian Science, he dismissed its cures – those to which "every quack charlatan appeals" – as due to little more than suggestion.

On November 23 the *Independent* published the results of its poll. Still won the Medicine or Physiology section by an enormous margin. In fact, with 22,061 votes he tallied more than all the other candidates put together.[24] "We recommend our osteopathic friends not be content with their present victory," the magazine's editorial stated, "but to take the necessary steps to bring their cause before the Nobel Commission, to be passed upon by the Caroline Medical Institute of Stockholm."[25] Protocol, however, dictated that nominations to the Karolinska Institute be made only through official channels – the medical profession – and the matter proceeded no further.[26] The prize went to Robert Koch.

Still took scant notice. He was busy working on a new project. On June 22, in fulfillment of the final pledge of the ASO's original charter "to improve our present system of surgery," he had laid the cornerstone of a seventy-five bed hospital adjacent to the infirmary at the corner of West Jefferson and Osteopathy streets. The facility would enable them to accept more serious cases previously needing referral to distant medical centers, where osteopaths were denied access and, in Still's opinion, surgeons were too eager to operate. "The great failing of many who enter surgical work is their too frequent use of the knife and anesthetics," he held. "Many are the sufferers who go through life disfigured, maimed or deprived of some essential organ who should have had their body restored to a perfect condition without being so mutilated."[27]

The policy of expeditious surgery derived from Rudolf Virchow's admonition that prompt excision of the diseased part would prevent it wreaking further havoc. "Cellular pathology demands, above all, local treatment," the German declared a decade earlier. "In surgery the consequence is the recommendation of early operation on, and destruction of, the focus of disease."[28]

Osteopathic principles pointed to a different conclusion. Though Still recognized the necessity of surgery as a last resort he estimated that, if begun early enough, judicious osteopathic treatment could avert the need for the knife in (among other conditions) three out of four cases of "so-called appendicitis" and ninety-five percent of "tumefactions, abdominal tumors, enlarged liver, gallstones, Bright's disease, diabetes and dropsy."[29]

The ASO Hospital was inaugurated on 25 May 1906 during the annual meeting of the Missouri Osteopathic Association. Frank Young was appointed chief surgeon, George Still assistant surgeon, and a circular room nicknamed the "pit" allowed undergraduates to observe operations in time-honored fashion. A new nurses college was created to train young women to care for patients in an osteopathic manner. Sanitation was emphasized, no drugs except anesthetics and antiseptics were used, and patients received daily osteopathic treatment before and after operations.[30]

The hospital's opening was marred by the death, on May 8, of Still's brother Ed, who had suffered a fall earlier that year. Still felt the loss keenly. In a heartfelt tribute he wrote that during the dark days of ostracism and abuse Ed had been "the only stake I had to lean on," a constant source of help and encouragement who urged him to keep on if he truly believed he had discovered a great truth.[31]

Eight days after Ed died Still asked freshman Hugh Russell to give him a haircut, and as he set about his task Charley and other faculty members gathered in the yard to poke fun at the poor job the inexperienced hairdresser was doing. The banter amused Still but upset Russell's ten-year-old daughter Ruth, who seized a lock of hair and ran away. Years later her parents found the lock stored in an envelope, tied with a ribbon, with a note attached: "On the 16th day of May, in the year 1906, in Kirksville, Mo., H. L. Russell served as barber to the 'Old Dr.' In after years we will be proud to say that we have been with the founder of osteopathy, and that we have a lock of hair which helped cover that wonderful head, wherein such deep thought had made its bed."[32]

Later that summer sophomore James Hegyessy accompanied Still to a dissection class. On the table lay a cadaver, perfect in form, but with no mind and no motion. All the wonderful physiology once wisely active in growth, repair and healing had ceased, abandoning the flesh to nature's laws of decomposition and decay. When the students settled Still pointed to the corpse and asked what they knew of the soul. There was a long silence, and when it became apparent that no answer was forthcoming he took Hegyessy by the arm and led him outside. "They do not understand me, Hegyessy," he said with tears in his eyes. "Since my brother died I feel like a lonely tree on top of a hill. I am all alone, none even of my own family understands me. You know what I mean."[33]

It was not a lack of friends but of kindred spirits. "There were always those," A. L. Evans explained, "who if they did not comprehend Still the philosopher, yet were bound to Still the man with hoops of steel; for there was that in him which commanded the love of his fellows." He cherished that love, but "it was in the realms of science, of prophecy that he suffered, though uncomplainingly, his greatest loneliness."[34] Few truly grasped the enormity of the philosophy, science and art he had termed osteopathy.

Perhaps he tried to contact his brother's spirit. An enigmatic message, signed with Ed's initials but dated after his death, bears Still's handwriting. "One lung exhales and inhales at a time," it states, "then the other exhales and inhales. Thus there is more time for chemical action with more space to expand by combination. E. C. S. July 31 1906."[35]

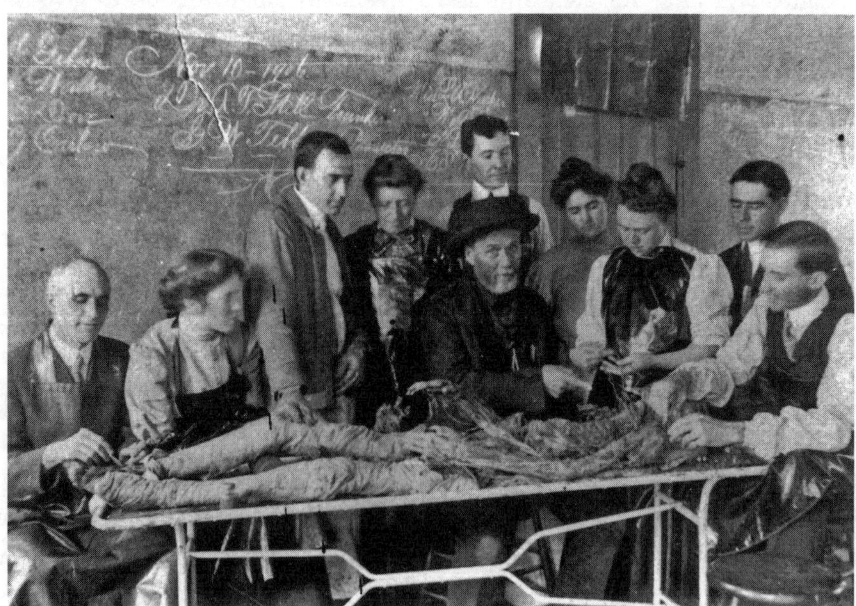

American School of Osteopathy dissection class, November 1906.

Still had recently been pondering why pneumonia presented more frequently in the right lung and tuberculosis in the left, and why in winter, when the weather was well below zero Fahrenheit, he always felt the sting of chilled air in his right lung. On examining his chest movements he arrived at the "probable" hypothesis that during relaxation and sleep we breathe with alternate lungs, since each is supplied by the "wholly independent" left and right vagus nerves. He believed that under normal conditions one lung fills with air as the other exchanges gases, but that during prolonged speaking or singing both lungs fill simultaneously. He further theorized that during bitterly cold weather we breathe only with the right lung. "Does it look reasonable to you that [the] lobes of the left lung, lying right against the heart would be filled with air at the temperature indicated?" he asked. "Do you think the left lung could take in atmosphere at such a temperature and not shock the nerves of the heart?" He wondered if the chilling might predispose to pneumonia in the right lung and, due to stasis of impure air in the smaller but warmer left lung (with two lobes compared to the right's three), to tuberculosis in the left.

Nature alone knew the truth. As with all conditions, what mattered was to find and fix the cause of nerve irritation and circulatory disturbance. "Since I began to treat the lung as a machine," Still lectured to one dissection class, "I have had results far beyond anything I could hope for in the treatment of asthma, pneumonia, croup, diphtheria, pleurisy and through the whole list of lung diseases. I find that Nature is a trustworthy leader, and there is much hope even for the consumptive."[36] One warm day that September he lay on his back on the lawn and invited a number of students and visitors to place their hands on his chest to feel the alternate breathing, but the demonstration came to an abrupt end when a young woman asked if he believed in hypnotism. "Do you want to see how I hypnotize?" he responded. He threw his arms around James Hegyessy and kissed him on the cheek. "Here you are," he said triumphantly, "I hypnotized him." The group laughed, but the young woman asked why he wasted his kisses on a man. "Because I love him," Still answered.

At five one morning Hegyessy was woken by a knock on the door. "Get up you lazy Dutchman," said a voice outside, "I've brought you something." The student leapt up to let in the caller. "This is no time to be in bed," Still said. "Dress quickly, I want you to take a walk with me." He presented Hegyessy with a copy of his *Autobiography*, signed *Comp's of your admiring friend, A. T. Still.*, and they went together on his daily stroll in the woods.[37]

Those accorded such a privilege spoke of private lessons illustrated by some natural observation. Still might stand next to an oak tree and discuss it from root to branches, teach how to navigate a way through the forest by a knowledge of the trees, or explain the blood circulation with the aid of a maple leaf.[38]

Nothing was "too small for his notice and study," Fannie Carpenter noted, "the blade of grass, the tiniest flower or insect, the smallest bit of creation was to him a source whence from he gathered wisdom, and so closely did he walk with nature that she led him into the very secrets of life itself, until to him the most complicated and wonderful of all the works of the Creator, the human body, was an open book."[39]

Freshman George Burton and a visiting friend, Bradley, went on one walk. As they stopped to catch their breath at the top of a steep knoll, Still asked Bradley if he could see something wrong with a nearby tree.

"No, I think not," the visitor replied.

"Look again," Still said.

"Well," Bradley reflected, "I cannot see anything wrong with it, unless you mean the dead end of the tip of the limb swinging nearest."

It was precisely what he meant. "Now, what caused it to die?"

They traced back, branch by branch, from the dead limb to the trunk until they found a little white spot where the bark had died, the work of wood-boring beetles. "Now I am going to give you your first lesson in Osteopathy," Still said:

> When you have a patient suffering, trace back branch by branch, or joint by joint, until you find the spot that is causing the pain or suffering. You will find the point of short-circuit or stoppage in nutrition somewhere between the peripheral point of suffering and the central point of issuance of the vital power. An insect probably stung the tree and killed it in the small spot where you dug into it with your knife, and that was way back on the trunk of the tree. That little interference was just enough to rob that particular tip-end of the limb of its natural nourishment, so it died. Just so you may have to trace pain or injury manifestations all the way back to the spinal nerve-center in order to find their cause.[40]

Carl McConnell was struck not only by the painstaking detail of Still's observations but also by the *way* he made them:

> He saw far beyond the mere objects. Everything to him seemed to be literally pulsing with life, of which the inner meaning was sought, analyzed and arranged after a certain order of cause and effect, and its relationship to the universe. Nothing was isolated.[41]

"All things in nature were to his perception but parts of *one great whole* and therefore essential parts of Infinity, or God," student Nettie Haight echoed. "Thus he understood and thus he revered the human body. And thus he was able to give to the world that message of love and harmony, that system of unity and strength, that philosophy of hope and health known as Osteopathy."[42]

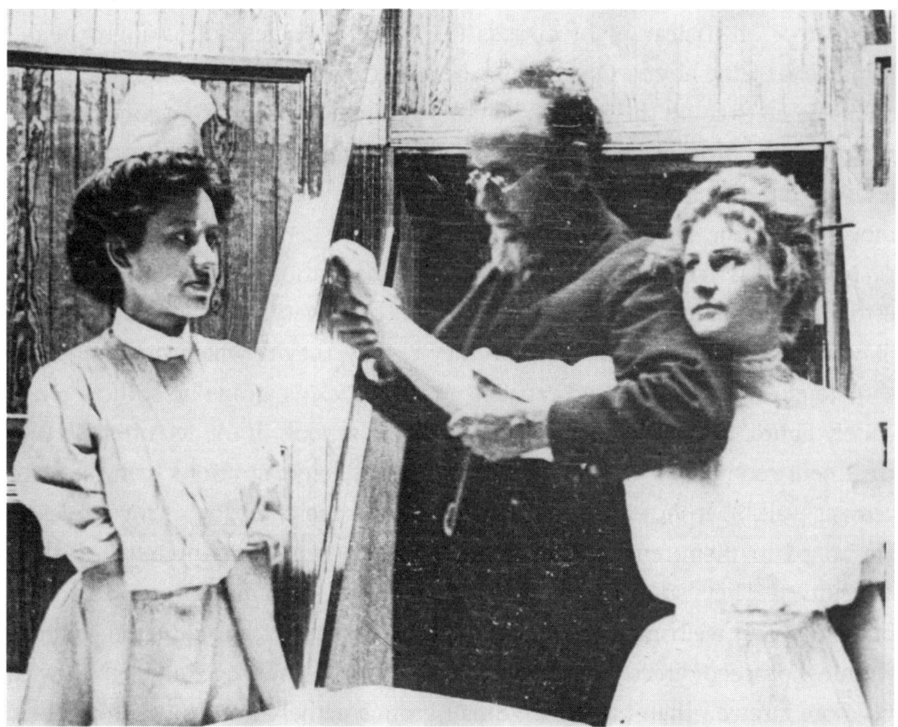

Still with nursing students in the ASO surgical pit. c. 1907.

To Still everything in nature, organic and inorganic, was the embodiment of absolute wisdom. "One observation on our surroundings this morning," he lectured one April in Memorial Hall,

> of budding trees, growing grass, opening flowers, plainly shows that intelligence guides, directs, and controls this wonderful creation of all animate and inanimate things. Nature, the great creator, made this mighty universe with such exactness, beauty, and harmony that no mechanical ingenuity possessed by man can equal or imitate the mechanism of that first and great creation. Botany, Astronomy, Zoology, Physiology, Anatomy, all natural sciences, reveal to man these higher, nobler, grander laws and their absolute perfection. Viewed through the most powerful microscope or otherwise, no defects can be found in the works of Deity.[43]

He might produce a pebble from his pocket and give an informal talk on geology, or on a clear night discuss the celestial bodies and changes in the firmament by the hour.[44] One evening he asked a group of students congregated on his porch to count the stars. When they hesitated he said, "Can you count the red or white corpuscles in a man? No!" "Right there I got my first osteopathic lesson," one listener wrote. "Man a miniature universe; health a proper, free movement of the corpuscle in its orbit."[45]

Nature was truth, a constant source of inspiration[46] – but Still's was no esthetic appreciation. "I'm not fond of flowers or flowery talk," he told a student. "My wife [is]. I like potatoes. Even if they're ugly, they're what I'm after."[47]

Though seventy-eight and carrying a rough stick as a cane he still cut a tall, stately figure. He was seen almost daily in the school, in the lecture halls and treatment rooms, or – the site of many practical demonstrations – on the large cement walk in front of the infirmary. He loved the company of the students. He talked to them, encouraged them, inspired them, and entered into their difficulties. They admired his great knowledge, high purpose and abiding humanity, and welcomed his visits to the classroom. He would enter without warning, proceed directly to the platform, deliver his message, and depart with no more farewell than greeting.[48] Small groups gathered on the railroad track or a pile of ties near the Wabash depot to listen to him philosophize, often until disrupted by an approaching train. He always had a few new points for them to think about, but the sublime could instantly switch to the ridiculous, an amusing anecdote, especially about someone he knew, provoking uncontrollable laughter to the point that they feared it would hurt him.[49]

Still gave treatment only informally now.[50] When Nettie Haight received a telegram from Oregon saying her mother needed an operation for glaucoma she sought his advice. He drew from his pocket a dollar and told the student to wire her mother to board a train for Kirksville immediately. Just after daybreak on the morning after she arrived a cane rapped on the front door and in walked Still blowing breath between his teeth in a suppressed whistle. "Where's Ma?" he demanded. He greeted Mrs. Haight with his customary curt "how-dy" and without further ado, in the middle of the kitchen floor, grasped her neck and performed a correction. He then removed a black silk handkerchief an MD had placed over her eye to expose an angry swollen mass. "The eye is an organ of light," he pronounced. "Would you expect a rose to thrive in the dark?" Then he turned and left. Daily treatment for two weeks averted the need for the operation, but irreversible damage left Mrs. Haight unable to discern anything but large objects with that eye.[51]

On a visit home from St. Louis, Arthur Hildreth looked on as Still, surrounded by a group of students, treated a woman with a swollen breast. Effortlessly correcting the fourth and fifth ribs on the affected side, he described how the lesions interfered with the sympathetic nerves to upset the circulation, and explained that the power within the body was the only means on earth potent enough to accomplish a cure. "His demonstration was so simple," Hildreth marveled, "yet it carried with it a weight of sacred knowledge that I liken to nothing other than a growth and unfolding of a beautiful flower."[52]

One day Still sat under a tree with Hugh Russell and related his long, lonely journey in trying to work out osteopathy. He uttered nothing bad about those who refused to listen, excusing them by saying they feared what they could not understand, but in speaking of those who had shown kindness, love or sympathy he poured out his very soul. "It is a wonderful thing to be truly loved by mankind and to love mankind," Still said, slipping an arm around the freshman's neck. "Remember you are a student in the University of the Infinite, in whose library there is but one book, and that book is Man. Study it."[53]

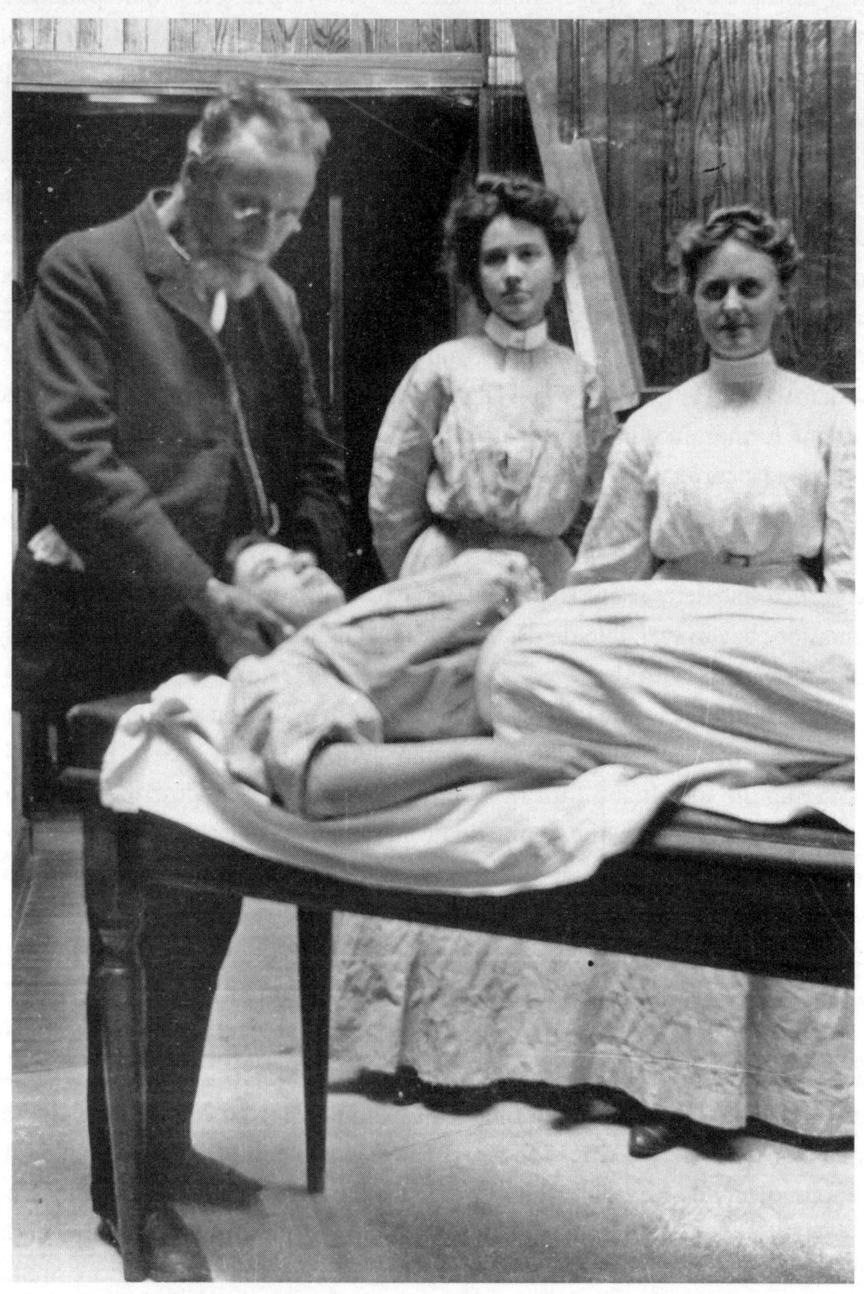

25

THE GREATEST ANTISEPTIC KNOWN

Despite Still's waning control over his now large and scattered profession, those in charge of policy-making continued to feel his influence keenly.

Many serving officers of the Associated Colleges of Osteopathy and the American Osteopathic Association had had little or no contact with the founder, had a poor grasp of his philosophy, and some were even graduates of schools whose standards he questioned. The American School of Osteopathy remained outside the ACO and without its cooperation the other schools struggled to find common ground. In 1906 the AOA tried to intervene by appointing a Board of Regents to secure uniform requirements for entry and graduation, but without success. The ASO, resenting any external control, saw the movement as an unwanted interference and, such was its standing, the scheme was allowed to "die of inanition."[1]

At issue was the purity of osteopathy. Still's fears over extending osteopathic courses to three years with added medical subjects proved well founded, as new graduates pondered whether an MD degree would help them in practice.[2] Even in Kirksville a strong medical influence prevailed, as evidenced when he ran into his nephew-once-removed Benjamin Still and asked him to describe what he had been learning. The student said "tonsillitis" and proceeded to reel off a train of facts learned from the book used in class. "Damn it, I don't want to hear that stuff," Still cut in. "I want you to tell me what the real change is in the throat and tonsils, and what nerves and structures cause the trouble, and then how you would go about correcting it, and forget all that Poll Parrot business that you have been reading in medical textbooks." The reproach stunned the student:

> For a moment I was speechless, and on regaining a fraction of my composure, it began to dawn on me what his meaning was; and right there he drove a great lesson into my brain, so accustomed, as it was, to following the medical textbooks in descriptions, etc., rather than grasping his great concept of what the real changes are in the body, called disease, and what are the methods of correction, or cure. He started my mind working in a different way from that the teachers and books had done, and I feel that whatever of success I have acquired in practice is greatly due to the shock above described.[3]

On 8 January 1907 Still's brother James died in Maryville, Missouri. The two had never been close, but Jim's death once again brought to the fore the deeper mysteries of man's existence. In the following months Still resorted to meditation, apparently without success, before reverting to spiritualist practices. From March 11 to September 13 he made entries in a small red pocket book advertising medical products. In it he jotted names of patients, charges for treatment, records of payment and recommendations on diet, interspersed with lines of poetry and philosophical musings listed under six headings: Psychic Force, Realization, Purpose, Subjugation, Concentration, and Continuity of Thought.

"Thoughts are units of the universe," he scribbled under *Concentration*. "They go far into making up the creatory force that rules said universe." He lamented the scarcity of prophets. "Where are the seers of today that we had in the past? There are none. This is the fault of distraction in which the world now dwells." He alluded to ancient diviners – "ever seeking to imbibe and partake of the grand and revelating utterances of thought that continually surrounded them" – and gave instructions on how to emulate them. "Hence seek ever for the door of concentration. When you have entered therein, let all else go, as the knowledge you seek is contained here and here only." *Continuity of Thought* detailed a formula for achieving success. "The first principle in continuity is a firm determinance along the will power, safe-guarded by a close concentrated watch over the slightest deviation. . . . Rehabilitate yourself with the raiment of continuity, carry a fixed purpose for the common good. Be brave, be courageous, be honest. To your heart ever be true."[4]

Meantime, in the absence of his aggressive leadership, the osteopathic profession was being swept along on a wave of politically motivated change. With many states still lacking protective legislation, the AOA, deeming it necessary to convey the right image to help sway the lawmakers, moved to purge the profession of the various tradesmen's terms that the founder had introduced with his mechanical analogies. DO should no longer stand for Diplomate but *Doctor* of Osteopathy, the osteopath or operator should be an *osteopathic doctor* or *physician*, who would not handle but *treat* a patient, and his business or work would be a *practice*. All these changes were adopted, with one exception: the word *osteopath* was retained, at least for now.[5]

At the end of the year Still traveled to Kansas to attend a fiftieth anniversary reunion of the Free State Territorial Legislature at the State Capitol in Topeka. The six surviving members were invited to meet on the evening of 6 December 1907 in the House of Representatives Hall during the annual meeting of the State Historical Society. For Still the visit evoked a flood of memories. "He sat in a rocking chair, a guest of Dr. Charles E. Hulett, one of the oldest osteopaths in Topeka," the *Topeka Daily Capital* reported. "Dr. Still crossed his hands over his lap and stared intently at the fire in the grate that was sputtering in front of him. 'I don't feel like talking tonight,' he said after a long pause. 'I shall make a short address at the meeting of the pioneers at the State house within an hour and I feel that I should save all my strength for that. I haven't a thing to say. What is there to be said?'

Still's countenance assumed a look of sadness. 'Baldwin, my old home, was never very kind to me. It was there you know that I lost my three children and decided that drugs were deficient in many things. I advocated bloodless surgery – that there was no efficacy in drugs – and they laughed at me. They called me a lunatic. I had been a physician and surgeon there, and when I deserted my profession my family and friends deserted me. I believe Baldwin has regretted that since. It has always hurt me though.'"[6]

The gathering was attended by Kansas governor Edward Hoch and two ex-governors (all three patients and advocates of osteopathy), but "the most unique, interesting and conspicuous figure," a journalist wrote, was Dr. A. T. Still.

In a short speech Still began by mentioning that he had first come to Kansas in 1853. "You must have lived with the Indians, there were no white people here then," ex-Governor Edmund Morrill interrupted doubtfully. "I did and I can speak Indian too," Still replied, waving his cane indignantly. He uttered something that sounded nothing like English and Morrill muttered grudgingly that he would take his word for it.[7]

Perhaps Morrill's challenge stirred memories of the Wakarusa Mission. Back at the infirmary, after helping a student treat magazine writer Grace Macgowan Cooke the three sat, legs swinging, on the tall treatment table. Cooke asked a question and was caught off guard by an incomprehensible reply, a "flowing, sonorous syllabification" with "a lilt like running water." "That's Shawnee," Still smiled and translated the words in answer to her question. "When I was a boy I was among the Shawnees. I learned all they could teach me about healing sickness. I have never forgotten their language. Pretty isn't it?"[8]

From 3 to 7 August 1908 Kirksville hosted the twelfth annual meeting of the American Osteopathic Association, and two thousand delegates crammed into a huge circus tent in De France Park for a program of lectures, practical demonstrations and social events. "Never before in the history of Osteopathy has there been a convention so large, so enthusiastic, and so harmonious," the *Journal of Osteopathy* exulted. "Representatives of all schools fraternized together, factions were forgotten, and apparently but one thought animated all." That thought was of the founder's eightieth birthday.

Mayor Hiram Selby proclaimed Thursday, August 6, a half holiday. The Normal School closed for the day, merchants decorated stores with memorabilia, and at eight in the morning a crowd assembled in the great tent to witness Charley's thirteen-year-old daughter Gladys unveil a portrait of Still painted by George Burroughs Torrey, whose previous sitters included Theodore Roosevelt, General Nelson A. Miles and King George of Greece. After lunch a procession led by the Novinger Band marched from the ASO to the marquee to attend a concert by the Normal School orchestra and listen to a marathon fourteen speeches.

Graduate J. L. Holloway delivered a nostalgic eulogy of the remarkable journey of the "supposedly addlepatted bone-setter with his sack of bones," a man who, despite a lack of sympathy or support, had uncomplainingly accepted professional and social ostracism rather than surrender his convictions of truth, and finally won through to popular acclaim and devotion.[9] Normal School

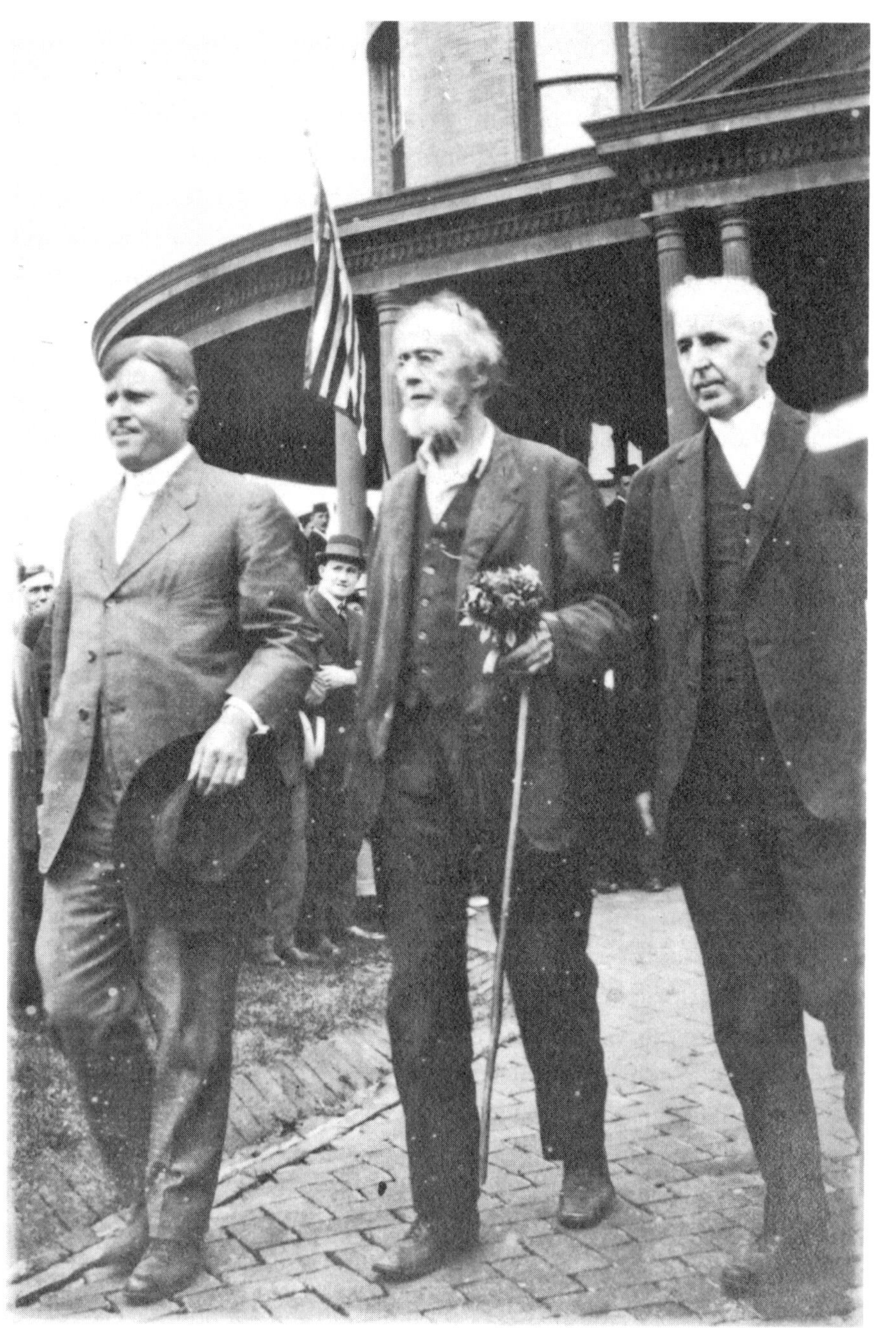

Still on his eightieth birthday flanked by Harry Still (left) and Arthur Hildreth.

president John R. Kirk, on behalf of the city, presented Still with a loving cup as a token of friendship.

Arthur Hildreth stepped onto the platform to solicit subscriptions for the funding of osteopathic research. The profession had reached a point where it felt a need to substantiate its methods, "to delve into the deepest recesses of the science underlying Osteopathy," as E. R. Booth put it, "to establish its claims so as to place it beyond the cavil of the faultfinder and make it convincing to the most scientific minds."[10]

The logical starting point was to investigate Still's fundamental principle of cause and effect. Carl McConnell, Louisa Burns and others had already conducted preliminary experiments, with encouraging results. Inducing spinal lesions in dogs, they found that even minor structural disorders produced acidosis in the cells and tissues around the lesion, in the spinal cord at the level of the lesion, and in organs neurologically connected to that level. They further found that correcting these lesions restored normal acidity and alkaline balance, and slides related to these studies were shown at the 1905 AOA Convention in Denver.[11]

Still repeatedly advocated research. He expected graduates to regard a diploma from the ASO as both a qualification to practice and "a commission to explore new fields and report the truth for the advancement of osteopathy."[12]

To that end he personally favored dissection. The tissues of the cadaver encoded a unique medical history: the sites of past disease (unresolved infections, fibrous adhesions, bony unions indicating past inflammatory conditions) and the lesions that predisposed to them. He personally examined every cadaver dissected at the school, sometimes sitting for hours studying a part,[13] seeking the subtle variations from normal that may have precipitated the person's demise. Frank Young, in charge of the ASO anatomy laboratory, kept careful records of 267 bodies dissected over a five-year period, noting probable causes of death and matching pathological findings to demonstrable lesions of vertebrae, ribs and sacroiliac joints. The results were striking. "When we consider what the disease process was in each instance, calling to mind anatomical relations, nerve and blood supply," he wrote, "we are almost forced to the conclusion that the theory of Osteopathy is proved."[14]

Sometime in 1908 Still dropped in on one of William Smith's classes (the Scot had returned to the ASO in June 1907 after five years practicing in St.

Louis) and compared osteopathy to a squirrel in a hole in a tree with its tail sticking out. "I've had a hold on that tail for thirty-four years," Still told the students, "and Bill's been trying to help me get the squirrel for a long time, and I want you to help me get it."[15]

But much of osteopathy was poorly suited to conventional scientific research. Finding and correcting lesions relied heavily upon subjective faculties, and success or failure depended in no small part upon the skill, knowledge and experience of the practitioner. A poor operator did not disprove the correctness of the approach.

Osteopathic research should therefore be conducted under its own philosophy – that of "matter, mind and motion, blended by the wisdom of Deity." A philosophy under which the word *science* assumed a more expanded, literal meaning, to include objective information, subjective *knowing,* and acknowledgement of the spiritual.

Still insisted that his was not the final word on osteopathy. "The river of intelligence is just as close to you and yours as it is to me and mine," he encouraged his followers. "Although by good fortune I dipped my cup first in the broad river of Osteopathy, the same stream flows for you."[16]

He appealed to the profession to investigate fully the injunction *Man, Know Thyself,*[17] to research not only the human body but also to "take up the human life, the human soul, solve as evidence of its durability and its truthful existence."[18] The physical formed only one aspect of the vast subject encompassed by the title *osteopathy*. "It is my hope and wish," he stated, "that every osteopath will go on and on in search for scientific facts as they relate to the human mechanism and health, and to an ever-extended unfolding of nature's truths and laws."[19] He quoted St. Paul in 1 Corinthians 3:16: *Know ye not that ye are the temple of God and that the spirit of God dwelleth in you?"*[20] "Ten thousand rooms of this temple have never been explored by any human intelligence," he added, "neither can they be without a perfect knowledge of anatomy and an acquaintance of the machinery of life."[21] Osteopathy's scope was boundless. "From the dry bone to the living man; from the living man to the bosom of Nature whence he came," he exhorted. "This is the text from which we expect to preach."[22]

Meanwhile, within mainstream science, the 1908 Nobel Prize for Medicine or Physiology was shared by two men for their separate contributions to

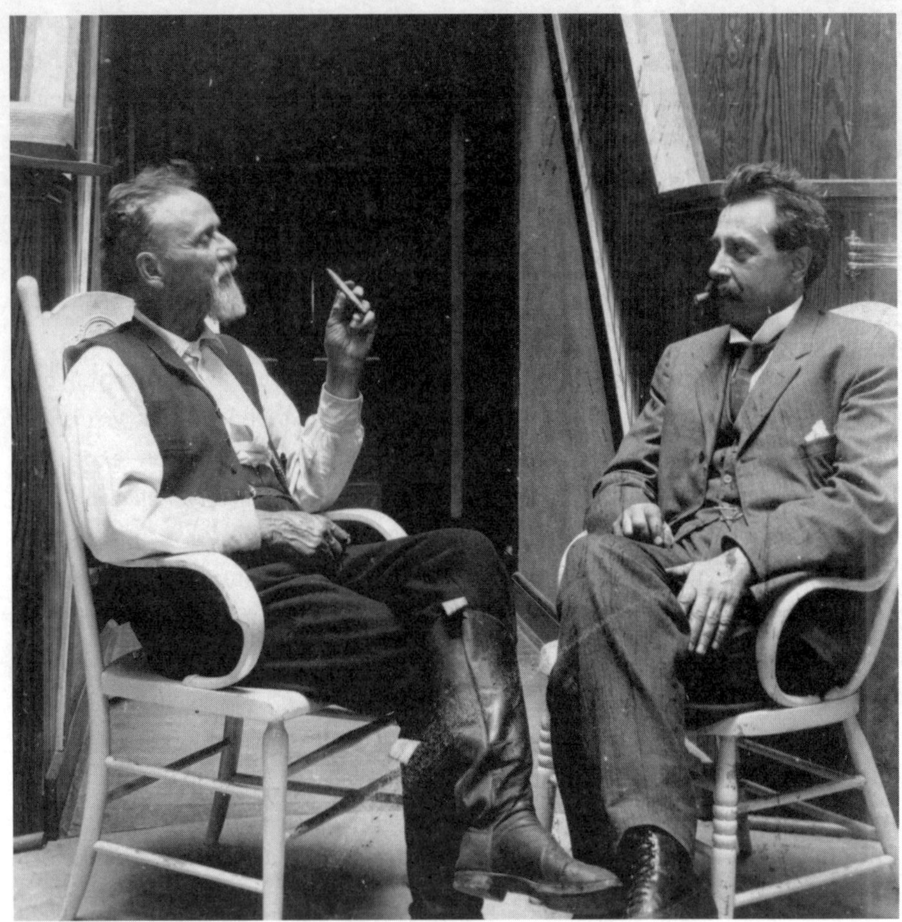

Still and William Smith in the surgical pit.

the field of immunology: the Russian biologist Elie Metchnikoff for his 1884 demonstration that blood and connective tissues contain *phagocytes*, amoeboid white blood cells that help defend the body against infection by ingesting bacteria and other harmful matter; and the German physician Paul Ehrlich for his 1896 "side-chain" theory of immunity.

When, in 1864, Still first articulated his crude insight that the body contains its own "drugstore" (the idea that later evolved into his concept of "body ferments"), no evidence existed to support his contention that when the body is attacked by infectious disease, the blood and tissues produce special and specific substances to meet the threat. He had simply reasoned, through common sense, that some mechanism must exist.

Ehrlich's side-chain theory provided a hypothesis to explain that very mechanism. Early in his career, staining animal tissues with aniline dyes, the German had discovered the mast cell, differentiated five types of white blood cell, and developed a technique for diagnosing tuberculosis from a patient's sputum. Staining worked because different cell types absorbed different dyes selectively. No one knew why, but Ehrlich theorized that the "mode of distribution" of a dye depended upon its "bond of union" with "receptors" he hypothesized to lie on the cell surface.

The side-chain theory derived from his application of the receptor idea to the problem of "active" immunity – the process by which the body, when exposed to a pathogen, mounts a strong response against it. Ehrlich coined the terms *antigen* for the invading microorganism and *antibody* for the protective substance in the blood, and proposed that each antibody possesses receptors for specific antigens, the two fitting as precisely as a lock and key. He further proposed that as the number of microorganisms increases, body cells are stimulated to manufacture more protective antibodies.

Still's supporters complained that once again the founder of osteopathy's contribution had not been recognized. They pointed out that whereas Ehrlich was honored for merely theoretical work, Still had not only anticipated the existence of the immune system by a generation[23] but also found a practical way of exploiting it for the effective treatment of nearly all diseases. ASO professor Michael A. Lane wrote,

> Dr. Still was the first to state outright, in unequivocal and clear terms, the great theory of immunity, or rather he was the first to perceive the fact that immunity applied not only to the diseases which, up to his time, were regarded as immunizing diseases but urged in clear terms the universality of this great modern biological principle in diseases of every kind. To him belongs the credit of having brought all diseases under one great law – that of body resistance; how, theoretically, the blood and the tissues themselves contained the *cure* for diseases of virtually every kind.[24]

Observation and experience had led Still to the same conclusions that followed years of patient laboratory work by Ehrlich, Koch, von Behring and others. "He said nothing about side-chains, phagocytes, amboceptors, antibodies and the rest of the classified agencies which today comprise the intricate science of immunology," ASO graduate Leon Page remarked. "By one clean stroke he cut to the heart of the problem and proceeded to demonstrate with direct evidence that his conclusions were right."[25]

Ehrlich had more recently been following a new line of inquiry. Over the previous two decades pharmacological divisions had appeared within the chemical industry, often as offshoots of dyestuffs businesses. Reasoning that drugs, like dyes, should be able to attach to his hypothetical receptors, Ehrlich embarked on a new search for chemical remedies to combat infectious disease.[26] Describing nineteenth-century medication as an imprecise science that dealt only with effects, and asserting that treatment should address not symptoms but the "cause" of disease, he set out to replace Osler's "popgun pharmacy" with weapons of precision and accuracy.

An obstinate problem stood in his way. All chemical drugs exhibited a fundamental characteristic: "side-effects" – a euphemism for direct but undesired effects. The French physiologist Claude Bernard had earlier established that all "biologically active" substances introduced into the body could be classed as either foods or poisons, and since all drugs were poisons Ehrlich sought to find chemicals maximally effective against microbes but minimally toxic to the body.

Not until the 1960s were Ehrlich's hypothetical "cellular receptors" found to be real structures: protein molecules on the cell surface whose purpose is to bind hormones, neurotransmitters and other natural substances. The chemical structure of each receptor type dictates not only which endogenous substances can bind but also which drugs, microorganisms and toxins. Nearly all cells possess a full complement of all receptor types, in different proportions depending on the cell, explaining not only the selective absorption of dyes in staining but also why drug uptake is indiscriminate and side-effects unavoidable.

In 1905 Ehrlich's Frankfurt laboratory found that trypan-red dye killed the protozoan parasite responsible for African sleeping sickness and, three years later, developed Salvarsan, an effective remedy for early-stage syphilis.[27] Salvarsan restored medicine's faith in drugs and created the hope that all infectious

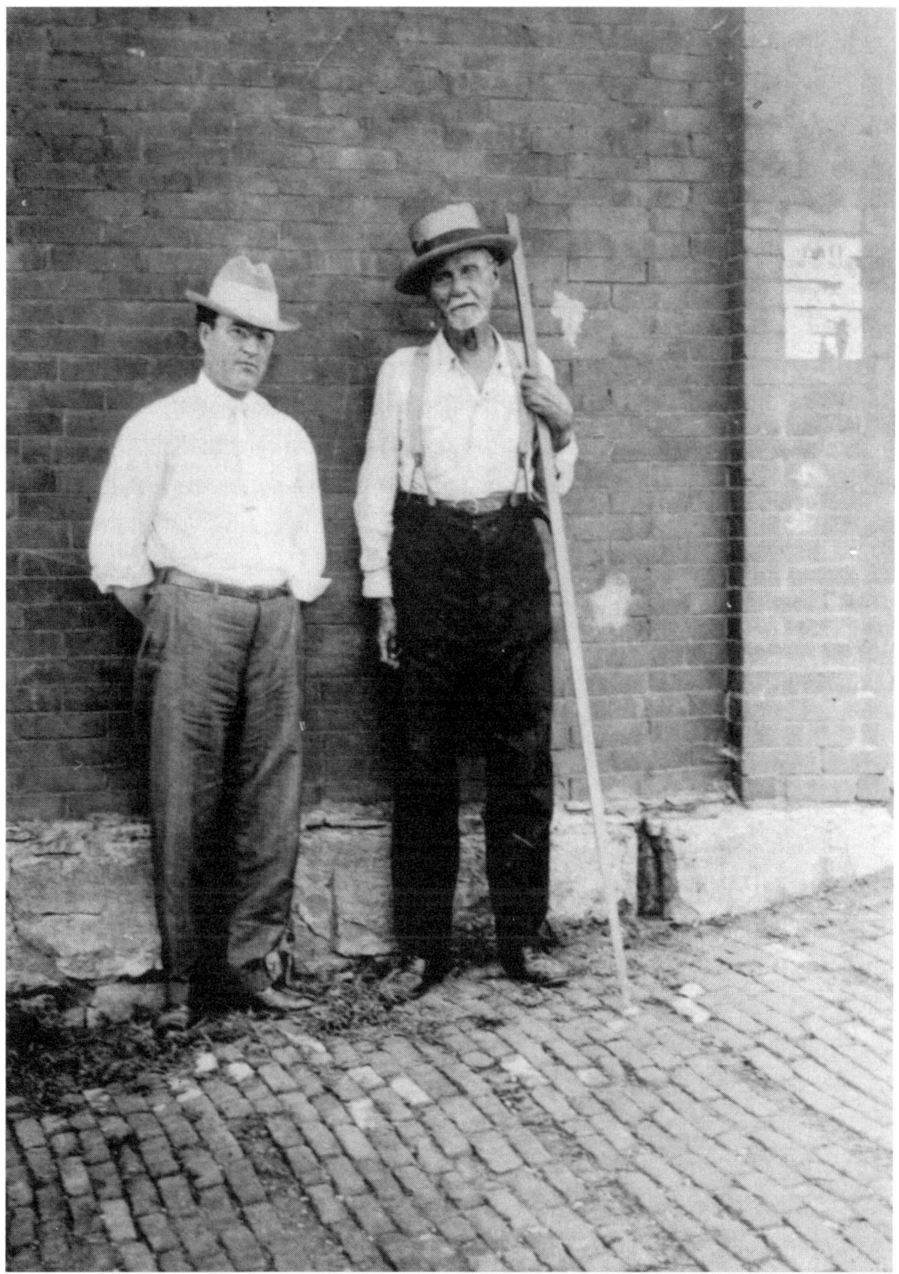

Still and anatomy professor Arthur D. Becker, 1909.

diseases might be eradicable by chemical means. The *doctrine of specific etiology* led medicine to regard *Vibrio cholerae* as the "cause" of cholera, *Corynebacterium diphtheriae* the "cause" of diphtheria, and so on, and inspired a hope that each disease could have a specific pharmacological cure.

The new doctrine ignored both Virchow's admonition that instead of looking for new drugs medicine should try "finding a way of strengthening the cells in their fight with bacteria,"[28] and Pasteur's conclusion that the proliferation of microbes was less the cause of infectious disease than the effect of lowered resistance. Science continued to vindicate their teachings. Research was showing that man had always coexisted with microorganisms. They were found ubiquitously in air, water and soil; the skin and digestive tract of healthy individuals always harbored the germs associated with certain diseases without causing harm; and at the time Koch discovered the tubercle bacillus most people in European cities were infected with the bacterium, yet relatively few developed tuberculosis.

The doctrine of specific etiology was nevertheless soon extended to other medical conditions. When it was found that various disease states could be induced experimentally by altering biochemical or physiological parameters, medicine came to regard metabolic disturbances, hormone imbalances, stress and other factors as "causes" of disease, and their cure a matter of finding the right drug.

Ehrlich's work charted the future course of medicine. It also illustrated the fundamental dichotomy between the medical and osteopathic approaches: to fight disease or to support the body's self-healing tendency. "Bacteria are only buzzards watching for something to die on which to feed," Still wrote:

> Different kinds thrive on different kinds of tissue. . . . The germs are not the real cause of the disease, so that the kind of bacteria developing will depend on the kind of tissue devitalized. Two people will nurse the same disease, inhale the same germs. One will contract the disease, the other will not; because in one was the area of lowered vitality, which furnished the suitable home and breeding place for that particular variety of germ. In the other, healthy tissues provided no germ food. A free flow of healthy blood is death to germs.[29]

"Pure blood flowing naturally is the greatest antiseptic known for internal conditions," E. R. Booth elaborated, "no germ can live long or multiply in it."[30] Though not impervious to microorganisms, a structurally normal body helps optimize blood circulation, resist invasion and hasten recovery. "You do not need drugs," Still said bluntly. "The blood has a hundred drugs of its own of which the doctor knows nothing. But the body's drugs actually cure the disease, whereas the doctor's drugs kill." And his followers raised a question: did primary osteopathic lesions and secondary lesions produced by microorganisms and their toxins compromise blood flow and thereby make it harder for not only the body's remedies but also medical drugs to reach the needful parts?

Ironically, as Ehrlich strove to find effective chemical remedies he stood in awe of the body's own healing system. "Antibodies are magic bullets," he famously declared, "which find their targets by themselves; but with chemicals we must concentrate all our powers on making the aim as accurate as we can contrive, so as to strike at the parasites as hard and the body cells as lightly as possible."[31] Despite his search for artificial remedies he recognized that the body's own defensive substances strike only at their enemies, with neither toxicity nor side-effects:

> All the greater then must be our admiration for the powers of nature in view of the fact that the living organism, when it takes upon itself the production of curative agents, does this in such a manner as to form ideal etiological remedies. The protective substances of the blood . . . completely fulfill the requirements of the case.[32]

"What a wonderful fluid blood is," Emil von Behring echoed, in admiration of its curative and immunological powers.[33]

Yet neither Ehrlich's awe of nature's remedies nor Behring's respect for the blood could shake the paradigm that disease was to be conquered and microorganisms destroyed. Though Ehrlich had used the term "magic bullets" to describe the body's own curative agents, medicine appropriated the term to nickname Salvarsan the "magic bullet."

Such was the power of philosophy.

26

THE FULFILLMENT OF LIFE'S DIVINE PLAN

On 6 August 1909 a party of forty well-wishers paid Still a surprise visit in celebration of his eighty-first birthday and found him sitting on the porch with Mary in the cooling evening air. They presented him with a bouquet of shell-pink Egyptian locust blossoms tied with satin streamers, the women served lemonade, punch and cakes, and Reverend Ben Jones of the First Methodist Church[1] delivered "an appropriately worded speech." Still responded in his "usual original and witty way." He proposed several toasts in the Shawnee language and, in reminiscent mood, recounted his pioneer days in Missouri, the fight for liberty, and the scientific discoveries made during his lifetime, emphasizing his points by poking his stick playfully into the minister's side, saying, "Eh – am I right boy?" He concluded by speaking of osteopathy, telling the group, "And if I should die before you do we can finish talking it over after we get to Heaven."[2]

Mary would precede him. Ailing for years since an attack of pneumonia and suffering from chronic nephritis, over the following winter her health progressively deteriorated and in the spring she took a turn for the worse. When it became apparent she would not recover, Arthur Hildreth paid them a visit from St. Louis. Late in the evening he sat with Still on the lawn and tried to offer consolation. "Daddy," he said (Hildreth always called him Daddy), "how your boys wish there was some way that they could bear a part, at least, of the great burden that now rests upon you in this trial hour of your life." Still's response surprised him. "You boys need not worry over me," he said directly. "For over twenty years I have been teaching natural law to you and to the world, and Mother's going is only the fulfillment of that natural law;

another step in the progress of her life from mortality to immortality. She has lived a good, useful life, and the time has come for her to pass on into greater usefulness. Her change is but the fulfillment of life's divine plan. I would be a rank coward to break down now."[3]

Mary died at 11 p.m. on Saturday, 28 May 1910, six months short of their fiftieth wedding anniversary, on the first day of the ASO graduation program.[4] Still insisted that the commencement, scheduled for Monday, go ahead, but as a quiet affair solely for graduates and their families. Before presenting the diplomas he spoke briefly of Mary's enduring support and encouragement, how she had always urged him to never turn back, and how he would never have survived the early days of ostracism and adversity without her optimism and faith in him.[5] At two that afternoon Reverend Jones conducted the funeral service in the house, the casket draped with a mantle of ferns and white carnations, but the interment was deferred until the following day as they waited for Mary's brother to arrive from Pennsylvania.[6] Next morning the graduates assembled at the grave in caps and gowns, and the pallbearers included William Smith, on his very last day in Kirksville. The ever restless Scot was embarking on yet another adventure, this time to open a practice in Portland, Oregon.[7]

Herman returned from Texas for the funeral and stayed on for a few months. When together he and Still acted more like two old pals than father and son,[8] and on this occasion they worked to market an invention Still had been working on intermittently for five years, whose patent had finally been granted that April. The device, a heating boiler to maximize efficiency and minimize pollution, aimed to solve the wintertime problem of the locally-mined low-grade coal begriming the town with a layer of soot. In describing the prototype the previous year the *Kirksville Daily Express* reported that "Dr. Still's Great Smoke Consumer" had reduced the ASO's annual coal consumption from between five and ten to two tons, and that "not a spot of soot has been found on the snow surrounding the power house this winter."[9] Still handed the design to a large manufacturer for further development, but the model they built (incorrectly, in his opinion) failed to perform properly and they lost interest. The project was eventually scrapped.[10]

During his visit Herman acted as agent for his father's last book, *Osteopathy: Research and Practice*, published the day before Mary died. Still described the simply worded text as “the body and soul of osteopathy.”[11] He had established principles, set them down as universal laws, and failed to disprove their veracity. “For thirty-five years,” he wrote, “I have observed man’s body with the eyes of a mechanic so that I could behold and see the execution of the work for which it was designed, and I have come to this conclusion: The better I am acquainted with the parts and principles of this machine – man – the louder it speaks that from start to finish it is the work of some trustworthy architect; and all the mysteries concerning health disappear just in proportion to man’s acquaintance with this sacred product.”[12] Only by applying osteopathic principles could medicine hope to fathom the numerous ailments it labeled *etiology unknown*.

A reviewer in the *Journal of Osteopathy* worried that readers used to the increasingly technical tone of medical publications might mistake Still’s unsophisticated style and aversion to scientific terminology for ignorance; that those not conversant with his philosophy might imagine he knew nothing of microbiology and perhaps even disbelieved in the existence of microorganisms. “Let no one imagine that the Old Doctor is ignorant of these things,” the writer stated. “He is acquainted with the ascertained facts concerning them, but in the light of his own discovery he places upon them what he thinks is their relative significance.”[13]

Blanche and George looked after him now, but the house always bustled with student lodgers, visiting graduates and spontaneously invited guests.[14]

“So keen and lively were Still’s interests,” lodger George Fulton noted, “that those in contact with him soon forgot to think of him as a very old man, for his strong personality, intellectual attainments, and incisive yet kindly humor marked him as a leader in any company.” A dominant figure who drew the love, respect and allegiance of both men and women. Time and again Fulton was impressed by the visits of early pioneers, those who Still had taught at first hand; how he affectionately referred to them as “his boys and girls in an unmistakable sense of deep gratitude,” and how they thanked him “for the spiritual, intellectual and moral help he had been to them.”[15]

Still always delighted in finding someone interested in talking about his favorite subjects, and when he did, Florence Gair related, “he would sit by the hour and discuss bit by bit, opening up his wealth of ideas as to the body mechanism, structure and life, the Universe, heavens, the Creator and the created." Gair lived in his home from 1907-11, and they developed a close bond. After supper, before her evening study period, she would spend an hour at his bedside listening to him reminisce about pioneer life, his intimate friendship with the Shawnee and how, through his prolonged study of nature, he eventually arrived at the conclusions upon which he developed osteopathy. He spoke over and over about nature. "Nature was the x of the algebraic problem," she noted, "the unknown quantity."

Still gave treatment infrequently now, but occasionally called Gair early in the morning to attend a patient downstairs. He showed her "how to treat the eye for cataract and other ailments; the feet, et cetera" – knowledge she later found invaluable in her work with "cripples" and "in normalizing deformed feet and hands from secondary contractures." Sometimes he treated her, too, once for a severe headache caused by an old atlas lesion. He rarely adjusted a joint twice in the same way. This time he asked her to kneel down and place her neck over his knee, and in a second she was freed of pain. When she returned home to New York, Still had her bring back the blue flannel shirts he liked to wear in the winter months, and he always requested she bring more for an old army pal. He continued to enjoy helping friends and needy neighbors. After his visits, some told Gair, they would find money under the clock or on the mantel. "No outsider knows what it meant to a student of this new science to be thrown in close daily contact with such an original mind," she wrote, "to absorb at first hand his ideas, to get the deep, fundamental truths he had had revealed to him from his long, tireless study of nature. To discuss his pet hobby over and over again with him was a privileged experience.[16]

Student John Deason liked to drop in and discuss the books in Still's collection, many provided by James Neal forty years earlier. One time he arrived to find the Old Doctor absorbed in rereading *Cellular Pathology*. "I think Virchow is right in stating that disease begins in Darwin's protoplasm," Still said. "But how does it start? What initiates these cellular changes?"[17] There were depths of knowledge he still craved to fathom.

Since Mary's passing he dwelled ever more on spiritual matters,[18] and on several occasions was heard to utter, "Ma knows it all now."[19] In spring 1912 his preoccupation with the afterlife intensified after receiving news of the untimely death, on February 15, of William Smith. After remaining only a short time in Portland the capricious Scot had practiced for an equally brief time in New York City before returning to his native land where, aged only fifty, he succumbed to pneumonia at his home in Dundee.[20]

On May 24, at a meeting of the Missouri State and Mississippi Valley Osteopathic Association, Still stood on the platform in Memorial Hall to deliver a now rare talk, one he entitled *Dr. A. T. Still's Philosophy of Immortality*. For half a century, he told the audience, he had sought a weapon to "slay the Black Wolf" – the fear of death – but had at last found solace:

> Today I have no more fear of death than life. I have a choice for death. Why? Because, when I am ripe and have been in the body long enough I wish to come out, being confident that it will be a higher step, which is necessary to man's spiritual perfection.

After failing to gain proof of the soul's immortality from the Church he had looked to nature – the henhouse, the stable, animal shows – and there seen innate, perfect knowledge: the newborn calf, colt or lamb going directly to its mother's teat; the two-day old chick carrying a piece of dry bread to a saucer of water to moisten it before eating; the chicken raised in an incubator possessing an instinctive fear of a hawk. "I learned more from an old hen than all the theologians have ever taught me," he said. "I learned the great lesson, which is that our lives are in the body which should be called an incubator, developing the spiritual man to make the step from mortality to immortality." He had concluded that the ephemeral, transitory body represents a "link in the ring which is connected to eternal life" and that at death the spiritual man breaks free, like a chick hatching from its shell, to a new and higher existence. "This philosophy has made me hope that at the mature hour of my development I will come out with that perfection which the Architect of all Nature intended," he beamed with radiant happiness:

> Every evidence that I have found in all Nature is that the God of Life is an architect, a builder, an engineer and no imperfection can be found – and there is no perfection short of completion, for which I think the spiritual

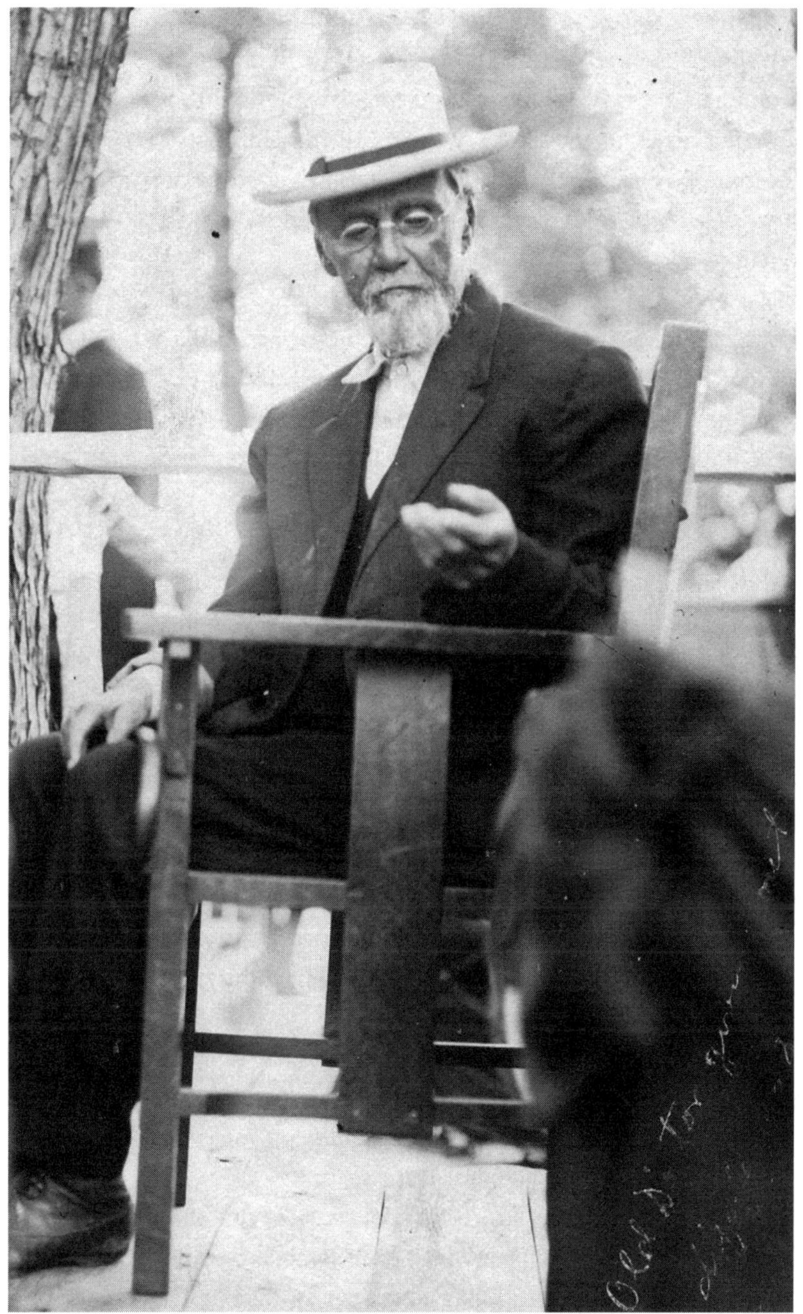

Still on ASO graduation day, 3 June 1912.

> man is retained in the physical body until Nature says it is finished, having absolute perfect knowledge of all requirements for his comfort and happiness. With me it has changed fear and dread to rejoicing at the perfect work of the Great Architect of the Universe, and I am ready to receive all changes that the Architect thinks are necessary to complete the work for which Man was designed. I will close by saying, 'Know thyself and be at peace with God.'[21]

They applauded warmly, but he sensed by the serious atmosphere that not all had understood him – he had perplexed some and saddened others – so in an instant he lightened the mood. "Now all that cheering is for my new hat," he quipped. "I won that off Charley. He said Roosevelt would not carry Ohio and I said he would."[22]

Theodore Roosevelt, alongside Lincoln, was his favorite American.[23] In turn Roosevelt, U.S. president from 1901-1909 and campaigning for re-election (to lose to Woodrow Wilson), was a firm advocate of osteopathy.[24] Still always wanted to hear what "Teddy" had to say, and every morning that summer he had Asa Willard, back for some dissection work, read to him from the St. Louis newspaper as they sat together on the lawn (with frequent interruptions as Still observed passers-by and pointed out signs indicative of physical problems or the trend of their health).

Before Asa returned home to Missoula, Montana, Still handed him a sheet of paper to show his mother. "Man on this earth is an egg," it read, "and if he is a good egg he will hatch out into the next world as a good chicken where, under happy circumstances, he will have the opportunity to do some especially worthwhile scratching."[25]

Those whose horizon extended only as far as the physical body might have blamed Still's *Philosophy of Immortality* speech on yet another spiritualist foray. They would have been right. He wrote Joe Sullivan:

> I will say that it was on the 16th day of last May that the angelic world gave me word for word what I wrote on Immortality. Since that hour I have been a happy man. Death has no terrors for me because I know we are in the hands of an intelligent loving architect who made the human race for

> a purpose, with whose work I have never found any variation from truth with all its wisdom from start to finish throughout all nature. Amen.[26]

That August he received a visit from Arthur Hildreth, en route to the AOA Convention in Detroit. Still seemed preoccupied. "Arthur," he said pensively, "do you suppose they will bring the convention to Kirksville next year?" Hildreth knew he was being asked to try and influence the committee and did not know if he would be able to. He replied that many in the profession had become very successful and were accustomed to holding the event in a large city. "In other words they like good quarters, good rooms and good food." Still looked away and there was a pause. "Well," he uttered at last, "I knew many of that bunch when they were glad to get a crust to eat and a blanket to sleep on under the trees."

He got his way. The 1913 convention was held in Kirksville, organized to coincide with his eighty-fifth birthday. An enormous marquee was erected near the school, citizens opened their homes to delegates, and churches assisted restaurants in serving meals.

Harry invited Hildreth, Margaret and their daughter Ina to stay. Arthur had purchased his first automobile and Margaret was looking forward to the trip, but the previous year, soon after the Detroit convention, she was diagnosed with cancer and as the time approached it became clear that she was too weak to travel by road. "I can go on the train," she told Arthur, "and you and Ina can go in the car, but we are all going to the convention."

"Little did she dream how we would all go to that convention," Hildreth wrote. Margaret died on Friday evening, August 1, three days before the meeting began.[27] "You are coming to our home just the same," Harry telephoned Arthur on receiving the news. "Bring your wife's body here and the funeral will be held from our house." Margaret was buried in Kirksville on the Sunday, and over fifty osteopathic physicians from across the Union acted as flower bearers.[28]

The convention began the next morning. Still, enfeebled by illness and a fall, had been judged too weak to appear at the event and it was understood he would not mingle with the crowd. But on the second day, as Hildreth delivered a speech in the tent, an unmistakable figure was seen marching towards the lecture platform leaning on a long staff. "With one accord the immense crowd rose to its feet in reverence and good will," one delegate wrote, "with cheer after cheer." Still proceeded to the lectern to give an impromptu speech. "Thirty-nine years ago I raised the flag and swore by the eternal that I would stand for the works of the Divine Architect of the Universe," he proclaimed. "God is an architect. He is a builder. He is an engineer, and all nature comes under the orders of that architect."[29]

The following day, Wednesday, August 6, an all-day celebration was organized to mark his birthday. Times were changing. On the country roads automobiles raised dust as they sped past farm wagons, carriages and buggies, and from early morning well-wishers disgorged from trains so packed that some traveled hanging on the steps. Trenches were dug for a gigantic barbecue on the Normal School campus and, in the largest gathering ever seen in Kirksville, fifteen thousand turned out to honor northern Missouri's most distinguished citizen.

Only two American medical schools could boast more students than the ASO. All but two states had legalized osteopathy and representatives of nearly all their associations were present. Still stood on a stand to acknowledge a parade of floats that took an hour to pass, and disappointed no one with his attire, casual to a fault, telling a woman standing next to him that he was saving his clean shirt for Sunday. But he was genuinely moved, and as he turned to go back to the house his eyes brimmed with tears.[30]

Three thousand dollars was raised as a birthday gift, but he refused to accept it. The present he would appreciate most, he had earlier told Hildreth, was for every dollar to go towards osteopathic research: "Tell them that my life efforts have been one continual battle for American freedom, freedom from the shackles of a medical monopoly. I have fought for the right of every free-born American citizen to be independent in all things, and that I want them to use their money to help carry on that great work."[31] The money helped found the A. T. Still Research Institute, established in Chicago later that year under the charge of John Deason.[32]

The day after the birthday celebrations Hildreth and Harry walked out to the pump in Still's yard for a drink of water. Harry, more suited to business than medicine, had quit practice in 1907 to become president of Kirksville's Citizen's National Bank.[33] He had a proposition to offer. He and Charley, recently elected Mayor of Kirksville, wanted to purchase the old Blees Military Academy just south of Macon to convert it into an osteopathic sanatorium for mental and nervous diseases, and they wanted Hildreth to run it.

The scheme had Still's full backing. Eminent psychiatrists and neurologists believed most forms of insanity incurable, but he had seen many psychiatric patients cured by osteopathy, from the girl in the State Insane Asylum in Nevada, Missouri, to the Sims case that so inspired Senator Foraker, while dissections of deceased mental patients in the ASO anatomy laboratory appeared to indicate that many confined in asylums might be similarly helped. In an undated manuscript Still wrote that spinal abnormalities capable of irritating vasomotor nerves and disturbing cranial blood circulation had been found in "all the insane subjects that we have examined in the last seven years."[34] With osteopaths generally denied access to state asylums their own facility would enable large scale testing of the hypothesis.

Despite his thriving St. Louis practice Hildreth accepted without hesitation. With Margaret gone and Ina about to be married it was a godsend. Besides, he felt he owed it to Still and to the patients who might benefit.[35]

The Still-Hildreth Sanatorium opened on 1 March 1914. The impressive four-story structure, with marble floors and high ceilings supported by columnar pillars, housed 120 bedrooms, twelve deluxe apartments and a four-hundred-seat dining room. In stark contrast to the notoriously barbaric state institutions it strove to provide sympathetic treatment for the mentally ill in an enjoyable relaxed environment favorable for healing. Landscaped grounds set in four hundred acres of rolling countryside offered walks and a small lake for fishing, swimming, boating and skating. Gardens, greenhouses and a herd of Holstein cattle provided the basis of a well-balanced, nourishing dietary regime with plenty of fruit and green vegetables. Patients had access to music and billiard rooms, a library, laundry and barber shop, and could attend entertainment programs (and, in later years, movies). Those requiring more restrictive care were housed in a building called the Annex.[36]

On March 4, Hildreth and ASO graduate Walter Bailey welcomed their first patient. After a month they had sixteen, and after a year seventy.

Such pioneering work proved an immense challenge. They took a complete case history and conducted thorough physical, neurological, mental and laboratory examinations. Over time a pattern began to emerge: all patients suffering from the various forms of insanity seemed to have experienced a previous mental or physical strain. Hildreth wrote:

> Physiological crises, such as puberty and menopause, inheritance of nervous instability, toxins or poisons, whether taken as drugs, formed by bacteria, absorbed from sluggish bowels, or formed in the tissues and retained in the blood through failure of elimination; all these are possible factors in the production of mental disorders. Of these, heredity is just a predisposing cause. Nervous instability is all that is inherited. Probably every case is the cumulative result of a number of causes acting in concert.

In 1939, after twenty-four years at the sanatorium, he would conclude that the most fundamental causes of nervous and mental problems were maladjustments of "bone, muscle or sinew." Every case was unique, but the commonest antecedent was altered cerebral blood circulation "due to vasomotor disturbances arising from lesions of the first to fifth dorsal vertebrae" and of the upper cervical region.[37] "A starved and poisoned brain cannot function well," Hildreth reasoned. "So the mind breaks down under a strain that normally would not affect it."

There could be other causes, too. Lesions affecting the kidneys might cause retention of urea and other poisons, predisposing the body to chronic infection and consequent absorption of bacterial toxins. Lesions affecting the endocrine glands might upset hormone production and balance. Lesions affecting the nerves to the gastrointestinal tract might affect digestion, absorption and assimilation of food or, by impairing elimination, allow poisons to be absorbed into the system. Laboratory tests verified autointoxication in many with long term constipation, and these patients, in addition to osteopathic treatment, received colonic irrigation and hydrotherapy (with baths and hot packs to calm nerves, induce sleep and stimulate elimination). It took years to build a body of knowledge on the most effective strategies for treatment and patient management, and to assemble a staff skilled in all aspects of the work.

Though too weak to visit in person Still took a vital interest in the institution and repeatedly asked Hildreth for detailed progress reports on the patients. "The treatment for insanity and results obtained at Macon in the last year seem to be nothing more than natural," Still wrote in August 1915. "I have always said that twenty-five percent of all insane cases could be cured by osteopathic treatment, and I am thankful to be able to live to see this truth demonstrated."[38]

In 1929 the sanatorium published statistics of all patients treated during its first fifteen years. Courses of treatment averaged between three to twelve months (though often much longer), with recovery rates of 35.5% in dementia praecox (schizophrenia), 66% in manic depression, 94% in infection, exhaustion and toxic psychoses, and 77% in "psychoneuroses."[39] Three years later Hildreth reported that in over 2000 cases treated to that date 55% had made full recoveries, and he asserted that "most types of insanity" could benefit from osteopathic treatment. By that time patients were being referred from nearly every state and, with so many passengers requesting that trains stop at a small building just outside the main gate, the Wabash Railroad marked on its map a station named "Hildreth." For many years every ASO graduate served a stint at the institution.

The purity of the founder's vision was kept alive at Still-Hildreth, but the profession at large struggled to maintain a coherent front. The American Medical Association remained obstructive to osteopathic legislation and, even in states that had achieved recognition, MDs often harassed DOs in petty ways: challenging their entitlement to sign birth or death certificates, practice minor surgery and obstetrics, treat infectious diseases, use antiseptics, anesthetics and antidotes for poisons, and even the right to use soap.

These challenges were irritating, but Still had long recognized that the greatest threat to his science came from within the profession itself. "You need not fear our enemies," he told Arthur Hildreth, "who have contested every advancement we have undertaken. They cannot harm us; their kicks are only blessings in disguise. Our great danger, in fact the only danger that could threaten the future of osteopathy, is the mistakes of those who profess to be our friends."[40]

Graduate W. R. Archer complained that the colleges were "drifting into channels of the least resistance" while practitioners, dissatisfied with being "only an osteopath," imagined they needed to attach a medical pedigree to their name before they became "really 'somebody' in the eyes of the public." And, with drug prescription more lucrative than manual treatment, he asked, "Is the greed of commercialism to play a part in the molding of the future of osteopathy."[41]

The schools argued about materia medica. Some offered optional courses on the subject without mentioning it in their catalogues; others asserted their right to teach whatever they wanted. In 1915 Henry Bunting declared in his Chicago-based journal *The Osteopathic Physician* that he favored the teaching of drug medication. Would you, he asked his colleagues, give morphine to a patient in the last agonizing stages of cancer, thyroid extract to a cretin child, the Pasteur treatment to someone bitten by a rabid dog, digitalis to a patient with a feeble pulse, iron to an anemic, adrenaline to a patient bleeding to death, pumpkin seed for tapeworm, mercury or Salvarsan to a syphilitic, or antitoxin to a child with diphtheria?[42]

These were questions the profession was finding increasingly difficult to ignore, especially after the tragic case of 1908 AOA Vice-president Frank Furry, an MD turned osteopath. When Furry's daughter contracted diphtheria he refused to administer antitoxin, insisting upon treating her osteopathically, but the girl died and a specialist who performed an intubation at the last accused him of being a criminal.[43]

Still consistently taught that medicines should be used only as antidotes for poisons, but *Osteopathy: Research and Practice* does contain a small proviso: "the world would be just as well off (with very slight exception) had there never been a system of drug medication."[44] And, in discussing the refractoriness of syphilis to osteopathic treatment, he once told Ellen Ligon, "Until we know something better I would make one exception in favor of drugs and give mercury."[45] Yet for most cases the best outcome demanded the application of osteopathic principles.

But with graduates clamoring to been seen as fully-fledged physicians and surgeons, and in numerous states demanding licenses to prescribe medicines,[46] many were abandoning and even disputing these principles. Still was angered and saddened by the development of schisms, arguments and different interpretations of his teachings, and he worried that the drift towards medical thinking would ultimately lead to the profession's demise.[47] But his views carried less weight now.

On 1 August 1915, before the AOA convention in Portland, Oregon, he drafted an impassioned appeal to "the thinking osteopaths of the profession," imploring them to take up the fight to keep osteopathy pure for he no longer possessed the strength to do so himself:

> There is an alarm at the door of all osteopathic schools. The enemy has broken through the picket. Shall we permit the osteopathic profession to be enslaved to the medical trust? . . . For a time I received hearty support from my friends, which I appreciate, but in my declining years my boys and girls have been on the defense rather than the offense. By winning this battle we have established the greatest truth unfolded to suffering humanity. Millions of lives can be saved annually. Osteopathy is yet in its infancy. I have only brought forth the principles and truth, which I have turned over to the profession, which has wisdom and enough moral back bone not to offer any compromise with the enemy. Stand behind all legitimate research institutes. Give them your support. . . . If we cannot have pure osteopathic principles taught in our schools, I hope the faithful will rally around the flag and we will build an international school that will offer no compromise unless it is the golden truth.
>
> D. O. means Dig On.[48]

The appeal failed. The AOA Board of Trustees, bowing to internal pressure, voted to allow the colleges to teach whatever they wanted.[49] The following year even the ASO extended its course from three to four years, regardless of Still's repeated warnings that the school was placing too much emphasis on specialized subjects and too little on osteopathic fundamentals.

That the profession should undermine its own foundations was all the more incongruous at a time when patient numbers were growing steadily and the practice drawing widespread comment. "Something unusually drastic and effective will have to be done with the osteopaths, if they continue to cure after the regular physicians have given them up," *Life* magazine joked in February 1916. "For the first offense there could be a moderate fine; if the offense is repeated, the fine could be doubled and a term of imprisonment added. The license could also be taken away and the wicked and reprehensible osteopath would thus not be permitted to practice any more, for it is quite obvious that if osteopaths continue to cure people, the regular medical profession, which now controls the laws and liberties of the majority, might eventually go out of business."[50]

In that October's *Osteopathic Truth* magazine Still tried again to shepherd his flock back to the fold:

> The Osteopath is one who has a mechanical knowledge of the human body, when normal and when abnormal; and he should know how to adjust all variations from the normal. The more mechanical knowledge you have of the physical body construction, the better your work will be. Bring your patient to normality, then go home. Plenty of good food and rest, and nature will effect the cure. Keep your knife in your pocket, and leave your drugs in the drug-store; give God credit for perfection in all things, as a Mechanic, Builder and Engineer.
> 'Life proves its perfection by its work.'
> A. T. Still.
> M. D. means More Drugs.[51]

Old age was slowly overtaking him, accelerated by a mild stroke the previous fall. He spent less time in the classrooms and clinic and sat for longer periods on his comfortable front porch at the top of Osteopathy Hill. From there he could gaze across the street at the activities of the school, the building accommodating thirty-five nursing students, and the surgical hospital where every patient was treated for post-operative complications solely by osteopathic means.[52] His eyes had grown dim, but he continued to have someone read to him for at least two hours every day.[53]

He enjoyed the visits of a stream of friends and admirers.[54] In 1915 these included the deaf, dumb and blind celebrity Helen Keller and William "Buffalo Bill" Cody, who credited his robust good health to regular osteopathic treatment.[55] When the Wild West Show came to Kirksville that August the famous showman was anxious to meet Still. They had both been early Kansas settlers and staunch abolitionists. In September 1854, when Bill was eight, his father Isaac was stabbed twice in the chest with a Bowie knife while delivering an antislavery speech. Isaac Cody survived the attack, though the wound was said to have contributed to his death three years later. Still remembered the incident well.[56]

On his occasional visits to the school he saw students manipulating strange chemical apparatus and peering through microscopes at microbes unknown when he was a young doctor. They now learned Ehrlich's side-chain theory of immunity from books that explained in scientific language the principle

Still had crudely expressed decades earlier, and he wondered why scientists bothered to tinker with guinea pigs, sheep and horses to manufacture artificial sera when the blood could be relied upon to supply the perfect remedies, in the right dosage and, with well-timed osteopathic treatment, distribute them to precisely where they were needed.[57]

Bodily strength failing, he rested for longer periods on the uncomfortable old leather-upholstered table in the center of the living room on which he had given the very first osteopathic treatments.[58] On the eve of his eighty-eighth birthday Harry Chiles and two colleagues came to visit and found him lying upon it. He was "the same independent, indomitable soul as he refused with the imperiousness of a king efforts to assist him in rising," Chiles related, "yet he was as kindly, as bright and humorous as in his best days. I say best days – I mean days of physical vigor, for Dr. Still saw to it that his spirit never grew

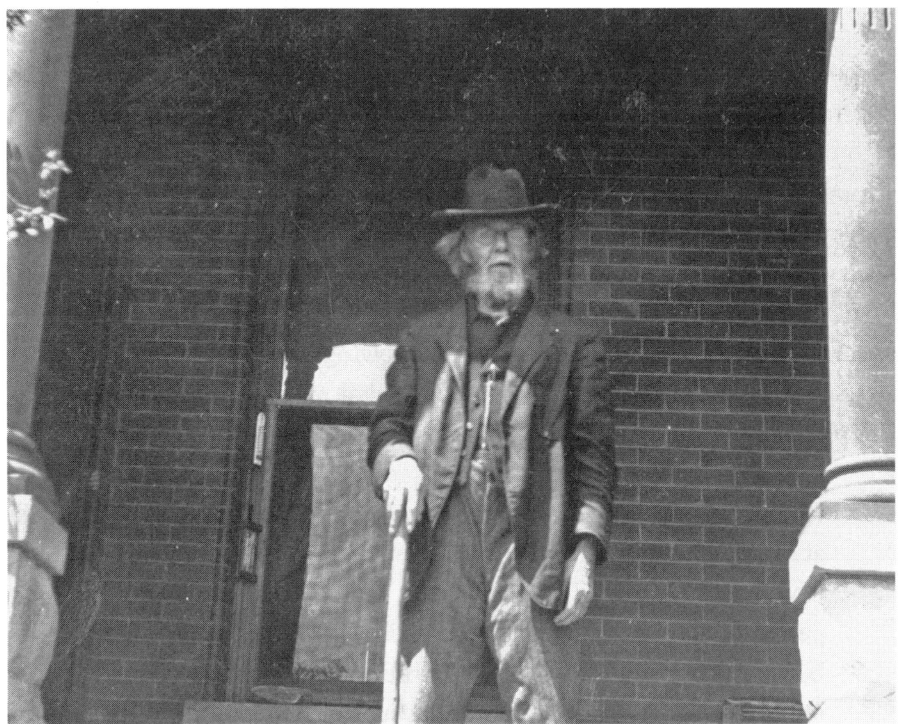

Still on his front porch, 1917.

old."[59] The last time Florence Gair saw him he confided that with most of his friends having already passed on he was anxious for the change to a "new and larger life."[60]

On 23 May 1917 a bronze statue commissioned by the Sojourner's Club and sculpted by the renowned George Julian Zolnay was unveiled on the ASO Hospital lawn across the street from Still's home. It depicted with faithful likeness the pioneer that Kirksville had for years written off as a dreamer and a quack, staff in hand and trousers stuffed into high cowhide boots. On its base was engraved the dictum *The God I worship demonstrates all his works*. That morning, as thousands crowded Jefferson and Osteopathy streets, Still walked across the lawn to Charley's house to watch the ceremony with 'two or three' friends.[61]

On Sunday, 9 December, a friend from Chicago, Oliver Foreman, brought to the house a young soldier, Private Harold Peat, wounded in the Great War and currently receiving osteopathic treatment. As Still reclined on the old treatment table in a threadbare coat he held up an arm to expose a big hole in the sleeve and joked that he belonged to the Holiness Church. He asked to hear Peat's experiences and to see his wounded arm, then instructed Foreman to place the fingers of one hand on the inner half of the soldier's clavicle, grasp the limb with the other hand, and perform a maneuver that resulted in a "pop" at the acromioclavicular joint. They were perhaps his last visitors. He kissed them goodbye and presented Peat with a signed copy of his *Autobiography* and a cut of his favorite chewing tobacco.[62]

At noon on Tuesday, Still suffered a stroke and an hour later lapsed into unconsciousness. At three-thirty the following morning, Wednesday, 12 December, he died. A dictation lay unfinished, a progress report on the Still-Hildreth Sanatorium. "Dear Boys and Girls," it read:

> I know you are keeping your eyes open on the progress that is being made at Macon, Missouri, in the treatment of mental and nervous disease. We have had a great deal of experience. My personal experience covers a period of something over fifty years in the treatment of mental cases, but until Arthur and the boys, Charlie and Harry, became interested in the Macon sanatorium, we never had a chance to look after this class of patients. I have always contended that a majority of the insane patients

> could be successfully treated by osteopathy and the success that the boys have been having in the last three and one half years bears out my faith, and I am very anxious for the entire profession to know of the work that is being done.[63]

Charley sent out the message, appended,

> The above is the Christmas Greeting that Father intended sending out to all of the boys and girls in the field practicing osteopathy. He has been so interested in the work at Macon that he felt like it was the crowning sheaf in his life's work. He, however, had his stroke of paralysis that terminated fatally before it was sent.

On Thursday, 13 December, Still's body lay in state at his home, the casket draped with the American flag and garlanded with flowers. Thousands called to pay their last respects. Among dozens of condolence letters was one from Reverend Ben Jones, the minister who had conducted Mary's funeral, now superintendent of the Methodist Episcopal Church in Cameron, Missouri. "Your father was a rare man in every way," he wrote Blanche:

> He was a pioneer of thought and investigation. He wanted to know for himself and, be it said to his credit, he never gave up until he did know. This attitude of investigation was carried out in the deeper things that have to do with the future, the eternal. I think I knew your father's attitude toward these things as few, if any, ministers ever did. At first he used to startle and even shock me with some things he would say about religious things, but after a while I grew to know and understand him, and I want to say here and now that the more I knew him and the better I understood his position, the more I was impressed by the sheer bigness of the man. Under that rough exterior which he showed more or less to everybody and especially to ministers, I found a heart of gold, and I loved him. I shall always be glad that it was my privilege to know him and feel that we were friends. I am in many ways a different manner of man than I was before I learned to know him.[64]

It was bitterly cold on Friday, the day of the funeral. Still had requested that Arthur Hildreth speak when this time came, and for the onetime farmer whose life had been so interwoven with his, this final task proved the most difficult to perform.[65] He knew the Old Doctor would not have wanted them to grieve but to rejoice with him in a change he welcomed as a natural step in life's divine plan. Hildreth stood before the bier to deliver a long, heartfelt address. He recounted Still's trials, burdens and hardships, his conviction and persistence, and his eventual triumph:

> His life should ever be a living example of what may be accomplished through unwavering, untiring efforts and devotion to principle and to truth. His success and what he has accomplished should be a lasting inspiration; our work given to us through him is one of service, and it has given to us a great privilege and most wonderful advantages. We have been blessed in having had given to us the opportunity of spending our lives in a field of such vast usefulness, and to him belongs the credit.

"The influence of his existence has been felt by more people and in more ways than any other man of this age," Hildreth continued, "and the beauty and the glory of it all is the far reaching effect of this influence, which has never failed to enrich the lives of those who came in contact with it. He has brought hope into hearts and health into lives where only despair existed." The prophet was gone, but his teachings would remain. "He has given mankind the simplest, most commonsense, scientific, rational treatment of disease ever discovered, a scientific method for the cure of disease." Society could be grateful for the comforts, conveniences, privileges and technological advances emerging in ever increasing rapidity but, Hildreth said, "what do privileges amount to, or all the wealth of the earth count, without health?" He predicted that time would prove Still to be "humanity's greatest benefactor."[66]

Reverend W. B. Christy offered prayers and a brief, sincere eulogy. "As I study his life and become familiar with his achievements," he addressed the mourners, "the conviction fastens itself upon me that he is one of the world's great men. Life is worthwhile when it touches some other life to brighten and cheer it. Dr. Still's life was a sacrificial life. He was unselfish in the extreme. He seemed to live for others. He never asked, 'how will this affect my standing or my welfare,' but 'the truth, justice and righteousness demand it.' Although a scientist and philosopher of the highest order he was the very embodiment of simplicity. This is the distinguishing mark of greatness."

Christy had often called to see Still and invariably left with a gift, on one occasion a copy of the *Autobiography* inscribed, *I love to love, and to be loved. Do you?* On a recent visit Still said to the pastor, "To some, departing from this life is a leap in the dark. To me it is no leap in the dark. It is the reverse. I am not afraid of God. I have thought the matter through. The future state is perfectly clear to me."[67]

The services at the grave were conducted by Kirksville's Masonic lodges under the charge of Judge Edward Higbee, Past Grand Master. Charley, Harry and Herman were all freemasons, though Still had never joined a lodge after returning to Missouri. Before leaving the house for the short walk to the Llewellyn Cemetery, Blanche's three-year-old daughter Mary Jane approached the coffin to kiss her grandfather goodbye. Speaking as though he were alive, she told him not to be lonesome when he got to heaven but to find Grandma.[68]

The osteopathic profession was now seven thousand strong, the fruit of its founder's long and unwavering pursuit of truth in the face of almost unimaginable odds. During these last years Ernest Tucker had listened as the old man traced his life's path from his earliest ideas to the national institution he created. "I did not dream that it would be anything like this," Still said with a kind of awe in his voice. "I guess it was sort of wonderful."[69]

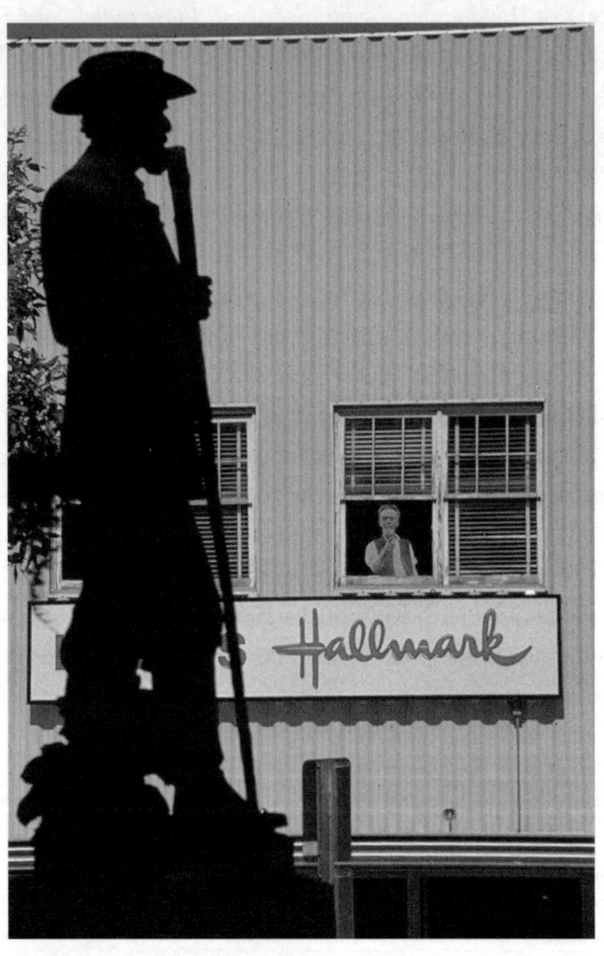
Hallmark

Epilogue

TEACH IT, PREACH IT, AND PRACTICE IT

> In years to come men will wonder what manner of man was Dr. Still, what it was like to have known him, to have walked and talked with him and have his personal instruction along the lines of his great discovery; and men will envy those of us who had the great privilege. They will wonder if they have received the message in its entirety and uncorrupted. For myself, I feel that it is a sacred charge to keep the faith as Dr. Still delivered it to me, and pass on its principles unchanged; as far as possible make others see the wonderful truth he had discovered and the limitless possibilities of its application to the relief of a suffering world. To those who did not know him there are no words that will give you a just estimate of this man who was a humorist, philosopher, seer, physician and philanthropist.[1]

So wrote Ellen Ligon in 1921. After years in practice Still's former students told of the lessons he taught returning with new force and significance, and of how they wished they could come under his instruction once more.

Yet his passing commanded little national attention, and his supporters blamed themselves for the lack of knowledge about the magnitude of his discovery and the integrity of his life.[2] "Those who knew Dr. Still only as a bone setter never really knew much of the real man," E. R. Booth elaborated. "Few fathomed the depth of his work or scanned the height of his attainments. Many caught a glimpse of him but few ever really knew him. His personal work is done but the force of the *idea* he gave the world permeates mankind and will become a greater force as the years go by if his followers live up to the high *ideal* he gave them and see the *vision* he saw."[3]

But the idea, the ideal and the vision were receding. In 1925 Asa Willard, then serving AOA president, was approached by a self-assured young undergraduate. "Of course, Doctor," the student said, "we realize that what Dr. Still gave us was rather crude, he being himself hardly what you would call a scientist, and it will be up to those of better training to develop it and dignify it."[4] This new breed sneered at the "religious fervor" and "prayerful devotion" of the early graduates, believing that the modern generation, with their more scientific attitude, had surpassed the Old Doctor's outmoded disciples.[5]

A year later Joe Sullivan complained of the "enormous list of desertions in our ranks, most of them due to the public's loss of faith in us as we apostatize from our original tenets." He spoke of the great heritage left by the founder and how, without Still's assertive leadership, the profession was wandering into "a sort of morass, a thicket, without a Moses to guide us."[6] Many new graduates regarded the early alumni as a lesser breed – "not qualified physicians, but something else" – and accused those who remained true to Still's teachings of "laboring under a delusion."[7] Sullivan found this hard to bear. After seeing his sick wife restored to health when given only three months to live, he had spent his first twelve years in practice treating both acute and chronic diseases in his busy Chicago office without once needing to call for regular medical assistance, and in a career spanning thirty years witnessed cures of gallstones, kidney stones, goiter, appendicitis, tonsillitis, gynecological conditions and at least twenty breast tumors simply by normalizing the structure of the body.[8] "I appreciate fully the convenience of possessing the right to prescribe Uncle Dam's booze," he acknowledged, "it means a tidy $100 a month towards the office rent.[9] If you think drugs of use, use them, but call yourself an M.D. not a D.O., else folks will think you want the dirty dollar not the advance of Osteopathy."[10]

Ed Pickler spoke of responsibility. "You must be either an asset or a liability to your profession and there is no middle ground. . . . If any of you are thinking of combining medicine with your osteopathy, that, of course, is your own business, but I will say to you candidly that I do not think it can be done. The systems are diametrically opposed to each other and I cannot see how the osteopath who is honest and who understands osteopathy can use them together."[11] For those who had forgotten the difference between the two approaches Still's nephew Turner Hulett offered a simple guide: "Every application, appliance, method or procedure used in the treatment of disease may be classified under one of two heads. If its effect is to modify the vital processes themselves, it is medical. If its effect is to remove conditions which are interfering with those processes, it is osteopathic."[12] Michael A. Lane cautioned that if the profession let go of the osteopathic lesion as the primary causative factor in disease it would cease to be, and any school that did not make it "the mainspring and purpose of its existence" could not be called osteopathic "without false pretense."[13]

Mark Twain expressed similar sentiments:

> An aspect that aggravates man's tragical situation is that he is so heady about his own devices that he fails to give ear to the Powers that move the Universe; in the matter of healing, to cooperate selflessly with Nature, the great healer. Indeed, the chief threat to the dignity of the profession of Osteopathy today is that it may turn too far to the side of the entrenched healing agencies and rely too exclusively upon shots and pills, departing from the original concept of Dr. Still: to make conditions favorable for the impulse of the body to cure itself.[14]

Ernest Tucker lamented that osteopathy had initially developed as "the lengthening shadow of Andrew Taylor Still, but the time came when persons who knew him only by narrowing tradition and a few selected epigrams gathered the reins of power in the profession. Then there was only the value of the idea to hold them."[15]

As the founder's teachings faded in the collective memory a new orthodoxy was established and with it came a change in attitude. Even the word osteopathy fell into disfavor, supplanted by "osteopathic medicine," careless of the inherent oxymoron. "It is incongruous for us to confuse some of our friends," Asa Willard disapproved, "and put a question mark in their minds by obtrusively tying the word 'medicine' or 'medical' to osteopathy every time it is mentioned."[16] Harry Chiles complained that without Still's "silent, unobtrusive influence" much of "the spirit, the courage and the willingness to be looked upon as unlearned and irregular because different" had disappeared. He observed that by the 1940s most in the profession lacked conviction of the truth of osteopathic principles and were simply "falling in line with what is done and going on around us."[17]

A dedicated nucleus kept the faith, but with some using hands, some prescribing drugs, and others a combination of the two it became increasingly difficult to convince the American public that osteopathy was a complete system of medicine sufficient in itself. As osteopaths themselves lost sight of its potential and measured its capacity by their own limited beliefs and abilities,[18] the public came to see it as a therapy for a narrowing range of musculoskeletal complaints.

In America a majority of DOs eventually discarded manual treatment altogether, becoming virtually indistinguishable from MDs in all but name. "It is disturbing . . . when too many people are saying the hardest thing to get in the office of so many Osteopaths is Osteopathy," Hugh Gravett wrote in 1948. "That when they are in need of an Osteopathic adjustment they go to a Chiropractor, and in the minds of the public a Chiropractor is a half-baked Osteopath, and in the minds of the masses most of the Osteopaths are only half-baked M.D.'s, and nobody likes their cake half-baked."[19] Gravett issued his colleagues a warning: "Teach it, preach it, and practice it, or you will not survive."[20]

As the medicalization of American osteopathy gathered pace Still's hope of an international school – not one single building but many institutions, "whether in this country or China"[21] – did eventually come to pass. J. Martin Littlejohn established the British School of Osteopathy in 1917 and osteopathic schools have since opened throughout the world. Outside America graduates are not entitled to prescribe drugs, but all continue to face political, legal and social pressures towards conformity with the dominant worldview and its political and economic imperatives.

The era of modern pharmacology did not begin until after Still's death. Had the new medicines been available might he have countenanced more "slight exceptions" to his drugless practice? In 1991 his grandson Charles Still, Jr. wrote:

> For several thousand like myself who practiced manipulative Osteopathy for years without the aid of drugs or antibiotics and successfully treated a variety of acute infections, did we in some way either free up or stimulate the immune system so that it could better the body's ability to resist infection? Was Andrew Still really being facetious in saying that there

> is no such thing as disease – only an inability of an individual's body to resist infection? While medical science finds more and more so-called diseases, while viruses change from year to year, and drugs and antibiotics lose their effectiveness, maybe it is about time to research any avenue that might lead us to a way to stimulate the body's immune system to more effectively resist infection.[22]

While medicine remains caught in the stream of social consciousness that draws it towards reductionist science and technological advance, where the search for cures continues along the path set by Descartes to investigate "the small parts of nature" to the minutiae of cells, molecules and genes, Still teaches that to find health we must consider the human organism in its entirety and in relationship to its environment. Instead of relying exclusively on science we must adopt the essentially American Indian philosophy of listening to, learning from and harmonizing with nature.

The continent's original inhabitants knew that health is maintained through interrelationships. They were guided not by science but by a universal principle: all is related. Harm the water, the air and the earth and you will ultimately harm yourself. "The whites, too, shall pass – perhaps sooner than other tribes," the respected Chief Seattle prophesied. "Continue to contaminate your own bed, and you will one night suffocate in your own waste."[23]

"I'm no normal professor," Still once told Asa Willard. "I don't pretend to know the finer points about pedagogy, but I do know you students have got to learn to think osteopathy."[24] The founder urges us to think for ourselves, seek truth, and challenge tradition, experts and authorities. He asks us to place principles above science, and to recognize that within every living cell resides an absolute intelligence we only dimly comprehend.[25]

Still leads us to the same fork in the road he reached on that momentous June day in 1874: try to control nature with limited knowledge; or humble ourselves in the face of the Great Mystery, acknowledge our ignorance, and remove obstructions to nature's unceasing self-regulation. "The one is man's way and is uncertain," he counsels, "the other is God's method and is infallible. Choose this day whom you will serve."[26]

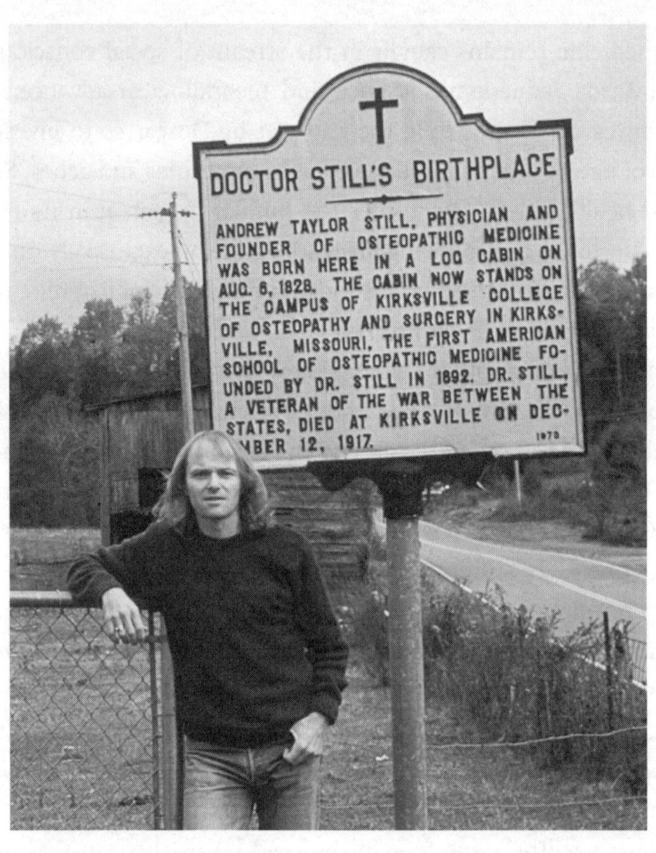
DOCTOR STILL'S BIRTHPLACE
ANDREW TAYLOR STILL, PHYSICIAN AND FOUNDER OF OSTEOPATHIC MEDICINE WAS BORN HERE IN A LOG CABIN ON AUG. 6, 1828. THE CABIN NOW STANDS ON THE CAMPUS OF KIRKSVILLE COLLEGE OF OSTEOPATHY AND SURGERY IN KIRKSVILLE, MISSOURI, THE FIRST AMERICAN SCHOOL OF OSTEOPATHIC MEDICINE FOUNDED BY DR. STILL IN 1892. DR. STILL, A VETERAN OF THE WAR BETWEEN THE STATES, DIED AT KIRKSVILLE ON DEC-
MBER 12, 1917.

Acknowledgements

The seed of this project was sown in 1991 when, as a first year student at the British School of Osteopathy in London, I read Dr. Still's *Autobiography*. Inspired by the timeless wisdom it contained and puzzled as to why it was not being taught, in May 1997 I travelled to Kirksville, Missouri, to investigate further. I remained there four years, immersing myself in the place, its history, and the archive collections of the founding school.

This book conveys the essence of Dr. Still's teachings. Weaving together biography, history and the evolution of his work, it is structured from birth to death, from not knowing to knowing, from the material to the spiritual. To ground it as closely as possible in the truth I have restricted my primary sources to the writings of the founder, his family and friends, and close students and colleagues.

During my initial research I visited Still's birthplace in Jonesville, Virginia, before interviewing many respected figures who helped guide my thinking about the unexpectedly difficult task I was about to embark upon: in North Attleboro, Massachusetts, Anne Wales, DO, who compiled and edited Dr. William Garner Sutherland's *Teachings in the Science of Osteopathy*; in Knoxville, Tennessee, Thomas F. Schooley, DO FAAO, a member of Dr. Sutherland's faculty in the 1940s, who I was told had the "best hands in America"; in Boulder, Colorado, Irvin M. Korr, PhD, who from the 1940s to the 1960s (initially with J. Stedman Denslow, DO) conducted the pioneering research on the neurological aspects of the osteopathic lesion; in Denver, Colorado, Harold Magoun, Jr., DO FAAO; at the University of North Texas Health Sciences Center, Fort Worth,

Jerry L. Dickey, DO FAAO (who also assisted with the book's revised edition), and David Vick, DO; at the Osteopathic Center for Children and Families, San Diego, Viola M. Frymann, DO FAAO. In Phoenix, Arizona, I spoke to Donald Snyder, DO, and in Scottsdale, Arizona, to Still's great grandson Gerry Still and his wife Paula. In Kirksville, I interviewed another great-grandson, Richard Still, DO, and Elizabeth Laughlin, whose husband George Andrew Laughlin, DO, was Still's grandson. Of those I spoke to, one had actually met Still, 100 year old Mabel Willbanks who, as a teenager, was treated by him on the counter of her father's store, Rinehart News Agency, at 112 South Franklin Street, Kirksville.

One person merits special mention: Miss Per (Priscilla) Brown, cousin of Harold Magoun, Jr., whom I interviewed in a residential home in Denver, Colorado. Previously a librarian, Per spent a decade (until the late 1960s) researching and writing a biography of Still that was never published. For three months during that period she had in her possession Still's elusive "diary," most of which she transcribed, but on the verge of publishing her book she suffered a breakdown and destroyed not only the text but also all her notes and papers. She was extremely pleased that I was intending to write Still's biography and wanted me to entitle it *The Lightning Bone Setter*. In her memory I have entitled one chapter just that.

Above all I am indebted to Dr. James J. McGovern, past president of Kirksville College of Osteopathic Medicine, through whose patronage I remained at KCOM for three years with unlimited access to the archive collections of what was then the Still National Osteopathic Museum (now the Museum of Osteopathic Medicine/International Center for Osteopathic History), the chief repository of Still's papers, historic osteopathic publications and other source material. I am grateful to the helpful and enthusiastic KCOM library staff from 1997-2002: Lawrence Onsager, Jean Sidwell, Cayrol Coffman, Karen Tannenbaum. Similarly to Cheryl Gracey, Jean Kenney, Devon Mills and, more recently, Debra Summers and Barb Magers at the museum which, before the collections were digitized, was an exciting treasure trove to explore.

I would like to thank the people of Kirksville and vicinity for their warm welcome, kind assistance, and for many invaluable "leads," since aspects of my research required a fair amount of detective work. A few deserve special mention: Al Srnka, for valuable advice and support, and for supplying me with early copies of the *Journal of Osteopathy*; John R. Roderick, DO, for his constant interest and encouragement; Bill and Patrice Shaw, who rented me the perfect rural house near Greentop. Thanks also to Matt and Sheri Farrell; Bret Ripley, DO; Mark Ferri, DO; Stephen Bergman, DO; Paul Simon, DO; Ellyn Herr; Audrey Johnson; and to Jamie Herd, who read and offered constructive suggestions on sections of a very early draft.

The staff of many institutions were immensely helpful. In Tennessee: Nashville Public Library. In Kansas: Kansas Historical Society, Topeka; Baldwin City Library; Lawrence Public Library. In Iowa: Glenda Wiese, archivist, Palmer College of Chiropractic, Davenport; Harvey D. Horstman of the Sunflower Spiritualist Church, Clinton; Clinton Public Library; Ottumwa Public Library; Bloomfield Public Library. In Missouri: The State Historical Society of Missouri, Columbia; Adair County Historical Society, Adair County Public Library, and Truman State University Library, all in Kirksville; Scotland County Memorial Library, Memphis; Macon Public Library; Hannibal Free Public Library; United States District Court, Hannibal. In addition I would like to thank Jimmie D. Oyler, Principal Chief, United Tribe of Shawnee Indians.

In the ten years since returning to Britain I owe special thanks to Voirrey Heath, who offered invaluable criticism and guidance through several revisions of the manuscript; my brother Chris Lewis who read it with time on his hands after breaking his leg; Jenny Lalau-Keraly for constant support and encouragement; Kirsty Macfarlane who read, commented and helped in the final stages; Josie Gritten for expert proofreading; Tim Albin of www.droplet.co.uk for graphic design and typesetting; Suzanne Boyes who assisted in innumerable ways.

I also want to thank the Sutherland Cranial College of Osteopathy, who remain true to the founder's vision.

I hope you learn as much from reading this book as I did in writing it.

MISSOURI

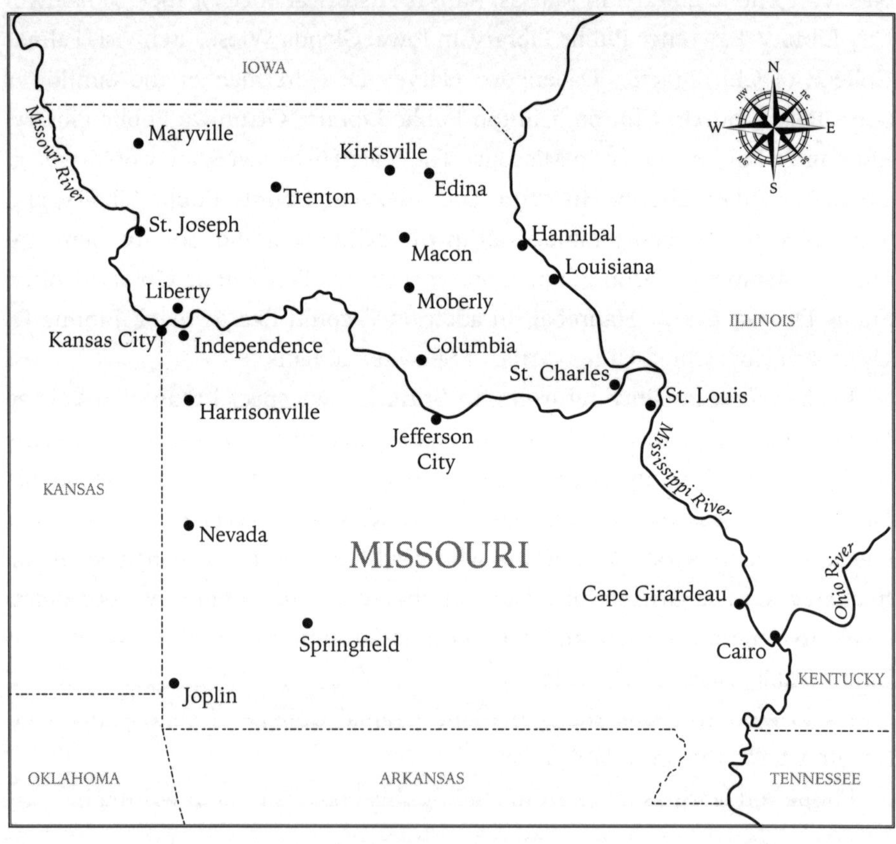

IOWA
Missouri River
Maryville
Kirksville
Edina
Trenton
St. Joseph
Hannibal
Macon
Louisiana
Liberty
Moberly
ILLINOIS
Kansas City
Independence
Columbia
St. Charles
St. Louis
Harrisonville
Jefferson City
Mississippi River
KANSAS
Nevada
MISSOURI
Ohio River
Cape Girardeau
Springfield
Cairo
KENTUCKY
Joplin
OKLAHOMA
ARKANSAS
TENNESSEE
N
S
E
W
nw
ne
sw
se

Sources

ABBREVIATIONS AND SHORTENED REFERENCES

AAO	American Academy of Osteopathy
AOA	American Osteopathic Association
AOHS	*American Osteopathic Historical Society Bulletin*
APC	Alice Patterson Collection, MOM
ATSP	Andrew Taylor Still Papers, MOM
CES	Charles E. Still Collection, MOM
CO	*The Cosmopolitan Osteopath*
DO	*The DO*
DJ	*The Diamond Jubilee of the Methodist Episcopal Church,* Baldwin, Kansas
DCHSN	*Douglas County Historical Society Newsletter,* Lawrence, Kansas
JAOA	*Journal of the American Osteopathic Association*
JO	*The Journal of Osteopathy*
KSHS	Kansas State Historical Society, Topeka, Kansas
MOM	Museum of Osteopathic Medicine, Kirksville, Missouri
NO	*The Northern Osteopath*
OM	*The Osteopathic Magazine*
OP	*The Osteopathic Physician*
OPR	*The Osteopathic Profession*
OT	*Osteopathic Truth*
SNOM	Still National Osteopathic Museum, Kirksville, Missouri
TKSHS	*Transactions of the Kansas State Historical Society*, Topeka, Kansas

STILL'S PUBLISHED WORKS

Auto 1897 *Autobiography of A. T. Still.* First Edition. Published by the author, Kirksville, Missouri. 1897.

Auto *Autobiography of A. T. Still.* American Academy of Osteopathy, Indianapolis. Reprint of Revised (1908) Edition. 1994.

PO *Philosophy of Osteopathy.* (6th Reprint of First Edition 1899.) American Academy of Osteopathy, Newark, Ohio. 1986.

PM *The Philosophy and Mechanical Principles of Osteopathy.* (Reprint of First Edition 1902.) Osteopathic Enterprise, Kirksville, Missouri. 1986.

ORP *Osteopathy: Research and Practice.* (Originally published 1910.) Eastland Press, Seattle. 1992.

OTHER PRIMARY AND SECONDARY SOURCES

Adams *In God We Trust* by Mary Still Adams. Buckingham Bros., Los Angeles. 1893.

Alford *Civilization* by Thomas Wildcat Alford. University of Oklahoma Press. 1936.

Anderson *The Methodist Episcopal Church in Missouri: Its Heroes, its Struggles and its Victories* by Rev. James W. Anderson. 1935.

Barber 1896 *Osteopathy: The New Science of Healing* by Elmer D. Barber. Hudson-Kimberly Publishing Co., Kansas City. 1896.

Barber 1898 *Osteopathy Complete* by Elmer D. Barber. Hudson-Kimberly Publishing Co., Kansas City. 1898.

Barclay *The Methodist Episcopal Church. Vol. 3: Widening Horizons, 1845-1895* by Wade Crawford Barclay. Board of Missions of the Methodist Church, New York. 1957.

Barry *The Beginning of the West* by Louise Barry. Robert Sanders Publishing, Topeka, Kansas. 1972.

Booth *History of Osteopathy and Twentieth Century Medical Practice* by Eamons R. Booth. The Caxton Press, Cincinnati, Ohio. 1924.

Bowcock *A History of Kirksville* by J. B. Bowcock. Booklet. Adair County Historical Society, Kirksville, Missouri. 1925.

Broomfield *Other Ways of Knowing* by John Broomfield. Inner Traditions, Rochester, Vermont. 1997.

Brown *The Captives of Abb's Valley* by Rev. James Moore Brown. New Edition. McClure Publishers, Staunton, Virginia. 1942.

Burtt *The Metaphysical Foundations of Modern Science* by E. A. Burtt. Revised edition. Doubleday, Anchor Books, Garden City, N. Y. 1954.

Bury *The Idea of Progress* by J. B. Bury. Macmillan, London. 1924.

Caldwell *Annals of the Shawnee Methodist Mission and Indian Manual Labor School* by Martha B. Caldwell. KSHS, Topeka, Kansas. 1939.

Clark Handwritten notes of Marovia Still Clark. KSHS, Topeka, Kansas. 1940.

Clendening *Source Book of Medical History* by Logan Clendening. Dover Publications Inc., New York. 1942.

Conner *The Mechanics of Labor: Taught by Andrew Taylor Still, M.D.* by Washington J. Conner. Privately published. 1928.

Cutler *History of the State of Kansas* by William G. Cutler. First published by A. T. Andreas, Chicago. 1883. Kansas Collection Books. www.ukans.edu

Deason *Dr. Still's Concept of Body Fluids* by Wilborn J. Deason. Manuscript in collection of author. Undated.

Dubos 1960 *Louis Pasteur: Free Lance of Science* by René Dubos. Reprint of 1960 edition. Da Capo Press, New York. 1986.

Dubos 1998 *Pasteur and Modern Science* by René Dubos. ASM Press, Washington, D.C. 1998.

Eaton *Descartes Selections*. Edited by Ralph M. Eaton. Charles Scribners Sons, New York. 1955.

Ebright *The History of Baker University* by Homer K. Ebright. Baldwin, Kansas. 1951.

Eckert *A Sorrow in Our Heart: The Life of Tecumseh* by Allan W. Eckert. Bantam Books, New York. 1993.

Endacott *The Story of the Bronze Tablet* by Rev. John Endacott. Privately published. 1925. MOM.

Eudora *Eudora Community Heritage 1776-1976*. KSHS.

Gaddis *Friendly Chats on Health and Living* by Cyrus J. Gaddis. AOA, Chicago. 1929.

Gevitz *The D.O.s: Osteopathic Medicine in America* by Norman Gevitz. Johns Hopkins University Press, Baltimore. 1982.

GHMC *General History of Macon County, Missouri.* Henry Taylor and Co., Chicago. 1910.

Gleick *Isaac Newton* by James Gleick. Fourth Estate, London. 2003.

Goode *Outposts of Zion* by Rev. William H. Goode. Poe and Hitchcock, Cincinnati. 1893.

HAC *History of Adair County, Missouri* by E. M. Violette. The Denslow History Company. 1911.

Hall *Ideas of Life and Matter: Studies in the History of General Physiology, Vol. 2: 600 B.C. – 1900 A.D.* University of Chicago Press, Urbana. 1969.

Haller *American Medicine in Transition 1840-1910* by John S. Haller. University of Chicago Press, Urbana. 1981.

Hancks *The Emigrant Tribes: Wyandot, Delaware and Shawnee, a Chronology* by Larry Hancks. Kansas City, Kansas. 1998. www.wyandot.org

Handbook *Hand-Book of Popular Quotations*. G. W. Carleton and Co., New York. 1877.

Harvey *History of the Shawnee Indians: From the Year 1681 to 1854, Inclusive* by Henry Harvey. Kraus Reprint Co., New York. 1971.

HASP *History of Adair, Sullivan, Putnam and Schuyler Counties, Missouri.* Goodspeed Publishing Co., Chicago. 1888.

Hildreth *The Lengthening Shadow of Dr. Andrew Taylor Still* by Arthur Grant Hildreth. Simpson Printing Company, Kirksville, Missouri. Second edition. 1942.

HMC *History of Randolph and Macon Counties, Missouri.* National Historical Company, St. Louis. 1884.

HNM *A History of Northeast Missouri.* The Lewis Publishing Company, Chicago. 1913.

Hulett *The Hulett-Turner Clan* by Ione M. Hulett. Columbus, Ohio. 1956. MOM.

HWCI *History of Wapello County, Iowa, Vol. 1.* The S. J. Clarke Publishing Company, Chicago. 1914.

Johnson *The Frontier Camp Meeting: Religion's Harvest Time* by Charles A. Johnson. Southern Methodist University Press, Dallas. 1955.

Kennedy *Ninety Years in the Nineteenth Century* by Barbara Vaughan Kennedy. 1933. MOM.

Lane *A. T. Still: Founder of Osteopathy* by M. A. Lane. Journal Printing Company, Kirksville, Missouri. 1925.

Lutz *The Methodist Missions among the Indian Tribes in Kansas* by Rev. J. J. Lutz. Ref: 970-7 pam v, 9. KSHS.

Müller *Elements of Physiology* by Johannes Müller. Lea and Blanchard, Philadelphia. 1843.

Nerburn *The Wisdom of the Native Americans*. Compiled by Kent Nerburn. New World Library, California. 1999.

Nuland *Doctors: The Biography of Medicine* by S. B. Nuland. Vintage Books, New York. 1988.

Oates *With Malice Toward None: A Life of Abraham Lincoln* by Stephen B. Oates. HarperPerennial, New York. 1994.

Page *The Old Doctor* by Leon E. Page. The Journal of Osteopathy, Kirksville, Missouri. 1932.

Porter *The Greatest Benefit to Mankind* by Roy Porter. Fontana Press, London. 1999.

Posey *Development of Methodism in the Old Southwest, 1783-1824* by Walter Brownlow Posey. Porcupine Press, Philadelphia. 1974.

Riedman *Portraits of Nobel Laureates in Medicine and Physiology* by S. R. Riedman and E. T. Gustafson. Abelard-Schuman, London. 1963.

Schnucker *Early Osteopathy in the Words of A. T. Still*. Edited by R. V. Schnucker. Thomas Jefferson University Press, Kirksville, Missouri.1991.

Semones *Doctor Andrew Taylor Still, Virginia and North Carolina Ancestors from Prerevolutionary Times to 1836* by Harry Semones. MOM.

Shryock *Medicine and Society in America: 1660 – 1860* by Richard H. Shryock. Cornell University Press, Ithaca and London. 1972.

Spencer *First Principles* by Herbert Spencer, *5th Edition*. Williams & Norgate, London. 1887.

Staab *When Shawnees die they go to probate court: Cultural practices of the Kansas Shawnees, 1830s-1860s* by Rodney Staab. KSHS.

Still C. E. *Frontier Doctor – Medical Pioneer* by Charles E. Still, Jr. Thomas Jefferson University Press, Kirksville, Missouri. 1991.

Sugden *Tecumseh: A Life* by John Sugden. Henry Holt and Company, New York. 1997.

Towne *Abram Still: Missionary to the West* by Ruth Warner Towne. MOM.

Trowbridge *Andrew Taylor Still: 1828-1917* by Carol Trowbridge.
Thomas Jefferson University Press, Kirksville, Missouri. 1991.

Truhlar *Doctor A. T. Still in the Living* by Robert E. Truhlar.
Privately published. Cleveland, Ohio. 1950.

Tucker *The Theory of Osteopathy* by Ernest E. Tucker and Perrin T. Wilson.
Journal Printing Company, Kirksville, Missouri. 1936.

Virchow 1863 *Cellular Pathology: As Based Upon Physiological and Pathological Histology* by Rudolf Virchow. (Reprint of second German edition 1863.)
Dover Publications, Inc., New York. 1971.

Virchow 1958 *Disease, Life and Man: Selected Essays by Rudolf Virchow*.
Translated by Lelland J. Rather. Stanford University Press, California. 1958.

Walter *The First School of Osteopathic Medicine* by Georgia Warner Walter.
Thomas Jefferson University Press, Kirksville, Missouri. 1992.

Ward *Notes on Dr. M. L. Ward and the Columbian School of Osteopathy*. MOM.

Waugh *Autobiography 5th Edition* by Lorenzo Waugh.
Methodist Book Concern, San Francisco. 1896.

Wernham *The Contribution of John Martin Littlejohn to Osteopathy* by T. Edward Hall and John Wernham. John Wernham School of Classical Osteopathy. Maidstone, Kent. Undated.

Wesley *The Works of John Wesley: Sermons (4 Volumes)* edited by Albert C. Outler. Abingdon Press, Nashville. 1985.

Wesley 1747 *Primitive Physick: or An Easy and Natural Method of Curing Most Diseases* by John Wesley. W. Strahan, London. 1747.

Genealogy

ANDREW TAYLOR STILL'S PATERNAL ANCESTRY

One branch came from England:

Samuel Still, b. ? England, d. 1782 North Carolina.
Son Boaz Still, b. 1765, d. ?

The other branch came from Germany:

Michael Hasserlin (or Haessler) married Barbara Roesheis.
Son Michael Hasserlin, b. 1699, married Magdalena Sihler.
Daughter Elizabeth (or Elisabetta) Hasserlin, b. 1718 Heningen, married Johann Andreas Leydig, b. 1715 Württemburg, d. 1762 Pennsylvania. On immigrating to America Johann anglicized his name to John Andrew Lyda.
Son Andrew Lyda, b. 1750 Washington, d. 1816, married Sarah Mackay.
Son Jacob Lyda, b. ? d. 1860 North Carolina, married Sarah Anne Wilkerson, a Cherokee.
Daughter Mary Lyda, b. ?, d. ?

Boaz Still married Mary Lyda. They had fifteen children, including Still's father Abram.

STILL'S MATERNAL ANCESTRY

Came from Northern Ireland:

James Moore II, Ulster protestant, b. Northern Ireland, married Jane Walker, b. County Down. They immigrated to America around 1726.
Son James Moore III, b. Pennsylvania c. 1740, married Martha Poage.
Son James Moore IV, b. 1770, d. 1851, married Barbara Taylor, b. 1777, d. 1832.
Daughter Martha Poage Moore, Andrew's mother.

Genealogy

STILL'S PARENTS

Abram Still 25 August 1796 – 31 December 1867.
Martha Poage Moore 28 January 1800 – 25 December 1888.

Abram Still and Martha Poage Moore married 21 August 1822. They had nine children.

STILL'S SIBLINGS

Edward Cox Still 15 January 1824 – 8 May 1906.
James Moore Still 5 February 1826 – 8 January 1907.
Andrew Taylor Still 6 August 1828 – 12 December 1917.
Barbara Jane Poage Still (Vaughn) 29 November 1830 – 4 March 1894.
Thomas Chalmers Still 6 July 1833 – 20 August 1922.
John Wesley Still 17 February 1836 – 7 February 1888.
Mary Margaretta Still (Adams) 10 September 1838 – 23 January 1920.
Marovia Marsden Still (Clark) 9 October 1843 – 8 August 1927.
Cassandra Elliott Still (McCollum) 10 October 1846 – 17 February 1888.

STILL'S CHILDREN

Still married Mary Margaret Vaughn (born ?) on 29 January 1849. They had five children:

Marusha Hale Still 8 December 1849 – July 1924.
Abraham Price Still 12 November 1852 – 8 February 1864.
George W. Still 9 March 1855 – 10 March 1855.
Susan B. Still 11 April 1856 – 7 February 1864.
Lorenzo Waugh Still 29 July 1859 – 4 August 1859.

Mary Margaret died on 29 September 1859.

Still married Mary Elvira Turner (born 24 September 1834 in Newfield, New York) on 25 November 1860. They had seven children:

Dudley Turner Still 12 September 1861 – 2 November 1861.
Marcia Ione Still 13 January 1863 – 23 February 1864.
Charles Edward Still 7 January 1865 – 6 July 1955.
Herman Taylor Still 15 May 1867 – 15 October 1941.
Harry Mix Still 15 May 1867 – 28 July 1942.
Fred Still 15 January 1874 – 6 June 1894.
Martha Helen Blanche Still 5 January 1876 – 19 October 1959.

Mary Elvira Still died in Kirksville on 28 May 1910.

Notes

Still's spelling is inconsistent. I quote mostly from his handwritten notes, misspellings included, but occasionally correct for the sake of clarity and readability. This book is written in American English.

Epigraph: ATSP 2009.10.880, 1-2.

A. T. STILL

1. Booth 476-7.
2. OP August 1934, 24.
3. JO 1929, 204.
4. PO 120.
5. Auto 201.
6. Page 41-2.
7. Booth 477.
8. OT January 1918, 84.
9. JAOA January 1918, 251.
10. JO July 1932, 401.
11. JO January 1918, 20.
12. CES 1997.04.92, 2.

1: PICTURES, EVENTS, FORCES, WHOLES

1. MOM 1979.289.02. Mary Jane Denslow (Still's granddaughter) to Harry Semones. 2 November 1949. Quoted in *Doctor Andrew Taylor Still, Virginia and North Carolina Ancestors from Pre-Revolutionary Times to 1836* by Harry Semones. Roanoke, VA, 1949. According to Denslow, Jacob Lyda "married Ann Wilkinson [Sarah Anne Wilkerson], whose one parent was full blood Cherokee." Their daughter Mary married Boaz Still.
2. Booth 1-2.
3. Towne 26.
4. Posey 36.
5. Endacott 3. Many Methodist ministers doubled as physicians. In his book *Primitive Physick: An Easy and Natural Way of Curing Most Diseases*, Church founder John Wesley advocated self-reliance in matters of health, advising simple traditional remedies and the preventive measures of exercise, personal hygiene, and temperance in food and drink. Regarding Abram's medical education, Still wrote that his "father was M.D. of the first Medical School that was in the State of Ohio." (Letter, Still to "E. D." "You can say from me A. T. Still that I am 65 years old...." MOM) Regarding Abram Still's medical training, in *Abram Still: Missionary to the West*, 27, Ruth Warner Towne writes, "While at Jonesville Abram Still began the study of medicine. He

explained this step as a way that he might minister to physical as well as spiritual ills and as a means of better providing for his growing family." According to John Endacott in *The Story of the Bronze Tablet, Unveiled in the Methodist Episcopal Church at Eudora*, 3, Abram obtained an MD degree from Rush Medical College, Knoxville, Tennessee. This is unlikely, since no medical schools existed in either Knoxville or Nashville in the 1820s. By contrast A. T. Still writes in ATSP 1985.1134.01, "My father was an M.D. of the first medical school that was in the state of Ohio." The first medical school in Ohio, the Medical College of Ohio, Cincinnati, was organized by Dr. Daniel Drake in 1819. However, private correspondence from Billie Broaddus of the Cincinnati Medical Heritage Center, December 3, 2002, reports no evidence of Abram Still having graduated from Cincinnati.
6. Auto 18.
7. Trowbridge 21-3.
8. Auto 53.
9. Booth 2, 7.
10. Auto 50-1.
11. Booth 2. HMC 1211.
12. HMC 702, 710, 786-7, 1211.
13. Adams 6. ATSP 2009.10.135, 3.
14. Auto 51-2. It took Harmon eight years to repay the loan, and then only $600 of the principal sum.
15. Adams 18.
16. HMR 110. HMC 920.
17. Adams 11. "And well did my elder brothers, Edward, James and Andrew heed this old adage by turning everything into account, bringing the most out of the least."
18. ATSP 2009.10.366, 1-4.
19. ATSP 2009.10.757.
20. Auto 39.
21. CES 1997.04.53, 2-3.
22. ATSP 1997.04.119, 15.
23. HNM 172, 592.
24. ATSP 1997.04.121, 20.
25. ATSP 2009.10.757, 4.
26. ATSP 2009.10.757, 12.
27. CES 1997.04.53, 2-3.
28. Auto 18.
29. HASP 241. HAC 115.
30. Auto 18-20.
31. Johnson 160.
32. Adams 12.
33. Booth 8.
34. Auto 21, 28-30, 52.
35. ATSP 2009.10. 820, 1.
36. Goode 253.
37. Wesley, Sermon 44, 185.
38. Wesley, Sermon 43, 158-60.
39. Adams 6.
40. Booth 3.
41. HNM 597.
42. Joseph Dennison, "Memoirs, Rev. A. Still." *Annual Minutes of the Kansas Conference, M. E. Church, 1868*, 28-9.
43. Towne 27-8, 31.
44. Brown, *Genealogical Index*, 44.
45. Adams 12-16, 99-101, 111.
46. JO May 1927, 279. Auto 221.
47. Auto 23-4.
48. Trowbridge 34.
49. GHMC 248.
50. Trowbridge 24.
51. Auto 53.
52. Auto 29-30.
53. Booth 16.
54. Auto 46.
55. Booth 8.
56. Auto 21, 29-30.
57. ATSP 2009.10.757, 2
58. Page 10.
59. CES 1997.04.119, 14.
60. CES 1997.04.119, 42.
61. Auto 40-1.
62. JO August 1898, 105.
63. Booth 8.
64. Booth 7.
65. Auto 43-4.
66. HMC 1211.
67. ATSP 2009.10.820, 2.
68. ATSP 2009.10.757, 3.

69. Auto 243.
70. ATSP 2009.10.370, 2-3.
71. CES 1997.04.121, 21.
72. Still wrote, "The old frontiersman knows more of the customs and habits of the wild animals than the scientist ever discovered." Auto 85-6.
73. Auto 56.
74. GHMC 408-9. ATSP 2009.10.757, 6-7.

2: WAKARUSA MISSION

1. Anderson 24.
2. Booth 2.
3. The Shawnee reservation was created by treaty in 1825 for the Fish Band and others of the tribe who relinquished a small tract at Apple Creek near Cape Girardeau in southwest Missouri. After the Indian Removal Act they were joined by a larger body of Shawnee from Ohio. The Kaw is also known as the Kansas River.
4. Goode 295.
5. Eudora 8.
6. Harvey 279.
7. Lutz 217.
8. Cutler, *Wyandotte County*, Part 6. See also Goode 296-7.
9. Eudora 6. Pascal Fish, Jr. (sometimes spelled Paschal) was born at Apple Creek in 1804. His father, Pascal, Sr., led a group of Shawnee to the new reservation in the year of Andrew Still's birth. When Pascal, Sr. died in 1834, his son assumed leadership of the Fish Band. *Douglas County Historical Society Newsletter* Vol. 3 No. 1, November 1973, 1-2. KSHS.
10. Trowbridge 40. Lutz 27, 32-3.
11. Barclay 345-6.
12. Barry 906.
13. Towne 35.
14. Barry 906, 988-9.
15. Booth 1-2. Originally of Scottish ancestry, Still's maternal great-great-grandfather James Moore emigrated from Northern Ireland "about the year 1726" and married "a Jane Walker, a descendent of the Rutherfords, of Scotland." Edward C. Still to E. R. Booth, 29 November 1904.
16. Brown 22-4. Shawnee "feelings towards the whites were bitter," Brown writes. "They had been much irritated by some of the occurrences of the [Revolutionary] war; they saw the settlements steadily extending westward; they had been driven from many hunting grounds; and many favourable districts which were formerly their dwelling-places, they saw in the possession of strangers." Black Wolf was "an inferior chief of the Shawnees . . . who took an active part in harassing the frontiers. . . . He was a man above the ordinary stature, possessing a large share of strength, activity, and courage; and was of the most stern and vindictive warriors of that tribe."
17. Booth 4-5.
18. Semones 1-2.
19. Adams 22. The unabbreviated story is told in Brown 42-9. See also Brown 30 (where he says James was bartered for $50), and Brown, *Genealogical Appendix*, 25.
20. Clark 7-13. Adams 30-2.
21. Clark 5.
22. Kennedy 4.
23. Eudora 8-11.
24. Adams 39.
25. Clark 48-9.
26. Clark 29-32, 48-9. Adams 9, 39. Pascal married Hester "Hettie" Zane, a Wyandot, in 1847. *History: Paschal Fish, Jr. 1804 – 1894* by Fern Long (KSHS). Hettie died, possibly during childbirth, two weeks after Abram arrived at the mission. By 1854 Pascal had remarried. That year's Shawnee census rolls lists Fish's family as Paschal, 50; Martha, 40; Obadiah, 12; Eudora, 9; and Leander, 7. DCHSN February 1974, 3.
27. Clark 13-17.
28. Clark 1.
29. Clark 4. "Black tongue" was possibly pellagra, a systemic disease caused by niacin

(Vitamin B3) deficiency. Still's sister Barbara Jane wrote that "hundreds" of Indians died of black tongue that winter: "Their tongues would turn black as human flesh could be and swell clear out of their mouths."
30. Clark 1, 4-5, 53-5.
31. ATSP 2009.10. 757, 5.
32. Inscription in Still's copy. MOM.
33. Eudora 15. ATSP 2009.10.757, 6.
34. GHMC 409.
35. JO March 1897, 6.
36. CES 1997.04.53, 3.
37. Adams 19-20, 39.
38. *Eudora Area Historical Society Newsletter*, No. 5, October 1984, 5.
39. Charles Bluejacket remained actively interested in the traditional life of the Shawnee, supplying stories and details of their culture and cosmology to Shawnee missionary Joab Spencer and ethnologist Lewis Henry Morgan.
40. DCHSN, November 1973, 2. Tecumseh's brother Tenskwatawa, also known as the "Shawnee Prophet," was undoubtedly acquainted with the Fish family in the early years of the reservation. See TKSHS 1905-1906, 166-7.
41. Booth 2-3.
42. Harvey 154.
43. Wesley, Sermon 69, 580. Andrew's sister Mary regarded the Shawnee as "semi-civilized." Adams 39. In the early years of the reservation some had tried to maintain a traditional way of life, venturing far to the west, hunting buffalo and trading with plains Indians. All eventually settled permanently in the eastern part of the tract on the banks of the Kaw and its tributaries, where they lived in log houses, increasingly adopted Western dress, and sent their children to school. They bred cattle, pigs and horses, raised corn and vegetables, planted orchards, and were known by travelers for the variety of their fruit. TKSHS Vol. X 1907-1908, 397.
44. Harvey 143-4.
45. Alford 18-20. Responsibility for Shawnee conduct traditionally extended only towards their own race, especially their own tribe, or others who acted kindly towards them. If they resorted to cunning or deception in their dealings with the whites, Thomas Wildcat Alford wrote, "it was pitted against something that the red man felt powerless to cope with on a common ground, something for which [they] had no name." To the white race they owed nothing, except to return in kind the treatment they received.
46. Clark 51-2.
47. See Alford 11-12. The Indians did not understand the white man's warring creeds and denominations, each claiming to be the true religion – how could one argue about God – nor how their spirituality could come from a book. Despite increasing acculturation most Shawnee clung tenaciously to their old customs, ceremonies and spiritual beliefs, and traditional ceremonies like the Bread Dance continued to be held each spring and fall. TKSHS Vol. X 1907-1908, 397.
48. Genesis 1:28.
49. Eckert, frontispiece.
50. Alford 23.
51. Alford 55.
52. Auto 260.
53. CES 1997.04.119, 15. Erysipelas is a streptococcal infection.
54. Auto 56-7.
55. CES 1997.04.119, 15. Still's student Ernest E. Tucker, who supplied this quote, wrote elsewhere. "He [Still] told of the growth of the general idea of bone-setting from his experience among the Indians. For instance, he said, when an Indian dislocated his hip, the limb was tied to a pony's tail, the Indian was placed astride of a young sapling, and the pony driven away, and ' Mebby-so leg come off, mebby-so hip get set.'" CES 1997.04.121, 18.
56. ATSP 2009.10.757. Handwritten note on reverse of page 7: "During the Autumn

of 1853 we returned to our old home in Missouri and remained until May 1855."

3: BLEEDING KANSAS

1. Adams 20. Clark 73-4.
2. Goode 251-5. See also Trowbridge 47.
3. Oates 113, 117.
4. Clark 78. S. C. Pomeroy to Mr. Blood, 3 February 1855. KSHS.
5. The Still Cemetery, as it is now known, lies near Chariton Ridge Church, three and a half miles from Elmer, Missouri.
6. Auto 61-2.
7. ATSP 2009.10.757. Handwritten note on reverse of page 7. F. P. Vaughn to Mr. Keeder (MOM undated): 'I came into the Territory of Kansas on the 26th of March, 1855 . . . .'
8. Trowbridge 69.
9. Auto 45.
10. Clark 140-2. Adams 62-4. ATSP 2009.10.757, 6-7.
11. ATSP 2009.10.757, 8. SNOM 1978.255.09, 1. In JAOA August 1923, 718, Herbert Bernard writes that Still's first successful manual "cure" was that of a Shawnee medicine man suffering from asthma, whose second rib he corrected.
12. Cutler, *Territorial History*, Part 8.
13. Trowbridge 58. Still was already acquainted with James B. Abbott as both were members of the Palmyra Town Company.
14. The term "Bleeding Kansas" was coined by Horace Greeley.
15. Cutler, *Territorial History*, Part 18.
16. J. B. Abbott Papers, KSHS. *Maj. Jas. B. Abbott's Account of Obtaining Sharps Rifles*,10-19. Though Still was implicated, conclusive proof is lacking that he was among the rescue party. See Trowbridge 59-64.
17. ATSP 2009.10.758, 2. TKSHS 1897-1900, Vol. VI, 225-31. Spiritualism began in 1848 when sisters Kate and Margaret Fox of Hydesville, New York, claimed communication with spirits through rapping sounds.
18. Auto 333-4. Still wrote that his father "was a sensitive man, and had an intuitive mind."
19. CO November 1898, 1.
20. ATSP 2009.10.758, 2. See also ATSP 2009.10.783, 4.
21. Cutler, *Territorial History*, Part 30.
22. Cutler, *Territorial History*, Parts 30 and 33.
23. Clark 116-7.
24. Clark 126.
25. Clark 128.
26. Clark 133. "So they hanged Haman on the gallows that he had prepared for Mordecai. Then was the king's wrath pacified." Esther 7:10.
27. Clark 139, 155, 158.
28. Clark 126-34. Cutler, *Territorial History*, Part 35.
29. Clark 79-92. Mary Margaret had returned from Missouri. In Clark 85, Marovia writes of a frightening incident during this period where they were warned of "a big company of Missourians coming & they were killing men women & children & burning houses. My father [Abram] was away from home as he was off preaching. My Bro. A. T. & wife & children were there that night." This incident likely preceded the 12 August Battle of Franklin.
30. Auto 63-5.
31. Still assisted in extracting a musket ball from James Lane's thigh. JO June 1897, 113.
32. ATSP 209.10.758, 3. CES 1997.04.119, 5. Booth 464.
33. Auto 84-5.
34. ATSP 2009.10.758, 1-4.
35. Ebright 5.
36. Auto 97.
37. Auto 65-6.
38. Auto 71.
39. Auto 55.

4: SERIOUS QUESTIONS

1. Hulett 16-18. Mary Elvira Turner was born on 24 September 1834.

2. CES 1997.04.56, 4-5. CES 1997.04.37, 1-2. CES 1997.04.54, 1-2.
3. JO June 1910, Supplement. Still C. E. 81.
4. Hulett 19.
5. Clark 204-5.
6. CO November 1898, 1.
7. ATSP 2009.10.855, 1-3. ATSP 2009.10.168, 7.
8. Auto 73.
9. Still C. E. 118.
10. ATSP 2009.10.941. Still's discharge papers from the Kansas infantry and application for a military pension list him as, "A. T. Still, Hospital Steward." On 17 December 1877, in applying for an army pension, Still wrote, "I was surgeon but the adjutant placed me on the roll as hospital steward and was paid as such. The whole regiment will testify to the truthfulness of the statement. I did the duty of surgeon." *Pension File of Andrew T. Still.* MOM.
11. Auto 186.
12. Military statistics show that whiskey and brandy, administered as stimulants, formed the only ingredients in over 60% of prescriptions. Trowbridge 92.
13. Auto 186.
14. ATSP 2009.10.814, 1.
15. Brown, *Genealogical Index*, 60, 67.
16. Hulett 21-2. Clark 216-7.
17. JO February 1929, 77.
18. JO November 1897, 198. Eudora, named after Pascal Fish's daughter, was built around the site of the Wakarusa Mission.
19. Auto 87.
20. ATSP 2009.10.758, 6.
21. ORP 191-2.
22. Still C. E. 64.
23. CO November 1898, 9.
24. Auto 86-7.
25. ATSP 2009.10.758, 6.
26. Auto 304.
27. Auto 322-3, 334. Deuteronomy 32:4: "He is the Rock, 'his work is perfect,' for all his ways are judgment."
28. Auto 87-8.
29. Auto 182.
30. ORP 188-91.
31. JO December 1986, 6.
32. ATSP 2009.10.932.
33. Auto 76.
34. Still C. E. 61.
35. Clark 209-11.

5: THE SECRET, IMPERCEPTIBLE CHAIN

1. Cutler, *The Era of Peace*, Part 1.
2. JAOA January 1934, 216. "Osteopathy was evolved in Baldwin by Doctor A. T. Still," *Baldwin Ledger*, 30 November 1933.
3. CES 1997.04.43, 1.
4. Auto 82-3.
5. Auto 264.
6. OT February 1920, 114.
7. ATSP 2009.10.759, 3.
8. OPR August 1934, 23.
9. JO December 1905, 351.
10. Tucker. CES 1997.04.119, 41. Still told his son-in-law George M. Laughlin that he attended the Kansas City School of Physicians and Surgeons immediately after the Civil War but, disgusted with the teaching, did not return for his diploma. OP January 1909, 8.
11. ATSP 2009.10.820, 2. John Deason writes that Still, "spent one year in a medical school but the school burned which, perhaps, was fortunate for him, because it left the young student more free to think independently." Deason 9.
12. *The Personal Library of A. T. Still* compiled by Lawrence W. Onsager. 1992. ATSU.
13. OPR August 1934, 22-5, 44.
14. Burtt 18.
15. Burtt 19.
16. Burtt 82, 75.
17. Burtt 116.
18. Eaton vi-vii.
19. Eaton xxi.
20. Quoted in Burtt 122. The conarium is now called the pineal gland.
21. Quoted in Broomfield, 34.

22. Burtt 223. Seekers of knowledge had two philosophical choices: *rationalism* and *empiricism*. Rationalism, derived from the Latin *ratio*, reason, used pure logical thought. It began with a premise, an assumption treated as a general law, and from it deduced other things. Rationalism had a serious drawback – if the initial premise was incorrect, so too was everything deduced from it. Empiricism, derived from the Greek *empirikos*, experience, relied on direct perception through the senses, without preconceptions or regard to science or theory. A picture gradually formed from experimental or observational data, from which a general law could be inferred or induced. The more times the result was confirmed, the more confidence could be placed in the law. The efficacy of many medicines had been determined in this way, by trial and error, but empiricism too had a drawback. While it gave the probability of an event it could not predict with certainty what would happen at the next observation. The scientific method, a process generally credited to Newton, combined rationalism and empiricism in a process involving observation, hypothesis, controlled experiment and conclusion. If experiment confirms the hypothesis a new scientific generalization can be established; if not, the hypothesis needs to be mended or abandoned.
23. Eaton xxvi.
24. Eaton xii.
25. Galen believed that blood passed from the liver to the heart to irrigate the body in two separate streams: venous blood carrying nourishment for "consumption" by the parts of the body, and arterial blood, mixed with *pneuma* – the breath of life – vivifying the body.
26. Porter 248.
27. Porter 266.
28. Haller 85-6.
29. Shryock 73.
30. Elisha Bartlett from his 1844 *Essay on the Philosophy of Medical Science*. Quoted in Shryock 117, 129.
31. Booth 341. Oliver Wendell Holmes in an 1860 address to the Massachusetts Medical Society.
32. JO August 1899, 92.
33. Hall 264-280.
34. Genesis 2:7.
35. Wesley, Sermon 103, 460.
36. Wesley, Sermon 69, 576.
37. Wesley, Sermon 69, 575. Psalm 139:14.
38. 1 Corinthians 13:9.
39. Wesley, Sermon 67, 540.
40. Booth 480. The girl was probably Pascal Fish's daughter Eudora.

6: VITAL UNITIES

1. Brown, *Genealogical Index*, 44.
2. ATSU 2009.10.24, 8. JO June 1912. (See Schnucker 373.)
3. Official Masonic record card. Andrew T. Still, Palmyra Lodge #23. MOM.
4. TKSHS 1897-1900, Vol. VI, 230. In late 1857 the Shawnee sold all their "surplus" land. Pascal Fish sold his allotment to the German Settlement Society, who founded the city of Eudora, named after his daughter. Pascal later moved to Oklahoma and died there on 15 February 1894, aged 91. Blind, he wandered out into a snowstorm and froze to death. Trowbridge 47.
5. DO July 1979, 22.
6. Auto 90-2. The McCormick "Old Reliable" Self-Rake Reaper, patented in 1858, also dispensed with the rake man. An automatic rake swept the cut grain off the platform, depositing it in heaps on the ground ready for binding.
7. ATSP 2009.10.759, 2-3.
8. Deason 9. In PO 14 Still describes Neal as, "a medical doctor of five years training, a man of much mental ability, who would give his opinions freely and to the point." Neal also sent to Edinburgh for a "large lens" that Still wanted for treating

skin growths. OPR August 1934, 25.
9. Trowbridge 202-3. The only surviving child of Still's first marriage, Marusha seemingly inherited a measure of her father's nonconformity, liking to "venture beyond the boundaries of the status quo." Marusha had twelve children, four of whom died in infancy. Two, Henry and Ralph, became osteopaths, graduating from the ASO in 1904 and 1906 respectively.
10. Virchow 1863, 5.
11. OPR August 1934, 25.
12. Virchow 1863 45.
13. Virchow 1958 163. A remnant of the historical concept of the fiber persists in the terms "muscle fiber" and "nerve fiber."
14. Virchow 1958 89.
15. Virchow 1958 230.
16. Virchow 1863 40
17. Virchow 1958 83-4
18. Virchow 1958 87.
19. Virchow 1958 40.
20. Virchow 1958 27.
21. Virchow 1958 xv. This served to disprove Schwann's theory that connective tissues contain "cytoblastema," a hypothetical substance from which he suggested arose new cells, inflammation, tuberculosis, and other pathological conditions by some form of spontaneous generation.
22. Nuland 325.
23. Virchow 1958 61.
24. JO December 1905, 354.
25. Virchow 1863 163.
26. ORP 14.
27. The sympathetic nerves adjust blood pressure and flow to the ever changing demands of the tissues, help regulate body temperature by adjusting the volume of blood brought to the surface and, by controlling sweating, play an important part in a host of other physiological mechanisms to ready the body for action: inhibiting the secretion of saliva, digestive juices, and the peristaltic movements of the gut; dilating the pupils and bronchial passages; and raising heart rate.
28. Virchow 1863 156.
29. Virchow 1863 147-9. Virchow described how any "pathological irritant" or "physiological stimulus" could trigger vessels into localized contraction followed by dilation as the circular muscle fibers fatigued.
30. JO December 1905, 354.
31. Virchow 1863 297, 305.
32. JO December 1905, 354.
33. The intervertebral foramen, surrounded by cartilage, ligament and muscle, is just large enough to accommodate the passage of the spinal nerve, the smaller recurrent meningeal nerve, and blood vessels to and from the spinal cord.
34. CES 1997.04.53, 5-6. JO February 1929, 77-8. In Auto 285 Still suggests that the displaced rib caused irritation of the phrenic nerve, perhaps through triggering diaphragmatic tension. "I myself was thrown from a horse and got a jolt, and that set my heart tooting, and they told me it was valvular disturbance. That noise indicates that the phrenic nerve and some of the muscles are not acting right."
35. CES 1997.04.119, 22. CES 1997.04.121, 18-9.
36. ATSP 2009.10.473.
37. Virchow 1863 28.
38. Auto 263.
39. John Deason wrote, "A failure of the tissue cells to function because of inefficient capillary, lymph and intercellular fluid circulation was Dr. Still's explanation of Virchow's theory that disease begins in the cell. Surely it is clear that his theory of venous and lymphatic drainage fully explains the mechanism by means of which stasis causes a perversion of the physiological environment of the tissue cells thus leading to the beginnings of pathological change." Deason 12.
40. Müller 596. It was later shown that paralysis of the *rima glottidis* (the opening between the true vocal cords and the arytenoid cartilages), also supplied by

the vagus nerve, allowed saliva to enter the air passages and the consequent inflammation was the true cause of death.
41. JO December 1905, 354.
42. Booth 55.
43. OT January 1918, 91.
44. CES 1997.04.43, 1.
45. CES 1997.04.37, 3-4.
46. DO March 1975, 29-30. CES 1997.04.37, 2-3.

7: PERFECTION

1. Auto 85.
2. CES 197.04.119, 5.
3. John Wesley, *Primitive Physick or An Easy and Natural Method of Curing Most Diseases*. 1747. Preface.
4. Wesley, Sermon 76, 72-3.
5. See Auto 271.
6. 1 John 4:16-17. Wesley, Sermon 40, 119.
7. Quoted in *The Illustrated Origin of Species*. Abridged by Richard E. Leakey. New York, Hill and Wang 1979, 223.
8. Spencer 546.
9. Quoted in Bury 340.
10. Spencer 549.
11. The naturalist Thomas Huxley, whom Still admired, argued that a solely material progress would never lead to the attainment of an ideal society. Bury 344.
12. Brown, *Genealogical Appendix*, 48.
13. ATSP 2009.10.785, 1. Still writes only that he was "in discussion with a brother." Jim was the only brother living in Kansas; Ed was in Missouri, Tom and John in California.
14. See Romans 2:15.
15. Wesley Sermon 34, 8-10.
16. ATSP 2009.10.777. An amended version of this address on 22 June 1896 (mistakenly dated 1895) can be found in Auto 258.
17. ATSP 2009.10. 801, 2-3.
18. JO June 1906, 225.
19. Romans 7:1.
20. JO September 1908, 526.
21. PO 258-9.
22. Booth 459-60.
23. OPR August 1934, 22.
24. Spencer 99-101.
25. Spencer 128.
26. Spencer 22.
27. Auto 250.
28. Auto 312.
29. Auto 258-9.
30. ATSP 2009.10.785, 1.

8: APOSTATE OF THE FIRST WATER

1. JO February 1929, 77. DO June 1975, 25.
2. Auto 93-4.
3. CES 1997.04.37, 4. CES 1997.04.103, 6. The Kansas State Medical Society was incorporated in 1859.
4. Auto 182.
5. ATSP 2009.10.759, 6-7.
6. Auto 304.
7. Auto 344-5.
8. ATSP 2009.10.759, 26.
9. JO November 1934.
10. Auto 167-74.
11. Hildreth 314.
12. Still C. E. 75.
13. OT January 1918, 91.
14. OPR August 1934, 23.
15. ATSP 2010.02.1227, 2. CES 1997.04.37, 4-6. CES 1997.04.43, 1. See also unreferenced document in the CES Collection beginning, "Dr. Still's treatments at the picnic and being read out of the church by black art." In different accounts of the story given by Charles Still, Sr., Viola Duboys is replaced by a Miss Vorhees. Which sister was "crippled," Anna or Jennie Hagler, is also confused.
16. ATSP 2009.10.759, 6. See also JO October 1928, 544. JO February 1929, 78. The identity of the minister is unclear. A booklet in Baldwin City Library, *First Methodist Church, Baldwin City, 1855-1863*, reads: "1873-4 No regular preacher. Rev. J. Boynton and Prof. S. S. Weatherby

supplied. 1874-5 Rev. R. A. Caruthers."

17. Booth 506.

18. JAOA June 1925, 750.

19. ATSP 2009.10.759, 6.

20. Auto 225.

21. JO February 1929, 78. According to Charley, Still was "the first worshipful Master of the Masonic Lodge. He organized that Lodge in Kansas. After being retained in the Lodge he kept his membership there until the time of his death." In an undated manuscript entitled *An Inquiry into the Masonic History of Andrew Taylor Still* (MOM), J. D. Raynesford relates that Still was initiated on 12 February 1868. His membership was suspended on 10 August 1875 for non-payment of dues, restored on 4 June 1879, and finally suspended for the same reason on 20 January 1886. Raynesford visited the Baldwin Lodge (previously Palmyra Lodge #23), but found no mention of any Masonic trial – a requirement for an eviction – though a number of early Lodge Record Books were destroyed in a fire.

22. Kennedy 7. Clark 227-9.

23. Adams 152.

24. Kennedy 7.

25. HMC 1211. JO June 1906, 202. AOHS Bulletin July 1961, 5.

26. Auto 98. At some point Ed suffered a broken neck that left it "permanently crooked." AOHS July 1961, 5.

27. CES 1997.04.37, 3. CES 1997.04.53, 8.

28. On 27 March 1874 the Missouri legislature enacted a new medical practice law that required a medical college diploma for registration, with no exemption for previous experience. Despite this, Still's name was entered on the Macon County Roll of Physicians and Surgeons on 29 August 1874 as a "Physician and Surgeon." See Hildreth 295. Paul Starr writes in *The Social Transformation of American Medicine* (1982, Basic Books), 104: "[Missouri] passed an initial law in 1874, but it required a doctor only to register a degree from a legally chartered medical school with a county clerk. The statute had little effect. Since lax incorporation laws permitted anyone to start a school merely by applying for a charter, Missouri soon had more medical colleges than anyone could keep track of. Many were simply diploma mills. The state's doctors were too disorganized to do anything about the situation. According to a survey by the state medical society, nearly five thousand people practiced medicine in Missouri in 1882; only about half of them were graduates of 'reputable' schools." It is possible that Still was entitled to call himself an M.D. in Kansas. See *Kenneth M. Ludmerer, Learning to Heal: American Medical Education in the Mid-Nineteenth Century* (Basic Books, Inc., 1985), 16: "Until after the Civil War, evidence that a student had spent time, usually three years, with a preceptor remained a standard condition to receiving the M.D. degree." Kansas enacted its initial medical practice law in 1870, which entitled any physician without a medical school diploma to be registered on providing evidence of 10 years of practice experience. Still would have qualified by dint of having been in practice for 15 years by that time. For an overview of the new medical licensing laws see also Samuel L. Baker. "Physician Licensure Laws in the United States, 1865–1915." *Journal of the History of Medicine and Allied Sciences* (1984) 39 (2): 173-197.

29. Auto 104-6, 198. On page 104 Still says he was walking not with Ed but with a Colonel Eberman.

30. Auto 198-9.

31. Auto 106-7.

32. SNOM 1978.255.09, 4.

33. Auto 107-8.

34. Auto 98. JAOA February 1921, 319. Deuteronomy 32:11: "As an eagle stirreth up her nest, fluttereth over her young, spreadeth abroad her wings, taketh them, bearing them on her wings. . . ."

9: KIRKSVILLE

1. HAC 109.
2. JAOA June 1906, 408.
3. Bowcock 3.
4. *The Tattler* 3 April 1875, 3, and 8 May 1875.
5. *The Tattler* 23 January 1875, 3.
6. Bowcock 2.
7. HAC 292.
8. Auto 240.
9. Booth 27.
10. Auto 108. HAC 149.
11. Booth 23.
12. JAOA September 1928, 30.
13. Booth 27.
14. ATSP 2009.10.49, 1.
15. Booth 514-5.
16. JO February 1895, 5.
17. *The Tattler* 6 February 1875, 2.
18. HAC 247.
19. Cynthia Short to Glenda Wiese, 8 October 1991, David D. Palmer Health Sciences Library, Davenport, Iowa.
20. *History of Wapello County, Iowa*, Vol. 1. 1914. Chicago, The S. J. Clarke Publishing Company, 236-8.
21. *North Missouri Register*, 18 March 1875, 2-3.
22. HAC 248.
23. CES 1997.04.105, 2.
24. CES 1997.04.117, 1. "The contact of these two minds produced stimulation and growth in both," George Tull wrote. "Dr. John's versatility and idealism appealing to and stimulating the profound and logical Dr. Still." They remained "great friends" until John's death sometime in the 1880s. On 15 April 1875 the *North Missouri Register* published an article by John on the immortality of the human soul: "Everything in nature is in a state of motion and seeks a state of harmony or equation – but never absolute rest – which state when applied to matter is termed equilibrium, when to organic life is instinct, and when applied to spirit as life expressed through mind is happiness. Man seeks continually this state and its ideal is Heaven; a state only to be attained approximately." In 1879 John delivered a series of lectures on psychic force, the Od law, mesmerism, somnambulism, instinct and, again, the immortality of the soul. *Kirksville Journal*, 14 August 1879.
25. HAC 149.
26. *Scotland County News*, Memphis, Missouri, 18 February 1875.
27. *North Missouri Register*, 10 June 1875. Mott was eventually arrested and charged with obtaining money under false pretenses. To the dismay of his attorney, Judge Edward McKee, the medium insisted his defense be argued not on a point of law, but solely on his powers to raise the souls of the dead. McKee was convinced that no witnesses would be found to corroborate this, but Mott produced a list of people of high standing, many of whom came to testify, and the court discharged him. *Memphis Democrat*, 19 August 1909.
28. *The Tattler* 15 May 1875.
29. *The Tattler* 27 June 1875, 2.
30. HAC 149.
31. CES 1997.04.37, 3.
32. JO February 1929, 79. JO October 1928, 544. Mary remained a Methodist but sympathized with spiritualists and objected to those who denigrated them. She and Still possessed a book entitled *Religious Denominations of the World* by Vincent Milner (Galesburg, Ill.: Bradley, Garretson and Co., 1872) with a section that gave undue prominence to a minority of spiritualists who advocated free love. "My good wife is an honest Methodist woman," Still inscribed inside, "and has torn out pages 47, 48, 49, 50, as she was satisfied they were a bill of slanderous lies on a good people. I agree with her." Still's copy, MOM, pages 546 and 551. Schooled in Poughkeepsie, New York, Mary would have been familiar with the

"Poughkeepsie Seer" Andrew Jackson Davis, whose books were standard reading for spiritualists. Still surely read Davis's books. During his first month in Kirksville he returned to Baldwin to spend Christmas with Mary and the children, and on 27 December 1874, co-signed, with Baldwin mayor J. G. Schnebly and two others, a letter to the spiritualist magazine *The Banner of Light*, published by the same company as Davis's books. *The Banner of Light*, 9 January 1875, 8.
33. Auto 98.
34. OM January 1918, 5-6.
35. JAOA August 1923, 718.
36. United Tribe of Shawnee Indians website.
37. OM January 1918, 6.
38. Booth 60.
39. CES 1997.04.102.
40. JO August 1907, 254.
41. JAOA January 1921, 244. As a boy James Bowcock also hunted for pebbles and Indian arrowheads along the local creeks. Sometimes he ran into Still who told him stories about what he had found and once explained how the locally mined coal was formed. Bowcock 1.
42. Booth 491-2.
43. MOM 2009.49.440. Undated article from *The Metropolitan Magazine*.
44. ATSP 2009.10.759, 3-5.
45. Hildreth 23.
46. NO February 1902, 29-30. Parker graduated from the ASO in 1895.
47. CES 1997.04.37, 3-4, 6-7.
48. MOM 2010.02.1227.
49. Booth 491-2.
50. DO April 1975, 38. Charley, who wrote this, identified Jim only as "one brother."
51. MOM 2009.04.102. Booth 443-4.
52. *Kirksville Democrat*, 28 September 1894, 1.
53. Auto 109.
54. Booth 25.
55. Auto 110.

10: LIGHTNING BONE SETTER

1. JO February 1929, 80.
2. NO February 1902, 29-30.
3. Hildreth 25-6. One day a man arrived on crutches asking to be examined. Still sat him on a bench, knelt down, lifted the leg, flexed the knee and rotated the hip, but found nothing amiss. He put the foot down and stared his patient in the face, demanding to know who had paid him to come. The embarrassed man welled up with tears and admitted that some doctors downtown had hired him to expose Dr. Still as a fake.
4. HAC 249. OT January 1918, 91.
5. Booth 55, 505.
6. AOHS December 1961, 1. Perhaps the title "Man's Lost Center" derived from Still's investigation of Spiritualism. In his *Harmonial Philosophy* Andrew Jackson Davis described how, in a mesmeric trance, "mighty and sacred truths" gushed up from the depths of his spirit. Davis claimed that these messages emanated from departed souls and contained moral exhortations on the spiritual importance of inwardly centering oneself in the universe.
7. JAOA June 1906, 408-10.
8. JO February 1929, 80. DO April 1975, 38. Still could not afford a horse and buggy.
9. Booth 29. Hildreth 1-2.
10. JAOA June 1906, 408-9.
11. Hildreth 1-3. Arthur Grant Hildreth was born on 13 June 1863.
12. Auto 118-20.
13. CES 1997.04.110, 8.
14. ATSP 2009.10.886, 1.
15. OPR August 1934, 22. Deason 10.
16. Still's students would later argue whether he was an evolutionist or a creationist. In JAOA May 1913, 503, Carl McConnell described osteopathy as "applied evolution," but insisted that Still himself

was not an evolutionist. "Let it not be thought that Dr. Still is an evolutionist," he wrote, "for the very statement that he considers man a perfect being precludes such an idea." JAOA March 1913, 350. John Deason declared that Still was "a creationist, not an evolutionist," but after citing Still's admiration for Antoine Béchamp and Alfred Russel Wallace ("his favorite biologist") stated it was "safe to class him with them as a creative evolutionist." Deason 10.

17. *The Independent*, New York, November 9, 1905. Reprinted in JO December 1905, 351.

18. Deason 4, 6, 9-10. Pasteur, too, had recognized this fact. See Dubos 1998 135.

19. Others before Pasteur had suspected that microorganisms might be responsible for infections and contagions. In the early 1700s the Dutch draper Antoni van Leeuwenhoek had seen miniscule organisms under his microscope and some speculated that if these "animalcules" multiplied within the body in the same way as large pathogenic parasites they might prove to be a cause of disease.

20. Deason 4.

21. OPR August 1934, 25.

22. Dubos 1998 90.

23. Dubos 1960 190.

24. Dubos 1960 196.

25. Dubos 1960 190.

26. Dubos 1960 233.

27. Dubos 1960 xxxiii. More recent research shows the cause of this disease, *flacherie*, to be viral, weakening the host and increasing its susceptibility to secondary bacterial infection.

28. Dubos 1998 137.

29. Quoted in Deason 12-13.

30. ORP 117.

31. ATSP 2009.10.774, 7-9.

32. Auto 280.

33. Auto 198-9.

34. Auto 343.

35. ATSP 2010.02.1227.

36. Auto 371-2. Still lists the families that made him welcome: William Novinger, William Hughes and Dr. Hendrix in the northwest of Adair County; his friend Dr. A. H. John and Andrew Linder in the west; Calvin Smoot in the east; and Sol Morris south of Kirksville.

37. Booth 56. OT January 1918, 91. Still C. E. 75.

38. ATSP 2009.10.760, 4. Auto 99. ORP 85-9. Page 28-9.

39. Booth 57.

40. HAC 248.

41. ATSP 2009.10.794, 1. Still C.E. 68.

42. Booth 57.

43. Auto 100.

44. ATSP 2010.02.1227.

45. Booth 32-3. OT January 1918, 91.

46. JO March 1903, 104.

47. Booth 506.

48. Booth 61, 64. In La Plata a hostile crowd ridiculed Still as he lectured in a church, and someone spoke out, demanding to be shown results. "One after another got up and 'spoke out at meetin'," a listener related, "saying that they had been treated at a certain time and no symptoms of their troubles had returned. After the lecture a howling mob, led by two physicians of the town, followed him to the hotel demanding to know how he performed the cures." JO March 1903, 104.

49. AAO Yearbook 1947, 7.

50. Booth 32-3.

51. JO February 1898, 415.

52. Booth 21, 32-3, 58. Charley's first trip with his father was to Holden in 1880.

53. Auto 100.

54. ATSP 2009.10.760, 5. Booth 56.

55. Booth 28, 57. JO February 1929, 80.

56. ATSP 2009.10.761, 1-4. 1899 ASO graduate Arthur L. Evans recalled Still calling to treat his father, confined to bed with sciatica and administering liberal quantities of St. Jacobs Oil for the pain. "Well," Still said, dismissing the nostrum, "St. Jakey can't reach this." After three or four treatments Evans senior

was well and asked for the bill. "I don't see how a man with two teams in the stable eating their heads off is in any shape to pay a doctor's bill," he said, "but if you have it, you might let me have a dollar or two." Booth 457.
57. OT January 1918, 91.
58. CES 1997.04.106, 4. When a farmer named McCartney went to his bank to withdraw some cash the banker surmised it was for Dr. Still: "Well, are you pretty well acquainted with him?" the banker asked. McCartney said he was. "Well, that's alright," he was told "I just wondered if you knew how his financial conditions were."
59. Booth 35.
60. JO February 1929, 80.
61. OP February 1918, 18.
62. Still C.E. 115.
63. ATSP 2009.10.934, 935 and 936.
64. Still C.E. 61. Still applied to the Commissioner of Pensions on 22 April, 1885, for a "rehearing," to no avail. Still C. E. 117.
65. Booth 28.
66. Booth 514. HAC 248.
67. CES 1997.04.115, 1-2. Kathryn Talmadge graduated from the ASO in 1904. Asked why she became an osteopath she replied, "[It] is answered out of my own experience."
68. Hildreth 23. EET 23. CES 1997.04.119, 23.
69. ATSP 2009.10.760, 6-8. Precisely when Still began using the title Lightning Bone Setter is unclear. He writes that these cards were printed in 1879, but his dates are often unreliable.
70. Psalm 139:14. "I will praise thee; for I am fearfully and wonderfully made: marvellous are thy works; and that my soul knoweth right well."

11: MIRACLES ARE STILL PERFORMED

1. JO February 1897, 7.
2. ATSP 2010.02.1227.
JO September 1901, 309-10.
3. ATSP 2009.10.39, 1-6. Still even drew patients from the families of physicians. One doctor's wife arrived with her face hidden by a veil, insisting he keep her identity secret. The daughter of another came disguised in rags, saying that if her father found out he would "whip her to death."
4. Hildreth 11-12. The Marion County court ledgers (held in the United States District Court, Hannibal) contain no record of the case, consistent with a policy of not entering details of cases that ended in acquittal. Later, when Charley was gathering material about his father's life for a proposed book (which never came to fruition), he wrote to Mahan requesting information about the trial. "He [Still] told me," Mahan wrote, "that he had a diploma from a college in the South which was burned down during the war, that he had lost the diploma and since the college was out of existence he could not produce a copy and I fully believed him." Mahan's typed letter has been corrected in handwriting (presumably Charley's) to read, "He told me he had a certificate from [unintelligible] in Kansas which was burned down during the war, that he, Dr. Still, later lost the certificate when his house burned and since the college was out of existence." George A. Mahan to Charles E. Still, 5 February 1923. The corrected version is likely the more accurate. In an undated letter to Arthur Hildreth, Mahan wrote, "It has been so long since the trial of Dr. Still, many things have slipped my memory."
5. JAOA February 1921, 318. Still's daughter Blanche relates that one of the council members, identified only as "Mr. S.," later became a firm supporter of osteopathy. In the *City of Hannibal Council Proceedings*, Book F, January 1882 to October 1887, the only member with a surname beginning with S is Alderman A. J. Settles. After Still's death "Mr. S." attended Kirksville's Laughlin Hospital for treatment. On the wall of the

waiting room hung a picture of Still and for Mr. S. it brought back memories of his first glimpse of the doctor, walking down a Hannibal street carrying a "large bone," stopping to talk to people and treating them where he found them. Mr. S. told a Laughlin Hospital doctor that he could never look at the picture without feeling what a fool he had made of himself for having helped pass the resolution. Booth 502.
6. Still's certificate of registration, dated 28 July 1883, reads: "I, S. S. McLaughlin Clerk of the County Court of the County aforesaid, do hereby certify that A. T. Still has this day complied with an act of the Legislature of the State of Missouri, entitled 'An Act to regulate the practice of Medicine and Surgery in the State of Missouri,' approved March 27th [1874] and that his name is duly entered on the 'Roll of Physicians and Surgeons,' in my office, as a Physician and Surgeon." See Hildreth 295.
7. Hildreth 28, 32. CES 2009.04.102, 1.
8. HMC 1211-12.
9. Booth 3.
10. Booth 57.
11. Booth 63.
12. JAOA January 1921, 246.
13. Booth 57. Still's nephew Charles E. Hulett reports that during his itinerant years Still travelled as far south as Webb City, Missouri. SNOM 1992.1456.02, 2.
14. OT January 1918, 91. See also JO September 1899, 147.
15. ATSP 2009.10.99A, 5-6. Booth 57.
16. JAOA March 1915, 348.
17. Booth 28.
18. ATSP 2009.08.05 10, 12, 23-4.
19. Hildreth 4-6. Booth 59.
20. Hildreth 5-10. Blue vitriol or "bluestone" is a pentahydrate of copper sulphate.
21. ATSP 2009.10.759, 4.
22. ATSP 2009.10.759, 13.
23. Booth 491.
24. AOHS December 1961, 7. Guttery wrote, "After several trials we struck on osteopathy, and he [Still] said, 'That is what I will call it.'" Ironically, Guttery later qualified as a medical doctor. Precisely when Still adopted the name osteopathy remains unclear. Hildreth dates it sometime in "the early eighties, soon after I was married [1884]. Still, he relates, "talked at length concerning his new theory of disease, which he told me at that time he had decided to call osteopathy." Hildreth 4. Still himself wrote, "By the year 1889 . . . I was urged to name my new science. After thinking over all the other 'pathies,' I decided that bone pathy expressed my idea. And as os means bone, I therefore adopted the name osteopathy." ATSP 2009.08.05, 12.
25. ATSP 2009.10.780, 1.
26. JO March 1901, 68.
27. *Kirksville Democrat*, 27 September 1895.
28. JO March 1899, 473-5. ATSP 2010.02.1227. JO February 1929, 79.
29. JO March 1899, 474.
30. SNOM 2009.49.440.
31. JO September 1908, 543.
32. ATSP 2009.10.760, 12.
33. JO December 1942, 26-7.
34. "Reminiscences of Effie Bell Koontz." Document in possession of author.
35. Hildreth 17.
36. Hildreth 24.
37. Hildreth 24-5. Booth 37.
38. Charley and Herman had returned home that month after serving three years in the 14th Infantry, stationed at Fort Leavenworth, Kansas. Trowbridge 204-5.
39. ATSP 2009.10.762, 1. Booth 61-2. In Ward 4, the incident is said to have occurred in December 1889 while Still was practicing from the home of Mrs. L. Mella in Schell City, Missouri. Ward is described as a "confirmed invalid, serious asthma."
40. CES 1997.04.56, 7.
41. J. O. Hatten to ASO, 14 January 1901. MOM. Dates are uncertain. ATSP 2009.10.762, 2 and JO December 1894, 2,

suggest that the class began on 1 January 1891, but this is likely incorrect.
42. JO December 1894, 2.
43. Hildreth 371. Booth 57-8, 72.
44. ATSP 2009.10.762, 3.

12: AMERICAN SCHOOL OF OSTEOPATHY

1. *Kirksville Democrat*, 15 and 22 January 1892.
2. CES 1997.04.98.
3. *St. Louis Republic*, April 1893, reproduced in Hildreth 34. A year later the paper persisted in describing Still as "an old Indian Doctor" and his treatment "a wild, miraculous, visionary affair." Even Charley doubted that he could learn to emulate his father. One day Still was called away, leaving his son in sole charge of a patient. Charley felt nervous about giving the treatment alone, while the patient doubted that anyone except Still senior could help him. "Son, if this treatment cures me," he said, "darned if I won't be surprised." To his astonishment Charley replied, "Darned if I won't too." NO February 1902, 31.
4. CES 1997.04.47, 1-2.
5. JO May 1894, 2.
6. *The Bloomfield Farmer* 13 February 1892, reprinted in *Kirksville Democrat*, 4 March 1892.
7. Hildreth 116-7. Beryl Franklin Carroll, an 1884 graduate of Kirksville Normal School, would become governor of Iowa from 1909-1913. While a student at the school he once came across Still sitting on the sidewalk on Normal Street. "An aged Negro was standing in front of him," Carroll recalled. "I stopped to see what was going on. The doctor was manipulating the bones of the man's wrist. The wrist apparently had been entirely stiff but the hand could then be moved a little. The doctor said some of the carpal bones were dislocated but that with another treatment or two he could entirely relieve the trouble."
8. Ward 1.
9. Letter, Dr. A. T. Still to Amos Steckel, 1 May 1892. MOM. Even now Still's stationery remained headed *Office of A. T. Still, Lightning Bone Setter*, appended in small print, *Discoverer of the Science of Osteopathy*.
10. DO May 1975, 28.
11. Booth 530.
12. Hildreth 5-11, 184.
13. Booth 499-500.
14. Hildreth 27-8.
15. Booth 72-3. Dobson later entered the ASO and graduated in 1902. From 1901 he taught chemistry and hygiene at the school.
16. Booth 447-9. CES 1997.04.37, 10.
17. JO September 1896, 6. See CES 1997.04.56, 8.
18. CES 1997.04.119, 29.
19. The Medical Directory, Scotland, 1903.
20. *Journal of the History of Medicine*, April 1967, 169-170. Flatbush, Long Island, is today part of the Borough of Brooklyn.
21. JO December 1897, 335-7. Smith had been inspired to study medicine through admiration for their family physician, Dr. George Keith, who believed the less drugs patients took the better they fared. All nine Smith children had grown up strong and healthy and the only remedies he remembered Dr. Keith prescribing, even for serious illness, were compound licorice powder and hot water. Keith himself had been an invalid until deciding to quit drugs and moderate his eating and drinking, and wrote a book about his recovery entitled *A Plea for a Simpler Life*.
22. Auto 127-9.
23. JO April 1908, 208-10.
24. CES 1997.04.56, 8.
25. JO September 1896, 6.
26. JO 1907, 210.
27. *Des Moines Sunday Register*, 19 January 1938, 2-3. The 1940 Iowa census 1940 states that Cuthbert was born in Kirksville in 1895.
28. Booth 447-9.
29. CES 1997.04.56, 9.
30. CES 1997.04.95, 1-3. JAOA January 1918, 250-1. JO September 1908, 568.

31. JAOA August 1921, 667. Since its inception the ASO was open to students of all races, but did not graduate its first black student until 1970. Walter 7.
32. JAOA January 1918, 251.
33. OP January 1903, 1-2.
34. Hildreth 30.
35. Booth 450.
36. CES 1997.04.119, 29.
37. CES 1997.04.47, 2.
38. Hildreth 31-2, 37. According to some sources the skeleton was called "Columbus." See Walter 7.
39. Auto 296-7.
40. *Kirksville Democrat*, 17 February 1893, 4.
41. Smith and Harry practiced in temporary premises at 1710 E. 8th St. before opening a permanent office at 430-434 Ridge Building in July. *Kirksville Democrat*, June 1983, 3. *Journal of the History of Medicine*, April 1967, 174.
42. Hildreth 38-9.
43. Hildreth 32-5.
44. ATSP 2009.10.762, 1-4.
45. *Kirksville Weekly Graphic*, July 28, 1893. Reply by J. B. Dodge to Marcus Ward's letter of June 30.
46. JO September 1898, 167. Still claimed that the Cincinnati medical school attended by Ward "was expelled from the national association on account of its low standard."
47. *Kirksville Weekly Graphic*, 30 June 1893, 2.
48. *Kirksville Weekly Graphic*, 28 July 1893.
49. ATSP 2009.10.63.
50. CES 1997.04.37, 11. CES 1997.04.55, 1-2. Hildreth 36.
51. Booth 58.
52. JO July 1894, 1.
53. CES 1997.04.55, 2-3.
54. Auto 266.
55. JO January 1895, 1. Virchow had written that in all types of inflammation, "we have in the main to deal with a change in the act of nutrition . . . in consequence to some cause or other external to the part which falls into a state of irritation," resulting in "the composition and constitution of this part undergo alterations which . . . enable it to attract to itself and absorb . . . a larger quantity of matter than usual, and to transform it according to circumstances." Virchow 1863 431.
56. ORP 258. Still followed a schematic method of reasoning: the "motor nerves" deliver blood to the proper place "for the convenience of the nerves of nutrition." The "sensory nerves" judge supply and demand and regulate blood flow. Sympathetic nerve irritation causes the arteries to bring an increased supply of blood, irritation of the "sensory" nerves (from inflammation) causes contraction of the veins, leading to congestion in the cellular environment, with retained fluids preventing the cell efficiently assimilating nutrients and excreting wastes.
57. CES 1997.04.55, 5. Governor Nelson and Senator Nelson were unrelated.
58. Auto 266-7.
59. *Kirksville Democrat*, 20 July 1894, 1.
60. ATSP 2009.10.763, 3-5. Auto 265-7. JO February 1929, 82. JO February 1898, 415-8. CES 1997.04.37, 11-15.

13: FIND IT, FIX IT, AND LEAVE IT ALONE

1. ATSP 2009.10.791.
2. JO January 1895, 1.
3. JO December 1894, 1.
4. Auto 250.
5. Hildreth 41.
6. JO July 1898, 73.
7. JO August 1907, 254.
8. Booth 493. JAOA January 1921, 247.
9. "Reminiscences of Effie Bell Koontz." Document in possession of author. In 1938 Koontz wrote that she had practiced osteopathy for forty-three years without resorting to drugs either for herself or for her patients. Tuition fees were $500 for men and $200 for women. HAC 262.

10. JO November 1897, 198-9. The *Journal of Osteopathy* reported that James Still was living in Trenton. In Brown, *Genealogical Appendix*, 48, he is said to have been practicing in Maryville, Missouri.
11. Auto 98. Two years after graduating from the ASO James Still wrote of osteopathy, "When it shall have the first chance at a patient instead of the last look at the cadaver then the death rate will experience a startling diminution, and the list of cures will be lengthened to most wonderful proportions." JO November 1897, 199.
12. JAOA June 1925, 749.
13. Recorded by H. H. Gravett, January 1896. AAO Yearbook 1948, 48-9.
14. AAO Yearbook 1954, 43.
15. PM 57.
16. Auto 229-30.
17. AOA Yearbook 1954, 38.
18. JO June 1925, 749.
19. PM 12.
20. PM 29-30. In his copy of Johannes Müller's *Elements of Physiology,* Still wrote on the front endpaper *A. T. Still Physiology Old Style of Reasoning*, and, at the back, *The end and the half has not been told*. At the bottom of the page, cryptically, he scratched the word *Angels*.
21. PO 17-18.
22. ATSP 2009.10.808 2.
23. AOA Yearbook 1954, 40. In distinguishing between osteopathic and medical lesions, Still wrote (paraphrasing Virchow), "barring accidents and specific poisons the primary [medical] lesions begin within the cells."
24. CES 1997.04.119, 3.
25. JAOA February 1929, 436.
26. Tucker 15. Tucker and Wilson wrote, "Experience has shown these lesions to be present in all persons suffering with any disease. It is further discovered that such lesions are also found in a majority of apparently well persons. This fact far from disrupting the theory of their relation to disease, leads to the interesting observation that few persons are operating at a maximum of efficiency."
27. SNOM 1980.373.10, 6.
28. JO September 1896, 4.
29. Lane 43.
30. JAOA December 1923, 238.
31. JO December 1920, 746-7.
32. JOAO December 1932, 140.
33. Hildreth 363-4.
34. JAOA September 1928, 22.
35. JO September 1902, 297.
36. Booth 82. AOA Yearbook 1954, 40.
37. JO July 1932, 400.
38. APC 1999.10.120, 1. Alice married ASO secretary Henry Patterson.
39. JAOA December 1923, 237-8.
40. JAOA September 1928, 22.
41. Booth 454.
42. AAO Yearbook 1947, 9.
43. OT February 1918, 102.
44. Booth 514.
45. JAOA June 1925, 749.
46. JAOA September 1928, 22.
47. "Reminiscences of Effie Bell Koontz." Document in possession of author.
48. Booth 81.
49. NO February 1902, 31.
50. JO April 1900, 469. A similar riddle featured a black horse: "We want no more words than just enough to tell what color a black horse is with four white feet, a bobtail, blind in left eye, kicks, balks, and runs away, and no good in any way. We do not think a history of the horse back to Babylon would do us any good. We want a horse we can use."
51. PM 17.
52. ATSP 2009.10.370.
53. Truhlar 131.
54. AAO Yearbook 1954, 40.
55. ATSP 2009.10.774, 2.
56. Hildreth 42-3, 184.
57. Hildreth 53-4. Hildreth explained Still's teaching, "The vasomotor center in the lower portion of the brain, which controls the function of contraction and dilatation of

blood vessels and consequently the circulation to the entire body may be influenced by lesions affecting the upper cervical region. Hence, in the cure of all forms of eczema, local or general, this center must be reached through that area." Hildreth 184.

58. JO November 1909, 799.
59. Untitled document in possession of author.
60. Booth 82.
61. JAOA December 1923, 238.
62. Gaddis 127.
63. ATSP 2009.10.695.
64. SNOM 1980.373.08.
65. ATSP 2009.10.802, 1.
66. JAOA August 1915, 643.
67. JAOA January 1921, 247-8.
68. PO 153.
69. Auto 208-12.
70. AAO Yearbook 1954, 39-40.
71. Hildreth 363.
72. JAOA August 1921, 671. A. L Evans wrote, "He no more demanded servile imitation of his technique than he would have required that the practicians of his therapy should all discard the necktie and wear flannel shirts and top boots, because in the simplicity of his nature it pleased him to wear that garb."
73. JAOA December 1923, 239.
74. AAO Yearbook 1948, 57.
75. Hildreth 362-3.
76. JAOA January 1918, 245.
77. CES 1997.04.110, 8.
78. JO December 1909, 886.
79. AAO Yearbook 1948, 50.
80. PO 42. Recovery demanded precise removal of the cause, as graduate operator Charles F. Bandel learned to his cost. A patient fell from a hay wagon and lost proper function of his left leg. After two weeks of treatment Still saw the man, propped up on crutches, leaning against the wall of a house and learned that treatment had so far yielded no benefit. Without further comment he escorted the patient to a treatment room and called for the junior doctor to report there too. "Say, Bandel, this fellow is no better," Still said, "why don't you do something for him." The graduate's explanation of the excellent treatment he thought he had given was greeted by silence. Still quietly examined the patient's abdomen, chest and back, stepped aside, and told Bandel to repeat the treatment he had given the day before. Still paced up and down the room observing intently as Bandel, anxious to create a good impression, relaxed every muscle in the patient's back, stretched the spine, eased the neck and, to be sure he had omitted nothing, concluded by treating the legs. He then raised the man to a sitting position, patted him on the back and said he hoped he would feel better tomorrow. "All done, Bandel?" Still asked. "Yes, Doctor," he replied proudly, anticipating compliments. None came. "Oh, Bandel," Still said, "you have heard me speak dozens of times, and I have talked with you privately; how long, in God's name, shall I have to be around you before you will comprehend our simple principle? Why, my son, the treatment you have given this man is nothing short of that done by an ignoramus; you are simply an engine-wiper; you rubbed, you pulled, you did everything under the sun except the right thing. An engine-wiper rubs up the whole machine when the trouble lies in one maladjusted part." The crestfallen graduate looked on as Still stepped behind the man, placed his thumb and forefinger on the second lumbar and performed a rotary movement that resulted in a pop, so loud it seemed incredible. "Now, Bandel," he said, "come round and pat your patient on his back and tell him he will be walking in three days." The lesson concluded with an allegory. "If I put my foot on a cat's tail, Tabby will cry with pain; presently you come along and rub Tabby's back and pull her legs about and say, 'There Tabby, you will feel better tomorrow.' But you are mistaken; she will not feel better. You must remove the pressure from the cat's

tail and then her nervous system will quiet down. I have just taken the pressure off this man's spinal cord, and nature will do the rest. Now, let this man alone, and if you can't grasp my principles, let all my patients alone." The following morning the patient was heard shouting with joy as feeling had returned to the leg. On the third day he was able to walk and two days later Bandel saw him ambling towards the railroad station, heading for home. Booth 510-1. See also Hildreth 411-2.
81. Auto 191.
82. JO September 1942, 17.
83. JAOA March 1946, 322.
84. AAO Yearbook 1948, 49-50.
85. Hildreth 184, 200.
86. AAO Yearbook 1954, 17.
87. JAOA December 1923, 239.
88. AAO Yearbook 1948, 57. Still did not call the work "manipulation," since to the public the word generally signified massage.
89. Auto 191-2.
90. AAO Yearbook 1954, 41-2.
91. Auto 225.
92. JAOA January 1923, 248.

14: A SECRET PROCESS OF TREATING HUMAN ILLS

1. JO May 1894, 1-2.
2. *Kirksville Democrat*, 4 May 1894, 1.
3. SNOM 1980.373.08, 1.
4. Booth 520-1.
5. American School of Osteopathy Record Book 1894-1898, 3. MOM.
6. JO February 1902, 81.
7. JO June 1894, 3.
8. HAC 252. JO June 1894, 3.
9. *Kirksville Democrat*, 1 June 1894.
10. *Kirksville Journal* 7 June 1894, 1.
11. ATSP 2009.10.49, 2-3.
12. *Kirksville Weekly Graphic*, 8 June 1894.
13. *Kirksville Democrat*, 22 December 1893, 5.
14. Fred Still to Harry Still, 23 March 1894. CES 1997.04.62.
15. JO June 1894, 1.
16. *Kirksville Democrat* 15 June 1894.
17. JO June 1894, 1-2.
18. Auto 380. Still apparently tried to communicate with his dead son through spiritualist practices. A long poem written by "Teddie" (undoubtedly Still's brother Ed) appeared in only the second issue of the *Journal of Osteopathy*. It told of Fred's spirit, "clothed with potent majesty," taking flight "to golden Summer Lands." [The "Summer-Land" was a term used by Andrew Jackson Davis for the afterlife.] The poem was accompanied by a verse, attributed to Fred, entitled "*A Message*":

> Dear Pa, write for me I 'died' loving all
> I am not dead, no not at all. . . .

"Could'st thou but stay," Still appended, "and close within thy father's arms take rest. May thy spirit voice speak unto him and cheer the passing days, until in Life he doth with thee rejoice." JO January 1895, 8.
19. *Kirksville Weekly Graphic* 22 June 1894.
20. JAOA September 1928, 58.
21. *Kirksville Democrat*, 24 August 1894, 5. HAC 254. The hotel was located at 500 West Pierce Street.
22. ATSP 2010.02.1227.
23. Hildreth 357-8.
24. Still C. E. 143.
25. Booth 478. Henry Patterson and Alice Shibley graduated from the ASO in 1895. Alice's mother had suffered from asthma for 47 years before being cured by Still.
26. ATSP 2010.02.1227. Hildreth 357-8.
27. JO August 1907, 253.
28. JAOA August 1923, 720. JAOA June 1925, 749. SNOM 1980.373.08, 3-4. Booth 34.
29. See ORP 206.
30. *Kirksville Weekly Graphic*, November 30, 1894, 3.
31. ATSP 2009.10.766, 1-2.
32. HAC 254-6. Booth 80.

33. JO December 1894, 6.
34. JO December 1894, 4.
35. JO January 1895, 4.
36. *Kirksville Weekly Graphic*, quoted in JO September 1895, 2.
37. JO January 1895, 2-3.
38. ATSP 2009.10.765, 5.
39. ATSP 2009.10.770, 2.
40. Hildreth 77.
41. ATSP 2009.10.773, 6.
42. Hildreth 71. Hildreth says the man was practicing not in Moberly but in Indiana.
43. Booth 500.
44. JO February 1895, 2.
45. Hildreth 77-80.
46. ATSP 2009.10.766. JO March 1895, 2, 4.
47. JO March 1897, 3.
48. Booth 30-1.

15: FLATULENCY AND PAUCITY

1. Booth 103.
2. *Kirksville Journal*, 28 March 1895.
3. JO April 1895, 5.
4. JO May 1895, 4.
5. Booth 43.
6. JO April 1895, 3.
7. JO May 1895, 4.
8. JO May 1895, 8.
9. Still told Ernest Tucker that where there is liberty everything acts according to its inherent wisdom and power, and we cannot surpass this nor substitute for it. JO May 1901, 159.
10. ATSP 2009.10.917, 1-2. The 1539 *Act for Abolishing Diversity in Opinions* obliged HenryVIII's subjects to accept and obey the doctrines of the Church of England, under penalty of imprisonment or burning at the stake.
11. ATSP 2009.10.778, 1.
12. SNOM 1980.373.08, 7.
13. JO December 1894, 6.
14. Still C. E. 143.
15. OM January 1918, 7.
16. JO May 1895, 8.
17. JO June 1895, 3.
18. *Kirksville Democrat*, 26 July 1895, 1.
19. Hildreth 367-8.
20. Reproduced in JO September 1895, 7.
21. Auto 274.
22. ATSP 2009.10.765, 3.
23. Booth 60.
24. James L. Holloway, "Some Salient Characteristics of Dr. Still," 1. Document in possession of author. "You are not any wiser to know the Latin, Greek or Choctaw names for such and such diseases unless you are a pill doctor," Still himself wrote. "Symptomatology leads you straight to a drug store." JO May 1900, 515-6.
25. Truhlar 123.
26. ATSP 2009.10.764, 5.
27. Auto 302.
28. Auto 187.
29. CES 1997.04.121. 12.
30. JO February 1898, 413.
31. Auto 275-6.
32. ATSP 2009.10.74, 5.
33. Hildreth 53.
34. SNOM 1980.373.08, 9.
35. AOHS July 1962, 3.
36. Auto 269.
37. AOHS July 1962, 3.
38. Auto 330.
39. JO February 1898, 440.
40. JO April 1899, 497-500.
41. *Kirksville Democrat*, 10 May 1895, 1. JO January 1898, 368.
42. JO September 1896, 5.
43. AAO Yearbook 1948, 49.
44. Hildreth 380. JO December 1897, 342-3.
45. ATSP 2001.10.781,.See also edited version Auto 276.
46. CES 1997.04.119, 31.
47. ATSP 2009.10.824. 1 Corinthians 3:16-17.
48. JO December 1900, 291.
49. AAO Yearbook 1948, 50.
50. AAO Yearbook 1954, 37-8, 41.

16: THE FIGHT FOR TRUTH

1. JO February 1896, 2.
2. JO May 1896.
3. ATSP 2009.10.762, 2-3.
4. ATSP 2009.10.765, 4-5.
5. JO June 1896, 4-5.
6. JO January 1895, 6.
7. ATSP 2009.10.766, 8.
8. JO May 1896.
9. JO July 1896, 8.
10. ATSP 2009.10.762, 4-5.
11. JO June 1896, 3, 8. Thomas Still was allowed to complete the course in one year and returned to California to practice osteopathy in San Luis Obispo.
12. ATSP 2009.10.773, 3. Mrs. Colbert was the infirmary matron.
13. Booth 444-5.
14. ATSP 2009.10.861, 1.
15. JO September 1896, 6.
16. JO January 1899, 415.
17. JO June 1895, 2. See edited version Auto 305.
18. OT February 1917, 80.
19. *Des Moines Daily News*, February 4, 1896.
20. JO November 1896, 5. Still abhorred animal experiments designed to test the fatal dose of a drug. "We read all about dead frogs, doves, cats and dogs. We know they have killed the live dog but failed to wake up the dead dog. We want a book that we can learn by its pages how to help the sick dog and the sick man. We want knowledge." ATSP 2009.10.802, 2.
21. JO February 1897, 6. Virchow also recognized the drawbacks of drug studies. He wrote. "The statistical aggregates which have been assembled in order to test therapeutic agents can never yield results, since we deal with the treatment of individual sick people rather than of masses. If, instead of assembling tables, we had carefully kept up individual case histories . . . then it would certainly have been possible to gather useful and convincing data." Virchow 1958 50-1.
22. ATSP 2009.10.928, 2.
23. JO November 1897, 285.
24. AOHS February 1963, 4-5.
25. JO October 1895, 3. The word "paralysis" indicated varying degrees of nerve interference from tingling, numbness or muscle wasting to frank loss of sensation or motion.
26. JO June 1896, 6.
27. AAO Yearbook 1954, 20-1. Booth 34-5. Joseph B. Foraker was Ohio governor from 1886 to 1890.
28. ATSP 2009.08.05, 1.
29. PM 205. Procidentia is prolapse of the uterus or cervix.
30. JAOA July 1924, 815-6.
31. ATSP 2009.10.838, 2.
32. ATSP 2009.10.770, 2.
33. ATSP 2009.10.838, 1-2.
34. Conner 11.
35. Conner 5-11. Washington Conner graduated from the ASO in 1896. He first met Still in 1874 after the Kansan grasshopper invasion, when he called at their farm to request provisions and seeds for planting crops to help destitute families in Baldwin City. Still had been a childhood friend of Conner's father, and Wash's mother Mary was an early patient. "A semi-invalid for many years," she was cured by adjusting a sacroiliac joint. Six family members, including Mary, became osteopaths. Wash entered the ASO after being healed (of an unspecified ailment) when medical doctors said that only an operation would help. As a farmer's son he had worried about whether he would be able to learn osteopathy, but Still assured him he would have no trouble since Arthur Hildreth had "gotten through all right."
36. Conner 31.
37. ATSP 2009.07.22, 4.
38. Conner also theorized that labor pains are caused not by muscle contraction but by congestion of uterine sinuses as they

engorge with blood preparatory to birth.
39. W. J. Conner to Dr. Mark O'Reilly. Copy of Conner's *Mechanics of Labor*, MOM.
40. Conner 22-4.
41. Conner 43.
42. ORP 173. Conner wrote of the squatting birth position adopted by American Indian women: "This is the position God instructed Eve to take when Cain was born and tradition has handed it down from generation to generation until the present day when man has interfered and tried to improve nature, and every time he has tried to improve on the natural position he has increased the hazards of labor. In this position the birth canal is made perfectly straight and shortened to the last degree." Conner 33.
43. Conner 12, 31-2.
44. Conner 17.
45. JO June 1899, 43.
46. JO October 1896, 5.
47. JO October 1896, 2, 5, 7.
48. JO January 1898, 373-4.
AAO Yearbook 1954, 15.
49. ATSP 2009.10.99A, 2009.10.767, 3-4.
CES 1997.04.37, 8. Another case was that of a stockman, brought in manacles, who became a "raving maniac" after being thrown from a horse. On having his neck adjusted he slept for hours and awoke sane. JAOA June 1925, 749.
50. ATSP 2009.10.99A, 6-7.
51. JO December 1896, 7.
52. During the next four years Herman opened further practices in Sherman, Texas; Brooklyn, New York; and St. Louis, Missouri. JO November 1898, 303.
March 1899, 493. August 1900, 119.
53. Hildreth 72, 97.

17: A BIG JOLLIFICATION

1. JO October 1896, 7.
2. Booth 107-8. JO November 1896, 4. Act No. 99 of the Laws of Vermont states: "It shall be lawful for the graduates and the holders of diplomas from the American School of Osteopathy at Kirksville, Missouri, a regularly chartered school under the laws of Missouri, to practice their art of healing in the State of Vermont."
3. Untitled document in possession of author.
4. JO February 1897, 6.
5. *Kirksville Democrat*, 22 January 1897, 1.
6. ATSP 2009.10.787, 3. Booth 593.
7. JO November 1896, 3. Despite the best medical attention Dr. Pratt had suffered from a "withered leg" that remained "practically useless for years." Impressed by a marked improvement after two months of osteopathic treatment, he visited the infirmary in November 1896 and lectured to ASO students on the sympathetic nervous system.
8. Harry was now running a second practice at 70 Dearborn Street, Chicago, dividing his time between there and his original practice at 1405 Benson Avenue, Evanston.
9. ATSP 2009.10.784, 1-9.
ATSP 2009.10.787, 1-4. Booth 110, 593.
The North Dakota law became effective on 1 July. Helen de Lendrecie suffered no more trouble with her right breast. Twenty-three years later, in September 1919, she wrote: "I know very well that the knife was never necessary in my case. I do not want to be understood as denying the use of the knife however, for in some cases I am sure it is necessary to prolong life."
10. Hildreth 94-7.
11. *Kirksville Democrat*, 12 March 1897, 1.
JO March 1897, 1.
12. Booth 38, 444. HAC 268-9.
13. *Kirksville Democrat*, 12 March 1897, 1.
14. JO July 1896, 3. Conger, president of the American Manufacturing Association, had been treated at the infirmary the previous year after suffering a stroke. Hildreth 383.
15. KSHS 1897-1900, 225.
16. ATSP 2009.08.06, 9.
17. CO November 1898, 2.

18: WHY, HE COULD BE RICH

1. Hildreth 392.
2. Booth 539, 593. Booth states that Still went to Fargo on May 10, but Helen de Lendrecie's letter is dated May 23, 1897, after he returned to Kirksville. See ATSP 2009.10.784, 11. Still returned to Fargo in October to find the practice flourishing. On 1 January 1898 Morris and de Lendrecie established the Northwestern College of Osteopathy.
3. Booth 250-2.
4. Hildreth 98-104.
5. Hildreth 92. Charles Hazzard became acquainted with Harry while a student at Northwestern University, Evanston. When Still came to visit Harry, who was practicing in the town, Hazzard attended a meeting at Harry's house along with a "considerable number" of patients and friends. Hazzard studied osteopathy while teaching at the ASO and graduated in 1899.
6. ASO Board of Trustees Records 1894-1898, 22 June 1897 entry. Those on the list were: Still, his brothers Ed and James, James's son S. S. Still, Charley, Harry, Herman, Blanche, Arthur Hildreth, William Smith, Henry and Alice Patterson, Carl McConnell, Nettie Bolles, Joseph Sullivan, C. E. Hulett, Washington Conner, J. W. Henderson, Frank Hannah, Mrs. L. J. Kern, E. B. Morris, A. A. Goodman, Ella Hunt, Effie Koontz, S. R. Landes.
7. JO June 1897, 96-8. Booth 450-2.
8. CES 1997.04.119, 12-13. CES 1997.04.110, 1.
9. JO July 1900, 52.
10. JAOA January 1918, 251.
11. Booth 483. AAO Yearbook 1954, 20.
12. OP February 1918. Charles Hazzard, "Reminiscences of the Old Doctor."
13. JO December 1894, 8.
14. JAOA August 1921, 663.
15. JAOA August 1921, 671.
16. CES 1997.04.119, 27.
17. CES 1997.04.113, 2.
18. Hildreth 361. See also CES 1997.04.94, 1-4.
19. Auto 223.
20. Hildreth 410.
21. Booth 444.
22. JO March 1898, 458.
23. JAOA August 1921, 667. See also JO October 1928, 545.
24. ATSP 2009.06.25, 11.
25. JO July 1898, 74.
26. See ATSP 2009.10.770, 2.
27. OT February 1917, 80.
28. JO December 1896, 3.
29. Booth 481-2.
30. AAO Yearbook 1954, 21.
31. Booth 36-7.
32. ORP 205.
33. JO November 1897, 299-300. ATSP 2009.10.643, 1-7.
34. JO November 1897, 290. JO December 1898, 334-5.
35. JAOA July 1924, 815-6. The innominate bone, Galen's name for the pelvis, is composed on each side of three fused bones, the ilium, ischium and pubis. The ilia articulate with the sacrum by means of the sacroiliac joints. Still taught that the sacrum forms the foundation for all the vertebrae. Anything that alters its position – whether originating from the feet, legs or pelvis – will affect the entire spinal column all the way to the skull, drawing it out of line as the body attempts to compensate for the shift in body weight. Hildreth, 183-4. Still laid great emphasis of the importance of proper pelvic alignment for women. "Many times Dr. Still called my attention to the immense importance of a perfect alignment in the pelvic bones," Ellen Ligon wrote, "because of the attachments of the broad ligament and the round ligaments to these bones brings about, through any disarrangement, a tension in the body of the uterus, pulling it out of line; or a disturbance

in the tension and circulation in the broad ligaments affects the ovaries, or the irritation of the anterior ends of the round ligaments, which are continuous with the structure of the cervix itself, affects the tension of the cervix and os, one way or the other, resulting in dysmenorrhea or metorrhagia; or by pulling on the coccygeal muscles, disturbs the position of the coccyx, with the evil consequences of a disturbed coccyx or irritated bladder nerves; or the sciatic, sacral, and lumbar nerves, resulting in either sciatica or lumbago." JAOA July 1924, 815-6.
36. JAOA August 1921, 665.
37. Hildreth 148.
38. DO November 1976, 35-50.
39. ATSP 2009.10.72.
40. ATSP 2009.10.23.
41. Hildreth 395.
42. NO February 1902, 32.
43. Booth 507.
44. William F. Englehart to C. E. Still, Sr., 3 April 1925. NCOH. CES 1997.04.98, 2.
45. Booth 33, 35.
46. JO 1929, 204.
47. JO February 1899, 436-9.
48. ATSP 2009.10.650.
49. Booth 209.
50. JO May 1894, 3. JO February 1895, 5.
51. Hildreth 373-4. Musick's wife Augusta was a 1900 ASO graduate.
52. ATSP 2009.10.761, 4-7.
53. Booth 522.

19: MATTER

1. Hildreth 366.
2. JO December 1920, 746-7.
3. Booth 466. "[Facts] might prove stepping stones to quick conclusions," Henry Bunting wrote, "but [Still's] thinking tarried only long enough upon instances, upon the data of sense, to afford him a sudden spring toward their interpretation with some sort of general theory; his ceaseless concern was to apprehend natural laws, give reasons for things, interpret facts, make theories to explain how nature operates."
4. CES 1997.04.121, 13.
5. JAOA January 1918, 246.
6. Booth 34.
7. JAOA January 1918, 253.
8. PO 149.
9. Conner 13.
10. Hildreth 184.
11. PM 44-5. Still wrote of the cerebrospinal fluid, "Unless the brain furnishes this fluid in abundance, a disabled condition of the body will remain. He who is able to reason will see that this great river of life must be tapped and the withering field irrigated at once, or the harvest of health will be forever lost."
12. PM 58.
13. PM 64.
14. PO 163.
15. PO 165.
16. Virchow 1863, 41.
17. Virchow wrote, "Every new tissue formation presupposes a cell from which its cells arise; this tissue is its matrix. There is no difference in principle between the descent of men and animals from one parent and the descent of pathological new formations from one matrix." He noted that not every living cell is capable of becoming a matrix. Once initially formed, some cells – for example nerve, muscle and red blood cells – divide no further or proliferate only in limited fashion, while other cells, particularly those of cartilage, connective tissue and skin, show great propensity for division. Virchow 1958 229.
18. Virchow added, "From this rule comparatively few pathological new-formations are excepted." He believed that inflammations arose from the multiplication and transformation of inflammatory cells ("pus corpuscles") in the connective tissue. In this Virchow was incorrect; in 1867 his pupil Julius Cohnheim showed

that the pus corpuscles were actually white blood cells that migrated from the blood vessels. Virchow 1863, 441-2.
19. PO 89.
20. PO 163-4. Virchow had noted that the cells of "cartilage, connective tissue, bone and mucous tissue" *anastomose* – connect with one another – by "a peculiar system of tubes or canals which must be classed with the great canalicular system of the body, and which particularly, forming as they do a supplement to the blood and lymphatic vessels." He believed that these anastomoses were significant because of "the greater energy with which they are capable of conducting different morbid processes." Virchow 1863 76.
21. PM 61.
22. PO 153.
23. PO 107-8.
24. Auto 279-80.
25. PO 42, 76.
26. JO December 1900, 314.
27. ATSP 2009.10.804, 1.
28. JAOA August 1921, 664.
29. JOAO December 1932, 140. Still had trained his hands in thermal diagnosis since 1874 after noticing the curious pattern of hot and cold on the boy with flux in Macon.
30. JO June 1899, 30-1.
31. JAOA December 1923, 238.
32. JAOA March 1948, 322.
33. JAOA July 1924, 815. Relaxing the muscles and correcting lesions of their attached bones reduced irritation, stopped convulsive coughs, normalized breathing, and freed the blood circulation to kill any germs. See also PO 89-90.
34. OM January 1918, 7. Still eventually decided that tuberculosis was related to bony obstructions irritating the vagus nerve, resulting in stagnation of blood, fermentation, and "cheesy matter" being deposited in the cells of the lungs. JO June 1909, 408-9.
35. Hildreth 185.
36. CES 1997.04.119, 23-4.
37. JAOA July 1924, 815.
38. SNOM 1980.373.10, 4.
ATSP 2009.10.769, 1-2.
39. ATSP 2009.10.774, 6.
40. PO 129.
41. APC 1999.10.111, 1.
42. CES 1997.04.116, 131.
43. PM 184-5.
44. OT February 1917, 80.
45. CES 1997.04.110, 7.
46. JO January 1898, 367-73.
47. JO February 1897, 3.
48. JO November 1897, 285-9.
49. JO September 1908, 526.
50. JO October 1898, 209-10.
51. JO January 1898, 397.
52. JO September 1898, 174-5.
53. JO October 1898, 209.
54. JO September 1898, 196.
55. 1 John 4:12.
56. JO November 1898, 271-2.
57. Booth 464.

20: WEEDS IN A FLOWER BED

1. Booth 251-2.
2. Booth 167.
3. Booth 271-2.
4. Barber 1896 11. "While it is our desire to give Dr. Still credit for the new science which he discovered," Barber wrote, "we must differ with him as to the true cause of the results reached by the Osteopath. While the good Doctor believes that nearly all diseases are caused by dislocated bones . . . in our practice we never find a great number of dislocations."
5. Ward 3.
Kirksville Weekly Graphic, 16 April 1897.
6. HAC 275.
7. M. L. Ward brochure, "True Osteopathy." MOM.
8. *Kirksville Democrat*, 24 August 1900.
9. Gaddis 125.

10. JO November 1898, 268.
11. ATSP 2009.10.836, 1-4.
12. ATSP 2009.10.238. The complete note reads, "S. S. leavs feb 13, lost all, goes to Graham with family 'busted' he is getting. . . ." Summerfield's parents lived in Graham, near Maryville, Missouri.
13. Booth 90-1.
14. CO August 1898, 36-7.
15. Booth 273.
16. Booth 684.
17. *Kirksville Weekly Graphic*, 30 November and 28 December 1894.
18. Hildreth 51-3.
19. *Kirksville Weekly Graphic*, 17 March 1899.
20. Booth 685.
21. *Chiropractic History* Vol. 7 No. 2, 1987, 5. Still's guest book has since become lost. Blanche's future husband, ASO graduate George M. Laughlin adds a measure of confusion by declaring, "So far as I know, Dr. Palmer was never in Kirksville." (Laughlin, however, was not in Kirksville in 1893.) In 1917 Laughlin conceded that the "better informed" chiropractors were doing good work, but declared that Palmer "became acquainted with osteopathy after taking treatments from Dr. Strother[s]" and that there was "no question but that their principle of treatment is stolen bodily from osteopathy." OT May 1918, 151. At the 1900 AAAO Convention, Northern Institute of Osteopathy graduate C. E. Achorn, who had visited Davenport, demonstrated the chiropractic mode of treatment. According to Hildreth, "the Palmer method was along the line practiced by Dr. Still for a number of years before opening his school in 1892 in Kirksville, only it was a very crude and very poor imitation." Hildreth 45.
22. OT May 1921, 1. Josephine de France graduated in 1900.
23. Truhlar 94.
24. CES 1997.04.119, 27.
25. CES 1997.04.119, 32.
26. JO November 1896, 2.
27. Hildreth 393.
28. Walter 28.
29. Conner 10.
30. JO May 1900, 515.
31. Hildreth 381. JO February 1898, 440.
32. AAO Yearbook 1948, 49.
33. JO July 1904, 258.
34. Hildreth 409-10.
35. Wernham 6.
36. ATSP 2009.10.165.
37. SNOM 1980.373.08, 9.
38. JO October 1898, 214.
39. Hildreth 409.
40. OT January 1918, 86.
41. Mabel Alexander to Lewis Chapman, 19 February 1972. MOM.
42. AAO Yearbook 1954, 23.
43. CES 1997.04.119, 11.
44. CES 1997.04.119, 34-5 and CES 1997.04.121, 21-2.
45. Hildreth 366-8.
46. SNOM 11980.373.08, 1.
47. ATSP 2009.10.799. ATSP 2009.10.800.
48. ATSP 2009.10.27.
49. *Kirksville Democrat*, 5 May 1899.
50. *Indianapolis Sentinel*, 28 April 1899, 1.
51. OT July 1920, 196.
52. JO August 1898, 117.
53. JO February 1899, 429-30.
54. American School of Osteopathy Record Book, 1897-1900, 22 March 1899 meeting. ATSP. A majority evidently consented to this idea, for it is recorded in the minutes of the next meeting on 8 April that the resolution "was ordered to be submitted to the trustees for approval with the strongest recommendation of the faculty that the Trustees authorize the proposed change in the Diploma." American School of Osteopathy Record Book, 1897-1900, 8 April 1899 meeting. ATSP.
55. J. Martin Littlejohn to ASO Board of Trustees, 6 June 1899. MOM.
56. JO July 1899, 84. During the visit J. Martin lectured before the Royal Society of Literature, London, on, "The Prophylactic

and Curative Value of the Science of Osteopathy." A transcription of this talk appears in JO February 1900, 365-84.
57. JO September 1899, 141.
58. Hildreth 118-9.
59. JO October 1899, 199.
60. JO January 1899, 419.
61. Hildreth 122.
62. "A talk by Dr. Charlie Still Before the Lower-Freshman Class, March 27, 1942," 2. STC-1 #3. MOM. A. G. Hildreth to Leslie D. Smith, Eugene, Oregon, 29 May 1900. MOM.
63. Hildreth 121.
64. CES 1997.04.119, 33.
65. ATSP 2009.10.654, 4.
66. ATSP 2009.10.650.

21: MIND

1. CES 1997.04.121, 2. CES 1997.04.119, 7-11.
2. CES 1997.04.121, 6. CES 1997.04.119, 8.
3. CES 1997.04.119, 7-9.
4. Walter 35.
5. CES 1997.04.119, 12.
6. ATSP 2009.10.133.
7. CES 1997.04.119, 1.
8. Perhaps he had learned this from the Shawnee. "They only wish to see a man," the tribe's Quaker missionary Henry Harvey noted, "to look him sternly in the face, and observe his manner for a few minutes; then it is no hard task to obtain from them their opinion of the man, and they are not often mistaken." Harvey 143-4.
9. CES 1997.04.121, 2-5. JAOA January 1918, 247.
10. CES 1997.04.119, 14.
11. Booth 517. George H. Fulton, who supplied this information, lodged in Still's house from 1911-13.
12. JO May 1901, 159.
13. ATSP 2009.10.890.
14. CES 1997.04.119, 54B.
15. PM 16-7. Still's terminology can be confusing. He used the words "motion," "spirit," "life," "soul" and "spiritual being," interchangeably. In his interpretation of Spencer's philosophical scheme ("Matter, mind and motion blended by the wisdom of Deity"), these terms represent the Knowable aspect, the material manifestation of the spiritual, the part capable of apprehension by human senses. "The spiritual," as used here, represents the Unknowable aspect, the "wisdom of Deity," incapable of sensory apprehension.
16. JO July 1898, reproduced in Schnucker 151.
17. JO November 1898, 267.
18. JO March 1895, 1.
19. ATSP 2009.10.769, 2.
20. ATSP 2009.10.92.
21. JO November 1898, 267.
22. ORP 252-3.
23. ORP 79. Still once placed a notice in the *Kirksville Democrat* asking patients not to board at places not favorably disposed to osteopathy as they did not seem to improve as quickly. *Kirksville Democrat*, 21 December 1894, 4
24. PO 13.
25. JAOA August 1921, 666.
26. Hildreth 181-3.
27. JAOA January 1918, 247.
28. CES 1997.04.119, 10.
29. CES 1997.04.119, 94.
30. JAOA September 1928, 22.
31. OP August 1918, 4.
32. Auto 1897 179.
33. HAC 266.
34. JO November 1898, 267.
35. Hildreth 194. JAOA December 1932, 140.
36. Auto 1897 413.
37. Booth 21.
38. Booth 468.
39. Auto 346.
40. JAOA July 1924, 814.
41. CES 1997.04.96, 2. Ellison had retired from the Circuit Court bench to act as legal advisor to the ASO and lecturer on medical jurisprudence.
42. JO September 1942, 17.

43. Hildreth 362.
44. JAOA January 1921, 244.
45. CES 1997.04.96, 1.
46. JAOA June 1925, 749.
47. Booth 468.
48. JAOA January 1921, 244.
49. CES 1997.04.93. 1-2. Puerperal or childbed fever is a bacterial infection of the genital tract following childbirth.
50. "The Founder of Osteopathy: Eighty Years Young" by Grace Macgowan Cooke. *The Delineator* (date unknown). STAT-24. MOM.
51. Auto 321.
52. ATSP 2009.10.540.
53. Booth 16.
54. Hildreth 382. The Spanish-American War resulted in Cuba's independence and the American acquisition of Puerto Rica, Guam and the Philippine Islands.
55. Booth 20. JO September 1942, 17. Cuba attained independence in 1902, but the United States established a perpetual lease of Guantanamo Bay.
56. CES 1997.04.119, 66. CES 1997.04.121, 8.
57. JO December 1921, 758-9.
58. Untitled document in possession of author.

22: THE SOW RETURNING TO HER WALLOW

1. Booth 87.
2. Barber 1898 27-8.
3. PO 3.
4. JO July 1899, 67.
5. ATSP 2009.10.656, 1.
6. PO 3-4.
7. ATSP 2009.10. 621.
8. ATSP 2009.10.656, 1-2. In another letter to Mrs. Orschel on 9 August 1899 Still wrote that he had applied for a patent for his latest invention, a "rig to take fat off people," and suggested she come and help him with "the fat business." ATSP 2009.10.652.
9. Booth 99.
10. Booth 130-5.
11. JO May 1900, 513-4.
12. OP November 1903, 1. George Laughlin was the younger brother of ASO anatomy professor Will Laughlin.
13. Trowbridge 213-4.
14. J. Martin Littlejohn eventually returned to Britain and, in 1917, founded the British School of Osteopathy in London.
15. ATSP 2009.10.658.
16. Hildreth 123.
17. Hildreth 134.
18. Hildreth 136-45.
19. CES 1997.04.47, 1.
20. DO October 1973, 31. George Helmer was treating Jean Clemens for severe epilepsy and "capricious changes of disposition" following a fall twelve years earlier. Clemens was familiar with medical prejudice. "To ask a doctor's opinion of osteopathy," he once wrote, "is equivalent to going to Satan for information about Christianity." Mark Twain, *Notebook*, Ed. Albert Paine, New York. Harper & Brothers, 1935, 344.
21. JO March 1901, 114-6. Reprinted from *Post Express*, Albany, Feb. 28. New York would not legalize osteopathy until 1907.
22. JO April 1901, 97.
23. *Milan Republican*, October 25, 1900, reprinted in JO November 1900, 273. Four months later the irrepressible Barber began to offer a correspondence course in "manual therapeutics." JO March 1901, 92.
24. Walter 47.
25. ATSP 2009.10.238.
26. Ward 2.
27. ATSP 2009.08.05, 9.
28. JO June 1901, 266.
29. Auto 295-6.
30. JO September 1898, 164. Still told a cautionary allegory. In a pasture stood a sturdy oak in whose branches he and a friend were ensconced for safety. Around the tree milled a herd of raging bulls, scraping and pawing the ground. The friend was agitated and asked if Still was afraid the bulls would

kill them. Still replied that they were safe biding their time as long as the tree remained standing, but if they climbed down they risked being gored to death. The tree represented osteopathic philosophy and principles, the bulls the medical profession. The moral: despite the aggression of the medical fraternity, the greatest threat to osteopathy lay within their own ranks. JO March 1901, 64-5.
31. JO August 1901, 256-8.
32. JO September 1942, 16-7.
33. JO August 1901, 271.
34. JO February 1902. See Schnucker 315.
35. Hildreth 130-2. Booth 130-8.
36. JO August 1904, 291.
37. JO November 1901, 357-9.
38. JO March 1903, 105.
39. JO January 1901, 23. Neither had Still complied with the ACO ruling of $500 as the acceptable level of tuition fees. Judging that the ASO had enough money and that some students could not afford the full amount, he reduced the fees first to $400 and then to $300. HAC 262.
40. Some speculated upon another reason for Still's withdrawal: the election at Milwaukee of Summerfield S. Still to ACO president. Animosity between Still and Jim's son had long been a public matter and sour relations between the two schools had at times threatened to irreparably damage the profession. OP October 1902, 7.
41. JO October 1902, 340.
42. OP October 1902, 1.
43. JO October 1902, 342. Still agreed with Pasteur that prevention was better than cure, but disagreed that vaccination was the best means to that end. (Perhaps this explains why John Deason wrote in *The Osteopathic Profession*, August 1934, 24, that Still "had little regard for the work of Pasteur.") Still's objection to vaccination stemmed from witnessing the detrimental effects of Edward Jenner's smallpox vaccine during the Civil War. Still believed the risks involved in injecting possibly impure equine and bovine products into the body were too great and that "instead of passing laws for compulsory vaccination, a law prohibiting the practice, with heavy penalties for violations, would prove a wholesome experiment. Simply take the fifty cents out of the 'dirty' practice and it would die out spontaneously with all doctors of average knowledge of the harm done by it."
44. JO September 1901, in EO, 297. JO September 1902, 314. Other suggested titles were *Treatment by A. T. Still* and *A. T. Still's Complete Work on Osteopathy*.
45. JO September 1901. See Schnucker 297.
46. JO July 1903, 209.
47. CES 1997.04.119, 70-1.
48. JO March 1903, 81.
49. OP May 1903, 8. After a short career as a traveling salesman Herbert Bernard entered the ASO in 1895.
50. JO September 1902, 302.
51. JAOA January 1903, 280, 283. After departing from the ASO at the end of 1899, Smith practiced briefly in Kansas City before serving a short stint as President of the Atlantic School of Osteopathy in Wilkes-Barre, Pennsylvania. In summer 1900 he left for Europe, visited medical schools in France, Germany, Belgium, England and Scotland, and returned to America in 1902. "Peripatetic Pioneer: William Smith, M.D., D.O. (1862-1912)" by E. R. N. Grigg. *Journal of the History of Medicine*, April 1967, 174-6.
52. JO November 1903, 361.
53. OP January 1903, 3. In May the *Journal of Osteopathy* published interviews with medical doctors who went on to qualify as osteopaths, asking why they had changed their allegiance. J. A. Vance of Chillicothe, Ohio, said he had taken a moral decision after hearing about Senator Foraker's son and seeing some of his own patients returning from Kirksville cured. For S. M. Pleak of DuQuoin, Illinois, an MD for thirty years, it was after witnessing its results on a patient he had been unable

to help. "I meet fewer disappointments in practice than when I practiced Allopathy," he said, "and none of the bad after effects we get with drug medication." W. D. Bowen of Washington, North Carolina, was swayed by the osteopathic cure of a chronic patient. An old medical school professor of his used to say that "a case correctly diagnosed is half cured," but only after studying osteopathy did he realize why his diagnoses had not always been correct. "I could not have benefited them with drugs, as drugs could not have removed the cause of the disease. I worked as faithfully then as I do now, but I can get good results now on the same persons that I totally failed on with drugs." JO May 1903, 154-9.
54. Hildreth 146-8. HAC 269.
55. JO November 1903, 366.

23: MOTION

1. JO August 1904, 290.
2. PM 250.
3. ATSP 2009.10.847, 1.
4. PM 256.
5. JO March 1900. See Schnucker 234.
6. JO September 1898, 163-5.
7. ATSP 2009.10.915, 2-4.
8. JO August 1901, 241.
9. ATSP 2009.10.540.
10. PM 16-17. Still wrote, "First, there is the material body; second, the spiritual being; third, a being of mind which is far superior to all vital motions and material forms, whose duty is to manage this great engine of life."
11. PM 256.
12. ATSP 2009.10.161, 6.
13. ATSP 2009.10.889, 1-2.
14. JO November 1901, 360.
15. Auto 241.
16. JO July 1901, 198.
17. ATSP 2009.10.856, 1.
18. 1 John 4:12.
19. Wesley, Sermon 69, 571.
20. ATSP 2009.10.24, 2. 1903 graduate Ernest C. Proctor told of meeting Still in the street. "Proc, are you learning anything?" Still asked, slipping an arm over the student's shoulder. "Sometimes I think I am getting a little," Proctor replied. "Well, if you don't learn anything more than this," Still said, "you will learn to understand your God and Creator better by learning of His handiwork." OT January 1918, 85.
21. JAOA January 1921, 244-5.
22. ATSP 2009.10.567.
23. *Webster's Revised Unabridged Dictionary*, 1913, defines *biogen* as "bioplasm" (literally "life form"); a word synonymous with protoplasm, "the material through which every form of life manifests itself."
24. PM 251. This metaphysical construct probably derived from St. Paul in 1 Corinthians 15:40: "There are also celestial bodies, and bodies terrestrial: but the glory of the celestial is one, and the glory of the terrestrial is another." In his 1823 *The New Testament of Our Lord and Savior Jesus Christ* (A. Paul Publishers, New York), Adam Clarke wrote, "The apostle certainly does not speak of celestial and terrestrial bodies in the sense in which we use those terms . . . the apostle speaks of human beings; some of which were clothed with celestial, others with terrestrial bodies. It is very likely, therefore, that he means by the celestial bodies such as those refined human bodies with which Enoch, Elijah and Christ himself appear in the realms of glory: to which we may add the bodies of those saints which arose after our Lord's resurrection, and, after having appeared to many, doubtless were taken up to Paradise." See also 1 Corinthians 15:44: "There is a natural body and there is a spiritual body."
25. JO July 1901, 198.
26. ATS Miscellany box. MOM.
27. ATSP 2009.10.915, 2-3.
28. Wesley, Sermon 43, 160-1. See also 1 Corinthians 2:9.
29. JAOA January 1921, 244.

30. Matthew 17:1-3.
31. ATSP 2009.10.24, 3-10. Still delivered the *Body and Soul of Man* talk in 1902 or 1903 ("I am getting old. I am seventy-four"). The Still family all believed in the soul's immortality. One day after Abram's death Still's sister Mary went to visit her mother (at the time living with Marovia) and said she intended visiting Cassie in California. "All right my child," Martha told Mary, "when I go to see my darling [Cassie] I will go the near cut and it will be upward instead of across the plains." Later Martha had a dream:

> I was walking out, and thought I had been very sick, and was only able to walk alone by the greatest care. As I slowly moved along . . . just in front of me, as I was about to take another step, there was what appeared to be a deep broad river, whose water was so very clear I could see myself; and my hair was white as snow. While I stood noting this fact, there appeared on the other side of the stream a man and woman. The man I noticed, and recognized at once to be father, whose hair had only a few threads of gray; and while I stood, rather wondering at your father's bloom of full manhood, I also wondered who the lady could be. I then thought I would try and wade the river and go to them, when, looking down, lo and behold! The river was not there at all; but I was with the two, and imagine my joy, when looking up to find it was our Cassie; at which glad surprise I awoke.

When Mary arrived in California she related the dream. "Oh! Sister," Cassie responded, her face suffused with radiance, "may it come true and father and I be together and be permitted to welcome mother on her arrival home." Mary added, "Might it not have been the lightning flash of coming events? Or was it her internal Christ externally revealed through her countenance? From what had happened and the finger prints in her Bible, I think it was both." The dream came true. Cassie died of tuberculosis on 17 February 1888; Martha on Christmas day the same year. Both were preceded by John, ten days before Cassie, struck by a limb of a tree he was felling at his home in Oakland. On the morning he died he told his family of feeling troubled by a dream a few days earlier that appeared to be a premonition: "I thought I had fallen asleep, and suddenly I awoke and seemed to be surrounded with angels, and in another state of existence." In later years Mary wrote of her parents: "They both have reached our Father's house, and telephone back, and this is what they say: 'The river of death, thought to be a monstrous flood, is but a narrow rill, and the task of death, the stepping over a thread, a hair; the curtain palpitates and the heart stops, and you are there.'" MSA 6, 192-6.
32. CES 1997.04.121, 10-12.
33. JO December 1921, 759.
34. ATSP 2009.10.863, 1. See also "Dr. A. T. Still's Visit to the Spiritualists' Meeting at Clinton, Iowa," *Bulletin of the Atlas and Axis Clubs*, September 1903.
35. *The Clinton Daily Herald*, August 26, 1903.
36. *Chiropractic History* Vol. 7 No. 2 1987, 5-7. B. J. Palmer *Fight To Climb*. Chiropractic Fountain Head, Davenport, Iowa, 1950, 57-8. B. J. Palmer does not mention the precise date. There is no reference to Still attending on any other occasion.
37. ATSP 2009.10.863, 1.
38. JO December 1921, 758.
39. CES 1997.04.119, 49.
40. ATSP 2009.10.125, 1.
41. ATSP 2009.10.170, 1.
42. ATSP 2009.10.61.
43. CES 1997.04.119, 49-54A.
44. ATSP 2009.10.162.
45. ATSP 2009.10.170, 1-2.
46. JO September 1908, 549. Booth 518.

47. ATSP 2009.10.892.
48. JO August 1903, 255.
49. OP November 1903, 1-2. Still was actually 75 years old.
50. ATSP 2009.10.785, 1-3. A rough draft of the speech reads, "Don't swallow old M. talk as something sweet and holy. Who run wireless teleg. to Heaven: Thousands of people over the earth that would surprise you. By ment teleg they can tell you exact words. Words of psychic and clairvoyancy." ATSP 2009.10.381, 6.
51. Booth 15.
52. Wesley, Sermon 71, 11. "An Evening Hymn" in *A Manual of Prayers* by Bishop Thomas Ken. 1709.
53. Wesley, Sermon 135, 224. Descartes believed he had been similarly inspired. The night after he discovered the foundations of his science, based on reason and mathematics, he dreamed of hearing a clap of thunder and interpreted it as the Spirit of Truth descending to take possession of him. Eaton xvii. The Shawnee also believed in guiding spirits who communicated with them through dreams. Sugden 116.
54. CES 1997.04.121, 19-20.
55. CES 1997.04.96, 1-3. Brewer suggests that the incident occurred in 1864 after the death of Still's children, but he appears to be mistaken.
56. ATSP 2009.10.712, 1. Still acted as a medium and invited sympathetic students to his séances. Interview with Dr. Anne Wales, May 1997.
57. CES 1997.04.119, 67. "A man who said he was J. H. Duvol came to me," Still once told Tucker. "I offered to shake hands, but he said 'Don't shake hands, it breaks the batteries and destroys the matter I have assumed. But give me a piece of paper and a pencil and I'll write my name' I did so and he wrote, J. H. Duvol. I have the card somewhere. He bore some resemblance to the form he had in school. The fingers were like rolls of cotton." CES 1997.04.121, 15.
58. CES 1997.04.121, 15.
59. CES 1997.04.119, 66-7.
60. CES 1997.04.121, 8-9 and 16. The measles virus was not isolated until 1954.
61. CES 1997.04.119, 63, 66-7.
62. CES 1997.04.121, 5-6. Thomas Edison was said to have rigged up a similar device.
63. CES 1997.04.119, 61.
64. Hildreth 125. "I shall never forget the ovation the Old Doctor received," 1900 ASO graduate D. E. McAlpin wrote, "every man and woman rose instantly. I was so full of enthusiasm it was almost overflowing; I jumped up, threw my hat, and cheered as loud as any man present. You see, I had been in the field a few years and knew through results what his teaching had meant to me and the reason for their enthusiasm when seeing Dr. Still." Hildreth 201.
65. ATSP 2009.10.928, 1.
66. Walter 49-51. The ASO's previous manager Henry Patterson had left to open a practice in Washington D.C. At the end of 1903 the ASO purchased the entire stock of S. S. Still's Des Moines College, which had already absorbed Fargo's Northwestern School and the Northern College of Minneapolis. See OP January 1904, 4-5. By 1905 the Denver, Ohio, and Atlantic schools had amalgamated with the ASO, and the Milwaukee School was forced to close after medical lobbying of the Wisconsin legislature.
67. ATSP 2009.10.928, 2-3.

24: TO THINE OWN SELF BE TRUE

1. JAOA August 1942, 506.
2. Quoted slightly incorrectly in JAOA December 1925, 279. (Quoted is the accurate version from the *Encyclopedia Americana, Vol. 10,* under the heading "Medicine.") The trend away from drug medication continued until the early 1920s. By then many doctors did not prescribe any drugs at all.

3. Booth 411.
4. Virchow 1958 181.
5. Lane 4. Michael A. Lane discovered and named the alpha and beta cells in the islets of Langerhans in the pancreas (producing, respectively, glucagon and insulin).
6. Lane 47.
7. JAOA December 1923, 238.
8. JO August 1905, 249. Still now reasoned that in meningitis microbial toxins caused spasmodic contraction of neck muscles and interfered with blood flow to and from the brain, resulting in stagnation and retention of blood within the skull, thus generating conditions favorable for fermentation and the proliferation of microorganisms.
9. JO December 1905, 355.
10. Booth 235-6. Before teaching pathology at the ASO, Michael A. Lane's work was cited by the English physiologist Ernest Starling in his book *Principles of Human Physiology*. Lane vii.
11. Page 17.
12. Booth 627-8.
13. Hildreth 254.
14. Behring showed experimentally that guinea pigs that had previously recovered from diphtheria thereafter remained unaffected by both the bacterium and its toxin. He took blood from recovered – "immunized" – animals, allowed the cellular elements to settle, mixed the straw-colored serum at the top with diphtheria toxin, and injected the mixture into guinea pigs who had never had the disease. They remained healthy. Not only that, but they were also able to resist ordinarily lethal doses of germs. Behring injected the blood serum – "antitoxin" – of these guinea pigs into human subjects. Though it did not kill the bacteria, it assisted them to resist the toxin and recover from the disease.
15. Trowbridge 207. Harry's patients in New York included the industrialist and philanthropist John D. Rockefeller.
16. AAO Yearbook 1954, 20. Still's speech was billed in the program simply as "A Friendly Chat."
17. ATSP 2009.10.879, 2.
18. ATSP 2009.10.845, 2.
19. Booth 474-5. OT January 1918, 97.
20. ATSP 209.10.170, 2.
21. JO June 1905, 189.
22. ORP 141.
23. Hildreth 155. JO December 1908, 765. On 6 December 1907, while visiting Topeka for the fifty-year reunion of the Kansas Free State Legislature, Still raised a hand to the front of his neck. "I have had so much trouble with my throat," he said. "I was in a wreck near Denver two years ago and I sustained an injury in my neck that has never completely healed." *Topeka Daily Capital*, 7 December 1907. ATSP 2009.10.969.
24. Booth 614-5.
25. JO December 1905, 351-64. George A. Still was Summerfield's son and James Still's grandson.
26. JO January 1906, 379.
27. Auto 324-5.
28. Virchow 1958 244.
29. ATSP 2009.10.796, 2.
30. Booth 741-2.
31. JO June 1906, 202. Ed had retired from medical practice through illness in 1900.
32. JAOA January 1918, 249.
33. OP December 1918. "Reminiscences of the Old Doctor" by James Hegyessy.
34. JAOA August 1921, 671.
35. ATSP 2009.10.02, 11.
36. ORP 71-4. ATSP 2009.10.02, 5-6.
37. OP December 1918.
38. CES 1997.04.100, 2.
39. OP February 1918, 15.
40. Booth 513-4.
41. JAOA January 1918, 244.
42. CES 1997.04.100, 2.
43. Auto 286-7.
44. JAOA June 1925, 749.
45. OT January 1918, 86-7.
46. Booth 529.

47. CES 1997.04.121, 24.
48. AOHS July 1961, 2.
49. JO November 1906, 344.
50. JO January 1906, 18.
51. CES 1997.04.100, 1.
52. JO January 1907, 6.
53. JAOA January 1918, 250. Both Russell and wife Sarah graduated from the ASO in 1906.

25: THE GREATEST ANTISEPTIC KNOWN

1. Booth 533.
2. ATSP 1980.373.10, 13.
3. Booth 507-8.
4. Still C. E. 223-7. The diary is now lost or possibly destroyed. It had been in the possession of Charles Still, Jr., Charley's son, who in a biography of his grandfather devoted four pages to the "little red book."
5. JO December 1907, 18.
6. ATSP 2009.10.969. (*Topeka Daily Capital*, 7 December 1907.)
7. TKSHS Vol. 10, 179. JO January 1908, 22. JO December 1907, 432.
8. "The Founder of Osteopathy" by Grace Macgowan Cooke. *The Delineator*, date unknown. MOM. STAT-24.
9. JO September 1908, 525-68.
10. Booth 555-7.
11. JAOA January 1918, 254.
12. ATSP 2009.10.799.
13. Booth 516.
14. JO August 1907, 263-5.
15. OT February 1918, 112. "I have but laid the foundations; you are to rear the complete edifice of the science of Osteopathy," Still said on another occasion. "I have but got the squirrel's tail of Osteopathy out of the hole and you must pull out his whole body." Booth 1925 467.
16. Auto 378. "While he often, indeed usually, spoke as one having authority," A. L. Evans wrote, "he did not expect his mere dictum to be accepted as law by those who followed him. Nor would he have us believe that when he had finished his contribution to Osteopathy it was henceforth to be regarded as a closed book, and that the fount of knowledge had been sealed. It was only in a few fundamentals that he proclaimed immutable laws." JAOA August 1921, 671.
17. Auto 222.. "Know then thyself, presume not God to scan; The proper study of mankind is man." *An Essay on Man* by Alexander Pope, 1733.
18. ATSP 2009.10.24, 6.
19. ORP 2.
20. 1 Corinthians 3:16.
21. Auto 164.
22. ATSP 2009.10.50.
23. Lane 183.
24. Lane 37. "Immunizing diseases" are infections that subsequently confer immunity for varying periods.
25. Page 28.
26. Sera and other therapies for infectious disease had met with mixed success. Effective sera had been developed for tetanus and diphtheria, but malaria, sleeping sickness and syphilis proved refractory, while Koch's *tuberculin*, a glycerin extract of tubercle bacilli produced in 1890 and touted as a cure for tuberculosis, had not lived up to its initial promise.
27. Riedman 66.
28. Virchow 1958 243.
29. JAOA July 1924, 814. "Buzzard" was the local name for the turkey vulture.
30. Booth 415.
31. Quoted in Riedman 65.
32. Clendening 408-9.
33. Riedman 25.

26: THE FULFILLMENT OF LIFE'S DIVINE PLAN

1. JO June 1910, Tribute. Mary had attended the First Methodist Church since 1876 and for the previous seven years assisted the

minister's wife in voluntary work for the Woman's Foreign Missionary Society.
2. JO September 1909, 688.
3. JAOA January 1918, 241. Hildreth had run a private practice in St. Louis for the past three years since severing his ties with the small ASO branch infirmary in the city.
4. *Kirksville Democrat*, 3 June 1910, 1. Mary died a day after Robert Koch died of a heart attack, aged 67, in Baden-Baden, Germany.
5. JO June 1910, Supplement.
6. JO June 1910, 561.
7. *Kirksville Democrat*, 3 June 1910, 1.
8. Booth 504.
9. *Kirksville Daily Express*, 22 March 1909, 1. "The furnace is patterned after the sun glass so far as the reason for the thing is concerned," the paper explained Still's innovative two-step design. "The fire-bricks in lining of fire-box are scientifically made and mathematically set, so that the flames are made to cross one another from opposite sides at a point just below the boiler, causing little loss of heat." Steam pipes, one for each fire box, "blew the fire into a livid flame, thus producing the greatest heat from a minimum amount of fuel."
10. JO February 1909, 112-5. Still C. E. 228-31.
11. JO June 1910, 564.
12. ORP 11-2.
13. JO June 1910, 649. "Still wrote in *Osteopathy: Research and Practice*, "All the bacteriology I want or need is a good knowledge of man's anatomy." ORP 8. In many autographed copies he inscribed the words, "Follow your guide and fear no danger."
14. Trowbridge 214.
15. Booth 517.
16. CES 1997.04.99, 2-4. Gair was introduced to osteopathy in 1898 when treated by Charles Bandel who, she wrote, "did miracles for a very much maimed body."
17. OPR August 1934, 24.
18. Booth 475.
19. ATSP 2009.10.957. Condolence letter from Frances Crowley.
20. Booth 447. HAC 262. Smith practiced at 229 East 39th Street in New York City.
21. JO June 1912. See Schnucker 373-5. Black Wolf was the Shawnee warrior who massacred Still's ancestors. Perhaps Still was thinking of the Shawnee orator Tecumseh, who said, "When it comes to your time to die, be not like those whose hearts are filled with the fear of death." United Tribe of Shawnee Indians website.
22. *The Bulletin of the Atlas and Axis Clubs*, September 1912, 13. MOM.
23. Booth 810.
24. Trowbridge 189. President Theodore Roosevelt and family were patients of 1905 ASO graduate Charles Green.
25. AAO Yearbook 1954, 20-6. Asa was a nephew of respected Kirksville physician and Johns Hopkins University graduate A. P. Willard. Asa's childhood ambition had been to follow in his uncle's footsteps and study medicine, but after witnessing Still cure Mary Mitchell and then his own asthma he changed his mind and entered the ASO instead. Dr. Willard had shunned Still ever since he came to town and, in abject dismay, accused Asa of ruining the family's reputation. In later years Still and Dr. Willard became good friends who would sit together exchanging reminiscences of practice, more often than not humorous. Hildreth 371.
26. ATSP 2009.10.142.
27. *Kirksville Democrat*, 5 August 1913, 8.
28. Hildreth 242-4.
29. JO August 1913, 460. Untitled document in possession of author.
30. *Kirksville Democrat*, 12 August 1913, 4.
31. JO June 1913, 332.
32. Booth 556-7.
33. Trowbridge 207-8.
34. STH-5. Still-Hildreth Collection. MOM.
35. Hildreth 243-4.
36. Walter 77-9. JO November 1913, 672.

Still commented of the state institutions, "Between you and me, as far as the lunatic asylum is concerned I would as soon go to a sausage mill as to enter one." And, "I have never yet pictured out a good old Methodist hell to be half as bad as an asylum. I would rather see my daughter shot and buried than taken to one." JO January 1895, 1. ATSP 2009.10.780, 5.
37. Hildreth 247-55. Bailey graduated from the ASO in 1912.
38. Booth 442.
39. *Fifteen Years at Still-Hildreth.* JO 1929, 518-21. In 1933 the sanatorium published results of 840 cases of dementia praecox treated over a nineteen-year period, with patients pronounced cured on leaving the institution routinely followed up to check if recovery was permanent. Statistics showed an overall recovery rate of 41.7%. Early treatment afforded a better prognosis: those admitted within six months of onset showed a recovery rate of 68%, tapering to 20% in those admitted more than two years after onset. This was significantly better than the 5% or less cure rate of the state institutions. Hildreth 272, 275.
40. Hildreth 211.
41. JO October 1909, 755-7.
42. OP June 1915, 5-6.
43. JAOA 1908, 90-1.
44. JAOA July 1924, 817.
45. ORP preface, xxii.
46. See Gevitz, 68-71.
47. OT January 1918, 83.
48. Booth 442.
49. OP August 1915, 1-3.
50. Booth 614.
51. ATSP 2009.10.107.
52. OT January 1918, 85.
53. OPR August 1934, 22-3.
54. Page 37-8.
55. Walter 85.
56. JO September 1915, 547-8.
57. Page 37-8.
58. Page 43.
59. JOAO January 1918, 254.
60. ATSP 2009.10.957. Condolence letter, Florence Gair to Blanche Still.
61. JO July 1917, 410-15.
62. Booth 504. OT January 1918, 90-1. ATSP 2010.02.1193.
63. ATSP 2009.10.86.
64. ATSP 2009.10.957. Condolence letter, Reverend B. F. Jones to Blanche Still.
65. Hildreth 279. JAOA January 1918, 242.
66. OT January 1918, 80. JAOA January 1918, 241-3.
67. JO January 1918, 20.
68. JAOA January 1918, 250.
69. CES 1997.04.119, 5-6.

EPILOGUE

1. JAOA August 1921, 664.
2. OT January 1918, 88.
3. OT February 1918, 109.
4. AAO Yearbook 1954, 22.
5. Hildreth 370.
6. SNOM 1980.373.10, 8.
7. SNOM 1980.373.10, 15.
8. SNOM 1980.373.08, 5, 10.
9. SNOM 1980.373.10. "Yes, fellow osteopaths, I am a standpatter. . . ." J. H. Sullivan.
10. SNOM 1980.373.08, 11.
11. JO July 1932, 400-3.
12. Booth 412.
13. Lane 17.
14. Quoted in JAOA September 1973.
15. CES 1997.04.119, 31.
16. AAO Yearbook 1954, 25. Hugh H. Gravett wrote similarly, "The mongrel terms we are applying to osteopathy, manipulative therapy, osteopathic medicine, are confusing to the masses. They think of manipulation as being massage, and medicine as drugs which, of course, it is." AAO Yearbook 1954, 37.
17. AAO Yearbook 1947, 9.
18. Hildreth 393.
19. AAO Yearbook 1948, 51.

20. AAO Yearbook 1954, 24.
21. OT February 1918, 109.
22. Still C. E. 280-1. Directly after Still's death the influenza pandemic of 1917-19 claimed 21 million lives. During it ASO graduate George W. Riley wrote to every State Health Commissioner in American cities with populations over 40,000 asking for data on both influenza and pneumonia, and received 148 replies. To this data he combined figures from the National Census Bureau and several insurance companies, and arrived at an "ultra-conservative" estimate that under regular medical care 5% of influenza cases and 33% of those that went on to develop pneumonia died. Official figures from U.S. Army camps corroborated his figures, recording fatalities from pneumonia as 34.5%. Riley sent blank report sheets to all practicing osteopaths in the United States and Canada asking for similar data, with instructions to report only well-developed cases and the number of fatalities. 2445 osteopaths, both in large cities and small towns, reported a total of 110,122 influenza cases with 257 deaths, and 6,258 cases of pneumonia with 635 deaths, giving statistics for patients treated osteopathically as less than 0.25% for influenza and around 10% for pneumonia. Additionally, around 50 of the pneumonia deaths occurred within twenty-four hours of the osteopathic physician being called, supporting Still's admonition to begin treatment early. Hildreth 418-20.
23. Nerburn 74.
24. Nerburn 23.
25. Still wrote, "Of God man has learned nothing; of his works but very little. When I behold man, I halt in the open field of crushing amazement." JO November 1901, 360.
26. Auto 235. Joshua 24:15: "And if it seem evil unto you to serve the Lord, choose you this day whom ye will serve . . . but as for me and my house, we will serve the Lord."

Index

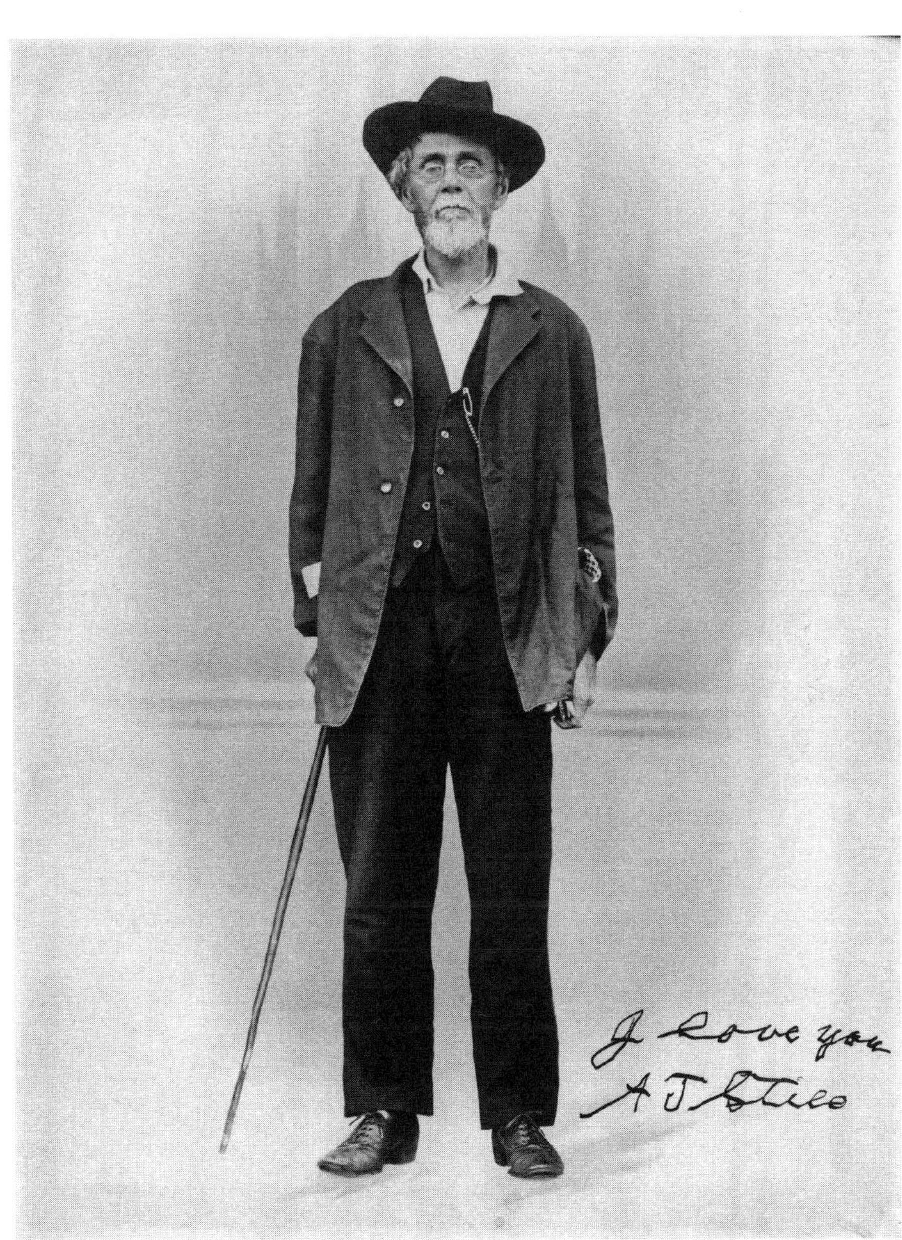
I love you
A T Still

(1)

~~Mental~~ Questions
arise. ~~Some pass away. others~~
~~remain. They~~ & wait ~~seem to Stand~~
for us to solve them. Some of ~~them~~
reach to the Infinite and
hold up lights to the traveller
and call aloud to the explorer
and ask his attention for a
time. among others was
this: Does [illegible] God [illegible] eve
play "hide and go seek"
I had been hunting for year
for some law by which we
could cure the afflicted.
their groans seemed to be
perpetual; misery appeared
to be a part of creation, a
much as a leg was a part
of a horse, and why could
not man find the reason
for these ills?